# Current Challenges in the Management of Vitreoretinal Conditions

# Current Challenges in the Management of Vitreoretinal Conditions

Editor

**Georgios D. Panos**

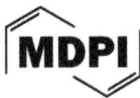

Basel • Beijing • Wuhan • Barcelona • Belgrade • Novi Sad • Cluj • Manchester

*Editor*
Georgios D. Panos
University of Nottingham
Nottingham
UK

*Editorial Office*
MDPI
St. Alban-Anlage 66
4052 Basel, Switzerland

This is a reprint of articles from the Special Issue published online in the open access journal *Journal of Clinical Medicine* (ISSN 2077-0383) (available at: https://www.mdpi.com/journal/jcm/special_issues/vitreoretinal_conditions).

For citation purposes, cite each article independently as indicated on the article page online and as indicated below:

Lastname, A.A.; Lastname, B.B. Article Title. *Journal Name* **Year**, *Volume Number*, Page Range.

ISBN 978-3-7258-0511-2 (Hbk)
ISBN 978-3-7258-0512-9 (PDF)
doi.org/10.3390/books978-3-7258-0512-9

© 2024 by the authors. Articles in this book are Open Access and distributed under the Creative Commons Attribution (CC BY) license. The book as a whole is distributed by MDPI under the terms and conditions of the Creative Commons Attribution-NonCommercial-NoDerivs (CC BY-NC-ND) license.

# Contents

About the Editor . . . . . . . . . . . . . . . . . . . . . . . . . . . . . . . . . . . . . . . . . . . . . . . . . . . . . . . . . . . . vii

**Georgios D. Panos**
Current Challenges in the Management of Vitreoretinal Conditions
Reprinted from: *J. Clin. Med.* **2024**, *13*, 1171, doi:10.3390/jcm13041171 . . . . . . . . . . . . . . . . . 1

**Filippo Confalonieri, Vanessa Ferraro, Gianmaria Barone, Alessandra Di Maria, Beáta Éva Petrovski, Josè Luis Vallejo Garcia, et al.**
Outcomes in the Treatment of Subretinal Macular Hemorrhage Secondary to Age-Related Macular Degeneration: A Systematic Review
Reprinted from: *J. Clin. Med.* **2024**, *13*, 367, doi:10.3390/jcm13020367 . . . . . . . . . . . . . . . . . 5

**Rodolfo Mastropasqua, Matteo Gironi, Rossella D'Aloisio, Valentina Pastore, Giacomo Boscia, Luca Vecchiarino, et al.**
Intraoperative Iridectomy in Femto-Laser Assisted Smaller-Incision New Generation Implantable Miniature Telescope
Reprinted from: *J. Clin. Med.* **2024**, *13*, 76, doi:10.3390/jcm13010076 . . . . . . . . . . . . . . . . . 64

**Naoyuki Yamakawa, Hiroyuki Komatsu, Yoshihiko Usui, Kinya Tsubota, Yoshihiro Wakabayashi and Hiroshi Goto**
Immune Mediators Profiles in the Aqueous Humor of Patients with Simple Diabetic Retinopathy
Reprinted from: *J. Clin. Med.* **2023**, *12*, 6931, doi:10.3390/jcm12216931 . . . . . . . . . . . . . . . . . 74

**Matteo Ripa, Georgios D. Panos, Robert Rejdak, Theodoros Empeslidis, Mario Damiano Toro, Ciro Costagliola, et al.**
Sympathetic Ophthalmia after Vitreoretinal Surgery without Antecedent History of Trauma: A Systematic Review and Meta-Analysis
Reprinted from: *J. Clin. Med.* **2023**, *12*, 2316, doi:10.3390/jcm12062316 . . . . . . . . . . . . . . . . . 83

**Aleksandra Sedova, Christoph Scholda, Thomas Huebl, Irene Steiner, Stefan Sacu, Michael Georgopoulos, et al.**
Effect of Changes in Surgical Strategies for the Treatment of Primary Rhegmatogenous Retinal Detachment on Functional and Anatomical Outcomes: A Retrospective Analysis of 812 Cases from the Years 2004 to 2012
Reprinted from: *J. Clin. Med.* **2023**, *12*, 2278, doi:10.3390/jcm12062278 . . . . . . . . . . . . . . . . . 102

**Raffaele Raimondi, Tania Sorrentino, Raphael Kilian, Yash Verma, Francesco Paolo De Rosa, Giuseppe Cancian, et al.**
Trans-Scleral Plugs Fixated FIL SSF IOL: A Review of the Literature and Comparison with Other Secondary IOL Implants
Reprinted from: *J. Clin. Med.* **2023**, *12*, 1994, doi:10.3390/jcm12051994 . . . . . . . . . . . . . . . . . 113

**Malik Merad, Fabien Vérité, Florian Baudin, Inès Ben Ghezala, Cyril Meillon, Alain Marie Bron, et al.**
Cystoid Macular Edema after Rhegmatogenous Retinal Detachment Repair with Pars Plana Vitrectomy: Rate, Risk Factors, and Outcomes
Reprinted from: *J. Clin. Med.* **2022**, *11*, 4914, doi:10.3390/jcm11164914 . . . . . . . . . . . . . . . . . 125

**Sławomir Cisiecki, Karolina Bonińska and Maciej Bednarski**
Encircling Scleral Buckling Surgery for Severe Hypotony with Ciliary Body Detachment on Anterior Segment Swept-Source Optical Coherence Tomography: A Case Series
Reprinted from: *J. Clin. Med.* **2022**, *11*, 4647, doi:10.3390/jcm11164647 . . . . . . . . . . . . . . . . . 137

**Cherng-Ru Hsu and Chung-May Yang**
Peripheral Circumferential Retinal Detachment after Pars Plana Vitrectomy: Complications and Management
Reprinted from: *J. Clin. Med.* **2022**, *11*, 4856, doi:10.3390/jcm11164856 . . . . . . . . . . . . . . . **144**

**Georgios D. Panos, Olyvia Poyser, Humera Sarwar, Dharmalingam Kumudhan, Gavin Orr, Anwar Zaman and Craig Wilde**
The Impact of the COVID-19 Pandemic and Lockdown on Macular Hole Surgery Provision and Surgical Outcomes: A Single-Centre Experience
Reprinted from: *J. Clin. Med.* **2022**, *11*, 3678, doi:10.3390/jcm11133678 . . . . . . . . . . . . . . . . **153**

# About the Editor

**Georgios D. Panos**

Dr. Georgios D. Panos is a Consultant Ophthalmologist specialising in Vitreoretinal Surgery and Medical Retina at the Queen's Medical Centre, Nottingham University Hospitals NHS Trust, U.K., and an Honorary Assistant Professor of Ophthalmology at the University of Nottingham. He graduated from the Faculty of Medicine, Aristotle University of Thessaloniki, Greece, in 2007, and earned his Doctoral Degree in Medicine (MD by research) from the University of Geneva, Switzerland, in 2013. He completed his Ophthalmology Residency in Switzerland and Greece, achieving board certification in 2014. Dr. Panos also holds a Professional Certificate in Medical Statistics from Stanford School of Medicine (2021). Following his residency training, he served as "Chef de Clinique" (Chief Resident/Junior Consultant) in Paediatric Ophthalmology and Neuroophthalmology at the Geneva University Hospitals. In 2015, he moved to the U.K., completing fellowships in Medical Retina, Cataract Surgery, and Vitreoretinal Surgery. Dr. Panos is active in academic circles, serving as Editor and on the Editorial and Advisory boards of ten international medical journals and reviewing for several others. He is a full member of the World Association of Medical Editors.

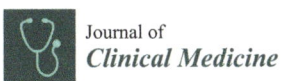

Editorial

# Current Challenges in the Management of Vitreoretinal Conditions

Georgios D. Panos [1,2]

1. Department of Ophthalmology, Queen's Medical Centre, Nottingham University Hospitals, Nottingham NG7 2UH, UK; gdpanos@gmail.com; Tel.: +44-115-924-9924
2. Division of Ophthalmology and Visual Sciences, School of Medicine, University of Nottingham, Nottingham NG7 2UH, UK

Citation: Panos, G.D. Current Challenges in the Management of Vitreoretinal Conditions. *J. Clin. Med.* 2024, 13, 1171. https://doi.org/10.3390/jcm13041171

Received: 31 January 2024
Accepted: 18 February 2024
Published: 19 February 2024

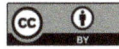

Copyright: © 2024 by the author. Licensee MDPI, Basel, Switzerland. This article is an open access article distributed under the terms and conditions of the Creative Commons Attribution (CC BY) license (https:// creativecommons.org/licenses/by/ 4.0/).

## 1. Introduction

In the dynamic realm of ophthalmology, the management of vitreoretinal conditions stands as a testament to both significant progress and ongoing challenges. These conditions, encompassing a diverse range of retinal and vitreous pathologies, are crucial in their impact on vision and in the complexity of their care. From diabetic retinopathy and age-related macular degeneration to retinal detachments and rare inherited disorders, the spectrum of vitreoretinal diseases poses unique challenges to clinicians and researchers alike.

The current state of the field is marked by rapid advancements and evolving practices. The past decade has seen considerable strides in diagnostic imaging, with technologies like optical coherence tomography (OCT) and OCT-angiography providing unprecedented insights into retinal structures [1]. Similarly, the advent of anti-VEGF therapies has revolutionised the treatment of conditions such as diabetic macular oedema and neovascular AMD, offering patients hope for preserved vision that was once inconceivable [2–4].

However, despite these advancements, the field continues to grapple with significant challenges. Diagnostically, the subtleties of vitreoretinal conditions often demand a level of precision that remains just beyond the reach of current technologies. The heterogeneous nature of these diseases, coupled with individual variations in patient response to treatment, further complicates the clinical landscape. Clinicians must navigate these complexities while also considering factors such as patient comorbidities, accessibility to care, and treatment adherence.

A critical challenge that has recently emerged is the impact of the COVID-19 pandemic. The pandemic has disrupted routine healthcare, leading to delayed diagnoses and treatments for vitreoretinal conditions [5,6]. Additionally, the potential direct and indirect effects of COVID-19 on the retina and its vasculature are areas of active investigation. The necessity for remote consultations and the limitation of in-person clinical interactions have accelerated the adoption of telemedicine, presenting both opportunities and challenges in the management of these conditions [7].

In terms of treatment, while anti-VEGF therapies have been a game-changer, their long-term efficacy, optimal dosing schedules, and systemic implications are areas of ongoing research [8]. Surgical interventions, though continually improving, still carry inherent risks and limitations, particularly in complex or advanced cases. Furthermore, the management of vitreoretinal conditions in paediatric populations presents an additional layer of complexity, given the differences in disease manifestation and treatment responses when compared to those of adults [9,10].

Moreover, the field is at a crossroads with regard to public health implications. As the global population ages, the prevalence of age-related vitreoretinal conditions is expected to rise, posing significant challenges in terms of healthcare resource allocation and patient management on a broader scale [11,12]. The intersection of systemic diseases such as diabetes with retinal health further underscores the need for an integrated approach to patient care, one that transcends the traditional boundaries of ophthalmology.

While the management of vitreoretinal conditions has advanced considerably, it remains a field defined by its challenges. These challenges span the spectrum from the molecular underpinnings of diseases to the practical realities of clinical care, public health, and the recent impact of the COVID-19 pandemic. As we continue to navigate this complex landscape, our focus must remain on the continued pursuit of innovation, improved patient outcomes, and the expansion of our understanding of these intricate conditions.

## 2. An Overview of Published Articles

Mastropasqua et al. (Contributor 1) conducted a study focusing on the short-term effects of a novel implantable miniature telescope (SING-IMT™) in patients with end-stage age-related macular degeneration (AMD) and cataract. They reported significant improvements in both distance and near visual acuity and manageable intraocular pressure increases, recommending intraoperative mechanical iridectomy for better post-operative management.

Yamakawa et al. (Contributor 2) identified immune mediator profiles in the aqueous humour of eyes with simple diabetic retinopathy (DR). Their research, comparing 15 eyes with simple DR against 22 control eyes, found ten immune mediators in higher concentrations in the DR group, suggesting the importance of monitoring these mediators even in early stages of DR.

Sedova et al. (Contributor 3) evaluated changes in surgical strategies for primary rhegmatogenous retinal detachment (RRD) treatment over eight years. Their retrospective analysis of 812 cases showed improved visual acuity and reattachment rates, with a shift from scleral buckling to primary vitrectomy and an increased preference for daytime surgeries.

Merad et al. (Contributor 4) focused on cystoid macular oedema (CMO) post pars plana vitrectomy (PPV) for primary rhegmatogenous retinal detachment repair. In their study involving 493 eyes, they identified risk factors for developing CMO, including worse presenting visual acuity and specific surgical techniques.

Hsu et al. (Contributor 5) investigated the treatment outcomes and complications of peripheral circumferential retinal detachment (PCD) following successful vitrectomy. They concluded that proper management, including peripheral retinectomy, is vital for preserving visual function in PCD cases.

Cisiecki et al. (Contributor 6) assessed the effectiveness of encircling scleral buckling surgery for severe hypotony caused by proliferative vitreoretinopathy-induced retinal detachment. Their retrospective study of six patients showed improved intraocular pressure and visual acuity post-surgery, suggesting the potential usefulness of this surgical technique in specific cases of severe hypotony.

Our research team (Contributor 7) reported on the significant impact of the COVID-19 pandemic on macular hole surgery. Our study compared pre-pandemic and pandemic-period data, highlighting a marked reduction in surgeries, increased waiting times, and poorer surgical outcomes during the pandemic, underscoring the need for better strategies to continue elective surgeries during such crises.

Raimondi et al. (Contributor 8) conducted a literature review on the FIL SSF (Carlevale) intraocular lens, comparing its outcomes with those for other secondary IOL implants. Their analysis revealed comparable outcomes and lower rates of post-operative complications with the FIL SSF IOL, indicating its effectiveness and safety in cases lacking capsular support.

Confalonieri et al. (Contributor 9) undertook a systematic review examining treatment outcomes for subretinal macular haemorrhage (SRMH) secondary to AMD. Despite various treatment approaches, there is no consensus on the best treatment modality, highlighting the need for further research.

Lastly, Ripa et al. (Contributor 10) performed a systematic review and meta-analysis to evaluate the incidence of sympathetic ophthalmia (SO) following vitreoretinal surgery in the absence of trauma. Their study indicated that VR surgery could be a trigger for SO, emphasising the need for careful patient counselling in VR surgery.

## 3. Conclusions

In conclusion, the articles featured in this Special Issue collectively underscore the multifaceted and evolving landscape of vitreoretinal conditions. The diversity of topics, ranging from advanced surgical techniques, as explored by Mastropasqua et al., to the intricate interplay of immune mediators in diabetic retinopathy investigated by Yamakawa et al., highlights the breadth and complexity of challenges faced in this field. The shift in surgical paradigms towards more effective and less invasive techniques, demonstrated in the works of Sedova et al. and Cisiecki et al., reflects a broader trend towards patient-centred care that maximises outcomes while minimising risks.

The impact of the COVID-19 pandemic, as discussed by our research team, has brought to light the vulnerabilities and resilience of healthcare systems, underscoring the necessity for adaptable and robust strategies to maintain high-quality care even in times of crisis. This is particularly pertinent given the time-sensitive nature of many vitreoretinal interventions, where delays can lead to significantly poorer outcomes.

The collective insights from these studies not only enhance our understanding of the current state of vitreoretinal management but also pave the way for future research and innovation. The need for continued exploration is evident, as seen in the systematic reviews by Confalonieri and Ripa et al., which call for more definitive research to establish optimal treatment protocols for complex conditions like subretinal macular haemorrhage and to better understand rare but serious complications like sympathetic ophthalmia post-surgery.

As we navigate the intricate interplay of clinical practice, research advancements, and healthcare delivery, the articles in this Special Issue offer valuable guidance and inspiration. They remind us of the importance of ongoing research, the need for the continued development of more effective and safer treatment modalities, and the critical role of adapting to new challenges, such as those presented by global health crises.

In summary, this Special Issue not only provides a comprehensive overview of the current challenges in the management of vitreoretinal conditions but also serves as a beacon, guiding us towards a future where improved understanding and innovative approaches can lead to better patient outcomes and a deeper comprehension of these complex conditions.

**Conflicts of Interest:** The authors declare no conflict of interest.

**List of Contributors:**

1. Mastropasqua, R.; Gironi, M.; D'Aloisio, R.; Pastore, V.; Boscia, G.; Vecchiarino, L.; Perna, F.; Clemente, K.; Palladinetti, I.; Calandra, M.; et al. Intraoperative Iridectomy in Femto-Laser Assisted Smaller-Incision New Generation Implantable Miniature Telescope. *J. Clin. Med.* **2024**, *13*, 76. https://doi.org/10.3390/jcm13010076.
2. Yamakawa, N.; Komatsu, H.; Usui, Y.; Tsubota, K.; Wakabayashi, Y.; Goto, H. Immune Mediators Profiles in the Aqueous Humor of Patients with Simple Diabetic Retinopathy. *J. Clin. Med.* **2023**, *12*, 6931. https://doi.org/10.3390/jcm12216931.
3. Sedova, A.; Scholda, C.; Huebl, T.; Steiner, I.; Sacu, S.; Georgopoulos, M.; Schmidt-Erfurth, U.; Pollreisz, A. Effect of Changes in Surgical Strategies for the Treatment of Primary Rhegmatogenous Retinal Detachment on Functional and Anatomical Outcomes: A Retrospective Analysis of 812 Cases from the Years 2004 to 2012. *J. Clin. Med.* **2023**, *12*, 2278. https://doi.org/10.3390/jcm12062278.
4. Merad, M.; Vérité, F.; Baudin, F.; Ghezala, I.B.; Meillon, C.; Bron, A.M.; Arnould, L.; Eid, P.; Creuzot-Garcher, C.; Gabrielle, P.-H. Cystoid Macular Edema after Rhegmatogenous Retinal Detachment Repair with Pars Plana Vitrectomy: Rate, Risk Factors, and Outcomes. *J. Clin. Med.* **2022**, *11*, 4914. https://doi.org/10.3390/jcm11164914.
5. Hsu, C.-R.; Yang, C.-M. Peripheral Circumferential Retinal Detachment after Pars Plana Vitrectomy: Complications and Management. *J. Clin. Med.* **2022**, *11*, 4856. https://doi.org/10.3390/jcm11164856.

6. Cisiecki, S.; Bonińska, K.; Bednarski, M. Encircling Scleral Buckling Surgery for Severe Hypotony with Ciliary Body Detachment on Anterior Segment Swept-Source Optical Coherence Tomography: A Case Series. *J. Clin. Med.* **2022**, *11*, 4647. https://doi.org/10.3390/jcm11164647.
7. Panos, G.D.; Poyser, O.; Sarwar, H.; Kumudhan, D.; Orr, G.; Zaman, A.; Wilde, C. The Impact of the COVID-19 Pandemic and Lockdown on Macular Hole Surgery Provision and Surgical Outcomes: A Single-Centre Experience. *J. Clin. Med.* **2022**, *11*, 3678. https://doi.org/10.3390/jcm11133678.
8. Raimondi, R.; Sorrentino, T.; Kilian, R.; Verma, Y.; De Rosa, F.P.; Cancian, G.; Tsoutsanis, P.; Fossati, G.; Allegrini, D.; Romano, M.R. Trans-Scleral Plugs Fixated FIL SSF IOL: A Review of the Literature and Comparison with Other Secondary IOL Implants. *J. Clin. Med.* **2023**, *12*, 1994. https://doi.org/10.3390/jcm12051994.
9. Confalonieri, F.; Ferraro, V.; Barone, G.; Di Maria, A.; Petrovski, B.É.; Vallejo Garcia, J.L.; Randazzo, A.; Vinciguerra, P.; Lumi, X.; Petrovski, G. Outcomes in the Treatment of Subretinal Macular Hemorrhage Secondary to Age-Related Macular Degeneration: A Systematic Review. *J. Clin. Med.* **2024**, *13*, 367. https://doi.org/10.3390/jcm13020367.
10. Ripa, M.; Panos, G.D.; Rejdak, R.; Empeslidis, T.; Toro, M.D.; Costagliola, C.; Ferrara, A.; Gotzaridis, S.; Frisina, R.; Motta, L. Sympathetic Ophthalmia after Vitreoretinal Surgery without Antecedent History of Trauma: A Systematic Review and Meta-Analysis. *J. Clin. Med.* **2023**, *12*, 2316. https://doi.org/10.3390/jcm12062316.

# References

1. Javed, A.; Khanna, A.; Palmer, E.; Wilde, C.; Zaman, A.; Orr, G.; Kumudhan, D.; Lakshmanan, A.; Panos, G.D. Optical coherence tomography angiography: A review of the current literature. *J. Int. Med. Res.* **2023**, *51*, 3000605231187933. [CrossRef] [PubMed]
2. Panos, G.D. Advances in intravitreal therapy and implants: Where are we now? *Ther. Deliv.* **2020**, *11*, 69–73. [CrossRef] [PubMed]
3. Fleckenstein, M.; Schmitz-Valckenberg, S.; Chakravarthy, U. Age-related macular degeneration: A review. *JAMA* **2024**, *331*, 147–157. [CrossRef] [PubMed]
4. Virgilia, G.; Currana, K.; Lucenteforte, E.; Peto, T.; Parravano, M. Anti-vascular endothelial growth factor for diabetic macular oedema: A network meta-analysis. *Cochrane Database Syst. Rev.* **2023**, *2023*, CD007419.
5. Carducci, N.M.; Li, K.X.; Moinuddin, O.; Besirli, C.G.; Wubben, T.J.; Zacks, D.N. Clinical presentation and outcomes of rhegmatogenous retinal detachments during the COVID-19 lockdown and its aftermath at a tertiary care center in michigan. *Ophthalmic Surg. Lasers Imaging Retina* **2021**, *52*, 593–600. [CrossRef] [PubMed]
6. Baudin, F.; Benzenine, E.; Mariet, A.S.; Ben Ghezala, I.; Daien, V.; Gabrielle, P.H.; Quantin, C.; Creuzot-Garcher, C.P. Impact of COVID-19 lockdown on surgical procedures for retinal detachment in france: A national database study. *Br. J. Ophthalmol.* **2023**, *107*, 565–569. [CrossRef] [PubMed]
7. Mahendradas, P.; Sethu, S.; Jayadev, C.; Anilkumar, A.; Kawali, A.; Sanjay, S.; Mishra, S.B.; Shetty, R.; Shetty, B.K. Trends in teleconsultations for uveitis during the COVID-19 lockdown. *Indian. J. Ophthalmol.* **2022**, *70*, 1007–1012. [CrossRef] [PubMed]
8. Xu, M.; Fan, R.; Fan, X.; Shao, Y.; Li, X. Progress and challenges of anti-vegf agents and their sustained-release strategies for retinal angiogenesis. *Drug Des. Devel Ther.* **2022**, *16*, 3241–3262. [CrossRef] [PubMed]
9. Agarwal, K.; Vinekar, A.; Chandra, P.; Padhi, T.R.; Nayak, S.; Jayanna, S.; Panchal, B.; Jalali, S.; Das, T. Imaging the pediatric retina: An overview. *Indian. J. Ophthalmol.* **2021**, *69*, 812–823. [CrossRef] [PubMed]
10. Lam, W.C.; Chan, R.V.P. Pediatric retinal diseases. *Asia Pac. J. Ophthalmol.* **2018**, *7*, 129.
11. Cioana, M.; Deng, J.; Nadarajah, A.; Hou, M.; Qiu, Y.; Chen, S.S.J.; Rivas, A.; Toor, P.P.; Banfield, L.; Thabane, L.; et al. Global prevalence of diabetic retinopathy in pediatric type 2 diabetes: A systematic review and meta-analysis. *JAMA Netw. Open* **2023**, *6*, e231887. [CrossRef] [PubMed]
12. Rosenblatt, T.R.; Vail, D.; Saroj, N.; Boucher, N.; Moshfeghi, D.M.; Moshfeghi, A.A. Increasing incidence and prevalence of common retinal diseases in retina practices across the united states. *Ophthalmic Surg. Lasers Imaging Retina* **2021**, *52*, 29–36. [CrossRef] [PubMed]

**Disclaimer/Publisher's Note:** The statements, opinions and data contained in all publications are solely those of the individual author(s) and contributor(s) and not of MDPI and/or the editor(s). MDPI and/or the editor(s) disclaim responsibility for any injury to people or property resulting from any ideas, methods, instructions or products referred to in the content.

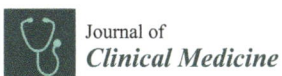

*Systematic Review*

# Outcomes in the Treatment of Subretinal Macular Hemorrhage Secondary to Age-Related Macular Degeneration: A Systematic Review

Filippo Confalonieri [1,2,3,4,*], Vanessa Ferraro [1,2], Gianmaria Barone [1,2], Alessandra Di Maria [1,2], Beáta Éva Petrovski [3], Josè Luis Vallejo Garcia [1,2], Alessandro Randazzo [1,2], Paolo Vinciguerra [1,2], Xhevat Lumi [3,5] and Goran Petrovski [3,4,6,7,*]

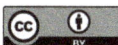

Citation: Confalonieri, F.; Ferraro, V.; Barone, G.; Di Maria, A.; Petrovski, B.É.; Vallejo Garcia, J.L.; Randazzo, A.; Vinciguerra, P.; Lumi, X.; Petrovski, G. Outcomes in the Treatment of Subretinal Macular Hemorrhage Secondary to Age-Related Macular Degeneration: A Systematic Review. *J. Clin. Med.* **2024**, *13*, 367. https://doi.org/10.3390/jcm13020367

Academic Editor: Georgios D. Panos

Received: 27 November 2023
Revised: 29 December 2023
Accepted: 4 January 2024
Published: 9 January 2024

Copyright: © 2024 by the authors. Licensee MDPI, Basel, Switzerland. This article is an open access article distributed under the terms and conditions of the Creative Commons Attribution (CC BY) license (https://creativecommons.org/licenses/by/4.0/).

[1] Department of Ophthalmology, IRCCS Humanitas Research Hospital, Rozzano, 20089 Milan, Italy; vanessa.ferraro@humanitas.it (V.F.); gianmaria.barone@humanitas.it (G.B.); alessandra.di_maria@humanitas.it (A.D.M.); jose_luis.vallejo_garcia@humanitas.it (J.L.V.G.); paolo.vinciguerra@humanitas.it (P.V.)
[2] Department of Biomedical Sciences, Humanitas University, Pieve Emanuele, 20090 Milan, Italy
[3] Center for Eye Research and Innovative Diagnostics, Department of Ophthalmology, Institute for Clinical Medicine, University of Oslo, Kirkeveien 166, 0450 Oslo, Norway; beata.petrovski@odont.uio.no (B.É.P.); xhevat.lumi@kclj.si (X.L.)
[4] Department of Ophthalmology, Oslo University Hospital, Kirkeveien 166, 0450 Oslo, Norway
[5] Eye Hospital, University Medical Centre Ljubljana, Zaloška Cesta 2, 1000 Ljubljana, Slovenia
[6] Department of Ophthalmology, University of Split School of Medicine and University Hospital Centre, 21000 Split, Croatia
[7] UKLONetwork, University St. Kliment Ohridski-Bitola, 7000 Bitola, North Macedonia
* Correspondence: filippo.confalonieri@humanitas.it (F.C.); goran.petrovski@medisin.uio.no (G.P.)

**Abstract: Background**: Subretinal macular hemorrhage (SRMH) secondary to age-related macular degeneration (AMD) is a relatively rare condition in ophthalmology characterized by blood collection between the neurosensory retina and the retinal pigment epithelium (RPE). Without prompt treatment, visual prognosis is poor. A plethora of treatment approaches have been tried over the past years ranging from intravitreal anti-vascular endothelial growth factor (anti-VEGF) monotherapy to direct subretinal surgery, with no conclusive superiority of one over the other. **Materials and Methods**: We conducted a systematic review of the outcomes and treatment modalities of SRMH from inception to 14 June 2022, following the Preferred Reporting Items for Systematic Reviews and Meta-Analyses guidelines (PRISMA). The level of evidence was assessed for all included articles according to the quality of evidence according to the Grading of Recommendations Assessment, Development and Evaluation (GRADE) system. **Results**: A total of 2745 articles were initially extracted, out of which 1654 articles were obtained after duplicates were removed and their abstracts screened. A total of 155 articles were included for full-text review. Finally, 81 articles remained that fulfilled the inclusion criteria. **Conclusions**: Even though there are solid results supporting a variety of treatments for SRMH, the best treatment modality has still not been conclusively demonstrated and further research is needed.

**Keywords:** subretinal macular hemorrhage (SRMH); age-related macular degeneration (AMD); vitreoretinal surgery; recombinant tissue plasminogen activator (rt-PA)

## 1. Introduction

Retinal hemorrhage is among the most common clinical signs in retinal disease and consists of a spectrum of blood collection differing in location, size, distribution, and etiology [1]. Fovea-involving subretinal macular hemorrhage (SRMH) is a sight-threatening condition defined as blood collection between the neurosensory retina and the retinal pigment epithelium (RPE) [2]. SRMH can be caused by a plethora of eye disorders, including neovascular age-related macular degeneration (n-AMD) and its variants such as polypoid choroidal vasculopathy (PCV), but also pathologic myopia, ruptured retinal artery macroaneurysms, presumed ocular histoplasmosis syndrome, and trauma [3–7]. SRMH can cause irreversible damage to the photoreceptors; if left untreated, a blood clot under the retina usually turns into a scar, causing permanent loss of central vision [8–10].

AMD is the leading cause of legal blindness in the industrialized world [11]. The real incidence of SRMH among patients with n-AMD is unknown [12], even though n-AMD has long been known to be a risk factor for submacular bleeding [8,13].

SRMHs larger than one disc diameter (DD) across in size have been reported in 24 people per million per year, according to a population-based study conducted in two UK centers, while SRMHs larger than two DDs have been reported in only 5.4 people per million per year in a study by a Scottish Ophthalmic Surveillance Unit (SOSU) [14,15]. Nevertheless, the population in many countries is ageing and the disease prevalence for AMD, and therefore SRMHs, is supposed to increase significantly in the coming years [16].

SRMH generally results in a severe and irreversible loss of vision, ranging from 6/30 to light perception, if left untreated [17]. Moreover, only 11% of the eyes in the control group of a submacular surgery study achieve a final best-corrected visual acuity (BCVA) higher than 6/60 [10]. The functional outcome may also be influenced by the duration and size of SRMH, as well as the etiology and location of the bleeding source. Persistent SRMH damages the photoreceptors through three main mechanisms: iron-related toxicity, impairment of diffusion of oxygen and nutrition, and mechanical damage due to clot contraction [18–23]. The natural history of SRMH typically leads to a central scotoma with a fibrotic macular scar (38%), atrophy (25%), or RPE rupture (22%) [17].

A variety of approaches have been employed in the treatment of SRMH, and even though ample literature exists, this is dispersive and predominantly made up of small, single-center outcome reports that do not encompass all the therapeutic techniques that have been described.

The purpose of this systematic review is to analyze and summarize the current therapeutic approaches in the management of SRMH while evaluating the level and quality of the research included.

## 2. Materials and Methods

A systematic review was conducted and reported according to the Preferred Reporting Items for Systematic Reviews and Meta-Analyses (PRISMA) guidelines [24]. The review protocol was not recorded in the study design, but a registration number will be available for consultation. The methodology used consisted of a systematic search of all available articles exploring the treatment modalities of SRMH secondary to n-AMD. To identify all relevant published articles, we performed a systematic literature search including papers published from inception until 14 June 2022. These were searched in Ovid Medline, Embase, Cochrane Register of Controlled Trials, and Cochrane Database of Systematic Reviews using controlled vocabulary and text words expressing (subretinal OR submacular) AND (hemorrhage OR haemorrhage OR bleeding). The search was not restricted by publication type, study design, or date of publication. The search was restricted by the English language. The complete search strategy is given in Appendix A.

Subsequently, the reference lists of all identified articles were examined manually to identify any potential study not selected by the electronic searches. After the preparation of the list of all electronic data, a reviewer (FC) examined the titles and abstracts and identified relevant articles. All the studies analyzing outcomes of the available treatment modalities of SRMH in n-AMD were considered as satisfactory for the inclusion criteria. Exclusion criteria were review studies, pilot studies, letters to the editor, case series with ≤12 eyes, case reports, photo essays, and studies written in languages other than English. Moreover, studies performed on animal eyes, cadaveric eyes, and pediatric patients were excluded as well. Exclusion criteria also included studies that were not specifically powered to detect a correlation between the treatment modality of either the anatomical or functional outcomes in SRMH treatment. SRMH secondary to diseases other than n-AMD was also excluded.

The same reviewer registered and selected the studies according to the inclusion and exclusion criteria by examining the full text of the articles. Any doubt was assessed by consensus with a third-party reviewer (GP), who was consulted when necessary. No further unpublished data were obtained from the corresponding authors of all selected articles, which were analyzed to assess the level of evidence according to the quality of evidence according to the Grading of Recommendations Assessment, Development and Evaluation (GRADE) system [25,26].

## 3. Results

A total of 2745 articles were initially extracted. Consequently, 1654 articles were obtained after the duplicates were removed and their abstracts were screened. Subsequently, 155 articles were included for the full-text review and more in-depth evaluation of the inclusion/exclusion criteria. Finally, 81 articles remained that fulfilled all the inclusion criteria.

Figure 1 summarizes the research approach applied here in a flowchart.

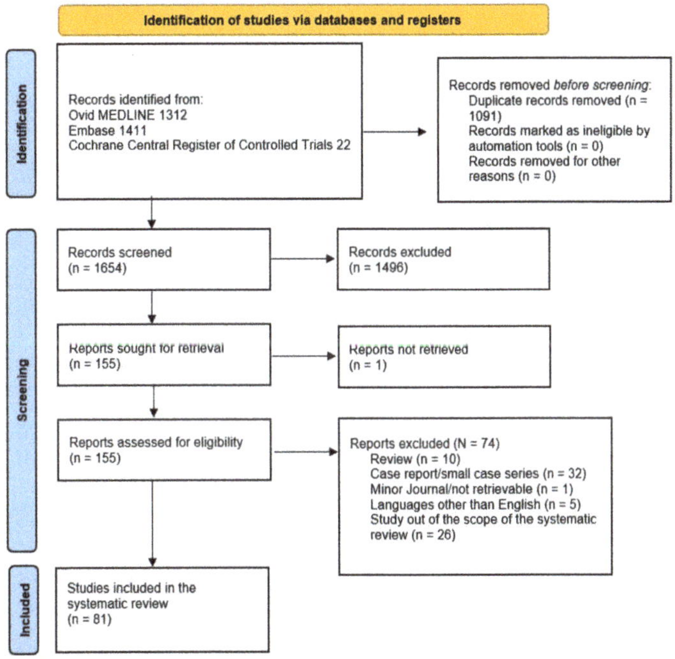

**Figure 1.** Flowchart of the literature search and selection according to Preferred Reporting Items for Systematic Reviews and Meta-Analyses guidelines (PRISMA) [24].

The determining reasons for inclusion or exclusion of the full-text reviewed articles are summarized in Appendix B. Furthermore, Appendix C summarizes all the studies extracted from the systematic literature search, with the relevant descriptive information.

In order to summarize the large amount of information derived from the systematic search, Table 1 was created to report on the studies that are prospective or randomized controlled trials (RCTs). These are in fact the most valuable studies, and they are the main source of evidence.

In Table 2, the studies were grouped according to the type of intervention that was applied, which were anti-vascular endothelial growth factor (anti-VEGF) only, intravitreal recombinant tissue plasminogen activator (rt-PA), and/or subretinal rt-PA.

Table 1. Prospective or RCT studies on subretinal bleeding.

| References | Year | Study Design | Study Sample (Eyes) | Type of Surgery | Mean Size of the Bleeding | Outcome Final BCVA | Mean Days from Onset | Complications | GRADE [1] |
|---|---|---|---|---|---|---|---|---|---|
| [27] | 2006 | Longitudinal PROSP | 101 | IVT PA | >1 DD | - | <4 weeks | None | Moderate |
| [28] | 2007 | PROSP, CONSEC, single-center, NComp, ITRV, case series | 20 | IVT C$_3$F$_8$ without rt-PA | N/A | Improved | Range from 1 to 30 days | 4 VH | Moderate |
| [29] | 2014 | PROSP, ITRV, case series | 23 | IVT ranibizumab | Occult choroidal neo-vascularization with flat large submacular hemorrhage > 50% of the entire lesion | Improved | N/A | None | Very low |
| [30] | 2015 | PROSP, NRandom, NComp, case series | 21 | PPV + 360° retinotomy + silicon oil (Oxane 5700) tamponade | N/A | Improved | N/A | 10 mild subretinal fibrosis | Moderate |
| [31] | 2016 | PROSP, NComp, ITRV, case series | 24 | Group A: PPV + gas + subretinal rt-PA; Group B: IVT rt-PA + gas | Group A: 11.1 DA (range 0.5–31.0); Group B: 9.7 DA (range 2.9–20.2) | Improved | Group A: 5 (range 1–11), Group B: 6 (range 1–14) | Group A: 3 increased IOP > 50 mmHg, 2 VH, 1 RD, 1 recurrence. Group B: 2 RD, 2 recurrences | Very low |
| [32] | 2016 | PROSP, ITRV, CONSEC, case series | 20 | IVT rt-PA + ranibizumab + gas without PPV | 11.1 ± 8.7 DD (range: 2–31) | Improved | 9.9 ± 9.8 days (range 2–30) | 3 VH, 1 RD | Very low |
| [33] | 2022 | Extended study of previous PROSP study | 64 | IVT rt-PA + ranibizumab + gas | 8 ± 6 (range, 2–27) disc diameters | Improved | 7 ± 7 days (range 1–30) | 46 recurrences | Low |
| [34] | 2021 | Secondary analyses of an RCT of image and clinical data | 535 | Randomly divided: monthly IVT ranibizumab, as-needed IVT ranibizumab, monthly IVT bevacizumab, or as-needed bevacizumab | 89% were < 1 DD | Improved | N/A | 1 RPE tear, 28 fibrosis, 10 atrophic scars, 6 geographic atrophies, 7 epiretinal membranes | Moderate |

Legend: CONSEC: consecutive series; IOP: intraocular pressure; ITRV: interventional; IVT: intravitreal; NComp: non-comparative; NRand: non-randomized; PROSP: prospective; RD: retinal detachment; rt-PA: recombinant plasminogen activator; VH: vitreous hemorrhage. [1] Grading of Recommendations Assessment, Development and Evaluation (GRADE) system [25,26].

Table 2. Studies on subretinal bleeding according to treatment strategies: anti-VEGF only vs. IVT rt-PA vs. subretinal rt-PA.

| References | Study Design | Study Sample (No. of Eyes) | Type of Surgery | Mean Size of the Bleeding | Outcome Final BCVA | Mean Days from Onset | GRADE [1] |
|---|---|---|---|---|---|---|---|
| [35] | NRand, Retro, ITRV, COMPR, CONSEC | 47 | PPV + IVT rt-PA + SF$_6$ (group A) vs. PPV + subretinal rt-PA + SF$_6$ (group B) | N/A | No significant difference | 6.6 days (group A), 5.9 days (group B) | Low |
| [36] | NRand, Retro, ITRV, COMPR, CONSEC | 38 | IVT rt-PA + SF$_6$ (group A) vs. IVT bevacizumab + rt-PA + SF$_6$ (group B) | >1 DD | Significantly higher in group B | 1–31 days | Low |
| [37] | NRand, Retro, COMPR, case study | 110 | rt-PA injection w/o gas injection (group A1: 50 μg of rt-PA; A2: 100 μg; A3: 200 μg) and with gas injection (group B1: 50 μg of rt-PA; B2: 100 μg; B3: 200 μg) | 12.5 (1–38) DD | Better in B1 and B2 groups | 10.0 (0.5–180.0) | Low |
| [38] | NRand, Retro, ITRV, COMPR, CONSEC | 45 | rt-PA (50 μg 0.05 mL) + SF$_6$ (group A); bevacizumab (1.25 mg 0.05 mL) + SF$_6$ (group B). Thereafter, all patients received bevacizumab | 1–5 DD | Better in group A | N/A | Low |
| [39] | Retro, single-center study | 46 | PPV + subretinal rt-PA (group 1); pneumatic displacement + IVT rt-PA + gas (group 2); PD + gas (group 3) | 5.6 ± 3.4 DD | No significant difference | 10 | Low |
| [40] | Retro, COMPR, ITRV, case series | 32 | PD (SF$_6$) + IVT bevacizumab (group A) vs. PD (SF$_6$) alone (group B) | >2 DD | Significantly better in group A | <10 days | Low |
| [41] | Retro, NComp, ITRV, case series | 46 | IVT bevacizumab (group A: 1–4 DD), group B (4–9 DD), group C (>9 DD) | 6 DD | Amongst groups, improvement of the BCVA in 57% (13/23), 53% (8/15), and 38% (3/8) of eyes, respectively. | 11.5 ± 19 days (range: 1–45 days) | Low |

Table 2. Cont.

| References | Study Design | Study Sample (No. of Eyes) | Type of Surgery | Mean Size of the Bleeding | Outcome Final BCVA | Mean Days from Onset | GRADE [1] |
|---|---|---|---|---|---|---|---|
| [42] | Retro, COMPR, ITRV, case series | 82 | PD ($SF_6$ or $C_3F_8$) + IVT anti-VEGF vs. anti-VEGF monotherapy | N/A | No significant difference; combination therapy group showed better BCVA at 1 month after initial treatment compared to monotherapy | 11.4 ± 10.4 days in the combination therapy group; 13.8 ± 11.5 days in the monotherapy group | Low |
| [31] | Prospective, NComp, ITRV, case series | 24 | PPV + gas + subretinal rt-PA (Group A); intravitreal rt-PA + gas (Group B) | Group A: 11.1 DD (range 0.5–31.0); Group B: 9.7 DD (range 2.9–20.2) | No significant difference | Group A: 5 (range 1–11), Group B: 6 (range 1–14) | Very low |
| [43] | Retro, case series | 39 | PPV + subretinal rt-PA (Group A); PD + IVT rt-PA (Group B); PD without rt-PA (Group C) | Group A: 9.1 mm²; Group B: 8.1 mm²; Group C: 9.1 mm² | Improved significantly in both Groups A and B, but not C | Group A: 5 ± 4.6; Group B: 6 ± 4.2; Group C: 6 ± 2.2 | Low |
| [44] | Retro, COMPR, ITRV, case series | 20 | Group A: subretinal rt-PA + PPV; Group B: or intravitreal rt-PA + gas to achieve PD. Additionally, combination treatment with either PDT or IVT of anti-VEGF was performed | 17.8 ± 19.2 disc diameter (DD) compared (2.64 DD) | Combination treatment with PDT showed significant efficacy in the improvement of BCVA | 14.3 ± 16.6 days | Very low |
| [45] | Retro | 18 | PD followed by IVT rt-PA if needed vs. PPV with subretinal rt-PA | N/A | ≥lines improvement at 1 year was 46% and 18% in the groups, respectively; no significant difference | N/A | Very low |

Table 2. Cont.

| References | Study Design | Study Sample (No. of Eyes) | Type of Surgery | Mean Size of the Bleeding | Outcome Final BCVA | Mean Days from Onset | GRADE [1] |
|---|---|---|---|---|---|---|---|
| [46] | Retro | 77 | Group A: anti-VEGF monotherapy; Group B: PD + anti-VEGF; Group C: PPV + subretinal rt-PA – gas tamponade | Three groups according to dimensions: small-sized (optic disc diameter (ODD) ≥ 1 to <4), medium-sized (ODD ≥ 4 within the temporal arcade), and large-sized (ODD ≥ 4, exceeding the temporal arcade) | Small-sized group: all treatments had gradual BCVA improvement; medium-sized group: PD and surgery were associated with better BCVA than anti-VEGF monotherapy; large-sized group: surgery showed a better visual improvement with a higher displacement rate than PD | 14.3 ± 25.8 | Low |
| [47] | Retro, NComp, ITRV, case series | 96 | IVT rt-PA + SF$_6$ for guiding the selection of additional treatments (anti-VEGF, PDT, or submacular surgery) or observation (CNV) | ≥3 DA involving the fovea | BCVA improved significantly | <14 days | Low |
| Asli [48] | Retro, case series | 54 | PPV + submacular rt-PA + 20% SF$_6$ or 14% C$_3$F$_8$; PPV + submacular rt-PA + 20% SF$_6$ or 14% C$_3$F$_8$ + anti-VEGF; PPV+ subretinal rt-PA without gas; IVT gas + rt-PA; PPV + subretinal rt-PA + drainage; IVT gas + IVT anti-VEGF | 31.5 ± 26.5 (2.8–145.3) mm$^2$ | BCVA improved | 13.7 ± 16.3 (1–95) days | Low |
| [49] | Retro | 29 | Group 1: IVT rt-PA + SF$_6$ Group 2: PPV + subretinal rt-PA + SF$_6$ with (2A) or without (2B) subretinal air | 9.45 ± 2.34 DD (Group 1) and 9.72 ± 2.02 DD (Group 2) | BCVA improved; Group 2: adding subretinal air gave no statistically significant difference in outcome | N/A | Very low |
| [50] | Retro | 30 | 13 eyes PD, 22 eyes IVT anti-VEGF, 4 eyes PPV | 17.0 ± 4.8 disc areas | BCVA improved | N/A | Low |

Table 2. *Cont.*

| References | Study Design | Study Sample (No. of Eyes) | Type of Surgery | Mean Size of the Bleeding | Outcome Final BCVA | Mean Days from Onset | GRADE [1] |
|---|---|---|---|---|---|---|---|
| [51] | Retro, CONSEC, case series | 31 | PPV + subretinal rt-PA + air displacement with or without IVT bevacizumab, respectively | $11.78 \pm 3.04$ mm$^2$ and $14.75 \pm 3.98$ mm$^2$, respectively | BCVA improved significantly | $3.3 \pm 1.6$ and $3.4 \pm 1.5$, respectively | Low |
| [52] | Retro | 54 | PPV + subretinal rt-PA + PD vs. anti-VEGF monotherapy | In rt-PA group: 5.0 DD; in anti-VEGF group: 4.2 DD | BCVA improved significantly for rt-PA group | 5 days (range: 1–13) | Low |
| [53] | Retro, COMPR, ITRV, case series | 25 | Group A: PPV + subretinal rt-PA + gas; Group B: IVT rt-PA + gas | $4.604 \pm 2079$ µm | BCVA improved significantly but did not differ between the 2 groups | $8.2 \pm 7.3$ days | Very low |
| [34] | Secondary analyses of an RCT of image and clinical data | 535 | Randomly divided: monthly IVT ranibizumab, as-needed IVT ranibizumab, monthly IVT bevacizumab or as-needed bevacizumab | 89% were <1 DD | BCVA improved | N/A | Moderate |
| [54] | Retro | 107 | Group A: IVT rt-PA + gas; Group B: PPV | 767 µm in Group A; 962.5 µm in Group B | Better improvement in the rt-PA + gas group | N/A | Low |

Legend: COMPR: comparative; CONSEC: consecutive series; DD: disc diameter; ITRV: interventional; IVT: intravitreal; NComp: non-comparative; NRand: non-randomized; PD: pneumatic displacement; RCT: randomized controlled trial; Retro: retrospective. [1] Grading of Recommendations Assessment, Development and Evaluation (GRADE) system [25,26].

In Table 3, a summary of the studies is provided according to the hemorrhage onset, as the timing of intervention seems to be crucial for the outcome of SRMH patients [55].

**Table 3.** Summary of the mean days from onset: less or more than 2 weeks from symptoms' onset in subretinal bleeding with references.

| Treatment < 14 Days from Onset (Mean) | Treatment More than 14 Days from Onset (Mean) | Treatment Both before and after 14 Days from Onset or Not Specified/Not Clear |
|---|---|---|
| De Jong et al. [31], Kitagawa et al. [32], Kitagawa et al. [33], Hillenkamp et al. [35], Tsymanava et al. [37], Rishi et al. [39], Kitahashi et al. [40], Dimopoulus et al. [41], Shin et al. [42], Fassbender et al. [43], Maggio et al. [47], Asli Kirmaci Kabakci et al. [48], Rickmann et al. [51], Sniatecki et al. [52], Tranos et al. [53], Ratanasukon et al. [56], Singh et al. [57], Yang et al. [58], Stifter et al. [59], Arias et al. [60], Cakir et al. [61], Kung et al. [62], Sandhu et al. [63], Treumer et al. [64], Cho et al. [65], Jain et al. [66], Moisseiev et al. [67], Kim et al. [68], Kimura et al. [69], González-López et al. [70], Lee et al. [71], Waizel et al. [72], Gok et al. [73], Waizel et al. [74], Bardak et al. [75], Sharma et al. [76], Karamitsos et al. [77], Lee et al. [78], Ali Said et al. [79], Avci et al. [80], Iannetta et al. [81], Kawakami et al. [82], Pierre et al. [13], Fukuda et al. [83] | Lin et al. [44], Jeong et al. [46], Juncal et al. [84], Olivier et al. [85], Kadonosono et al. [84,86], Kim et al. [87], Caporossi et al. [88], Ura et al. [89] | Mozaffarieh et al. [27], Gopalakrishan et al. [28], Mehta et al. [34], Guthoff et al. [36], Mayer et al. [38], Yang et al. [58], Iacono et al. [29], Wei et al. [30], Bell et al. [45], Kishikova et al. [49], Matsuo et al. [50], Tiosano et al. [54], Ura et al. [89], Thompson et al. [90], Ron et al. [91], Meyer et al. [92], Fang et al. [93], Fine et al. [94], Mizutani et al. [95], Han et al. [96], Shienbaum et al. [97], Chang et al. [98], Kimura et al. [99], Plemel et al. [100], Helaiwa et al. [101], Wilkins et al. [102] |

Finally, Table 4 groups all the included studies on the basis of SRMH size in an attempt to simplify the understanding for prognostic purposes.

**Table 4.** Studies on subretinal bleeding according to the size.

| References | Mean Size of the Bleeding (Disc Diameter (DD)) |
|---|---|
| Mehta et al. [34], Tiosano et al. [54] | <1 DD |
| Mozaffarieh et al. [27], Guthoff et al. [36], Fassbender et al. [43], Asli Kimarci Kabakci et al. [48], Rickmann et al. [51], Arias et al. [60], Kung et al. [62], Jain et al. [66], Meyer et al. [92], Shienbaum et al. [97], Ura et al. [89] | 1–3 DD |
| Iacono et al. [29], Rishi et al. [39], Dimopoulos et al. [41], Ratanasukon et al. [56], Kung et al. [62], Sandhu et al. [63], Treumer et al. [64], Kimura et al. [69], Avci et al. [80], Maggio et al. [47], Iannetta et al. [81], Pierre et al. [13], Thompson et al. [90], Ron et al. [91], Stifter et al. [59] | >3 DD |
| Iacono et al. [29], De Jong et al. [31], Kitagawa et al. [33], Mayer et al. [38], Kitahashi et al. [40], Jeong et al. [46], Kishikova et al. [49], Sniatecki et al. [52], Tranos et al. [53], Kimura et al. [69], Lee et al. [71], Gok et al. [73], Sharma et al. [76], Karamitsos et al. [77], Lee et al. [78], Kawakami et al. [82], Kim et al. [87], Juncal et al. [84], Helaiwa et al. [101], Ueda-arakawa et al. [103], Kim et al. [104] | <12 DD |
| Mozaffarieh et al. [27], De Jong et al. [31], Kitagawa et al. [32], Tsymanava et al. [37], Lin et al. [44], Matsuo et al. [50], Rickmann et al. [51], Cho et al. [65], Kim et al. [68], Sharma et al. [76], Juncal et al. [84], Plemel et al. [100], Bae et al. [105] | >12 DD |
| De Jong et al. [31], Ali Said et al. [79], Caporossi et al. [88], Fine et al. [94], Han et al. [96], Wilkins et al. [102] | Other (>2 quadrants; N/A) |

## 4. Discussion

SRMH poses a formidable challenge in the realm of retinal pathology, given its potential to cause irreversible damage to central vision. Despite its clinical significance, the optimal treatment strategy for SRMH remains to be an ongoing debate, largely due to the scarcity of comprehensive prospective studies and the consequent absence of a widely accepted best practice.

This systematic review critically assessed the existing literature on SRMH treatment modalities, focusing on prospective studies to elucidate the current landscape of therapeutic interventions. The number of prospective trials specifically targeting SRMH is limited, thus underscoring the need for further robust investigations to guide evidence-based decision-making. Within the sparse collection of prospective studies, various treatment options have been explored, ranging from conservative observation to surgical interventions. Notably, only retrospective studies by Ueda-Arakawa et al. [103] and Maggio et al. [47] have explored the merits of a watchful waiting approach, positing its suitability for cases marked by minimal visual impairment and self-resolving hemorrhages. Nevertheless, due to the relatively small sample sizes and inherent variability in hemorrhage characteristics, these studies have not been able to definitively establish the superiority of observation over the active therapeutic interventions.

Pneumatic displacement, an innovative approach, has gained attention for its potential to physically displace subretinal hemorrhage away from the macula. The prospective investigations by Gopalakrishan et al. [28] and De Jong et al. [31] unveiled encouraging results, suggesting improved visual outcomes. However, the limited number of patients and the absence of long-term follow-up data cast a shadow over the sustainability of these positive findings.

Anti-VEGF agents, with their established efficacy in various retinal pathologies, have been examined as a potential treatment modality for SRMH. Iacono et al. [29] conducted prospective studies probing the impact of anti-VEGF injections on neovascularization and inflammation associated with SRMH. Despite the promise showcased in this study, the lack of consensus in the treatment regimens and the modest sample sizes hinder the establishment of a definitive therapeutic role for anti-VEGF agents.

Surgical interventions, specifically vitrectomy with or without rt-PA injection, have been a subject of exploration through prospective studies by Wei et al. [30], Mozafarieh et al. [27], Kadonosono et al. [86], Kimura et al. [69], and De Jong et al. [31]. These studies have shed light on the potential benefits of surgical intervention, particularly in cases of larger and dense or recurrent hemorrhage. However, the invasiveness of the procedure, coupled with concerns regarding complications, necessitates judicious patient selection and cautious consideration of risks and benefits.

Photodynamic therapy (PDT), a modality with established efficacy in other retinal conditions, has also found its way into the discourse surrounding SRMH treatment. Notable retrospective studies by Lin et al. [44] have ventured into investigating PDT's potential role in addressing neovascularization in SRMH. Nevertheless, the existing body of evidence is marked by its infancy and a lack of consistent findings, impeding the establishment of PDT as a definitive treatment avenue.

Our work sums up all the available treatment modalities of SRMH. As the management of this condition is a complex and challenging task, several treatment modalities have been developed to address it, each with its own set of advantages and limitations. We will further highlight the various treatment modalities for SRMH below.

Intravitreal Anti-VEGF Therapy: Intravitreal injection of anti-VEGF agents, such as ranibizumab and bevacizumab, has gained popularity in recent years. These drugs can resolve SRMH by inhibiting abnormal blood vessel growth and leakage in conditions like CNV. The advantages of this approach include its minimal invasiveness and relatively rapid resolution of the hemorrhage. However, it may not be effective in all cases, and multiple injections over an extended period of time may be required. The long-term safety profile of these agents also warrants the ongoing and further research.

Pneumatic displacement involves the injection of expansile gases, such as sulfur hexafluoride or perfluoropropane, into the vitreous cavity. This gas displaces the SRMH, moving it away from the macula, allowing for improved vision. Pneumatic displacement is less invasive than other surgical procedures and can be an effective treatment option. However, it may be associated with complications, such as subretinal blood displacement, which necessitates careful patient selection and follow-up.

Vitrectomy is a surgical intervention that involves the removal of vitreous gel from the eye. This procedure allows direct visualization and access to the subretinal space, enabling the removal of blood and other substances. Vitrectomy is effective in a wide range of cases, particularly when the hemorrhage is extensive, the fibrosis has occurred, or when other treatment modalities have failed. However, it is an invasive procedure with potential surgical risks, longer recovery times, and need for careful postoperative management. Potential complications from pneumatic displacement during vitrectomy can include vitreous or choroidal hemorrhage, hyphema, RPE tear and cataract formation, retinal detachment, increased intraocular pressure/glaucoma, full-thickness macular hole formation, and endophthalmitis (Appendix C).

Subretinal injection of rt-PA followed by the injection of an expansile gas, such as sulfur hexafluoride or perfluoropropane can facilitate the mechanical displacement of the SRMH and potentially improve visual outcomes. However, it is a surgical procedure and requires experienced surgical skills to minimize risks.

The choice of treatment for SRMH should be individualized, considering factors such as the extent and location of the hemorrhage; the patient's overall health, including blood pressure and cardiac status, use of blood thinners, and INR level where applicable; the visual acuity goals; and the potential risks and benefits associated with each option. A multidisciplinary approach, involving ophthalmologists, vitreoretinal surgeons, and the patient, is often crucial in making the most informed decision.

A flow chart on the clinical diagnostics, management, and treatment of patients with acute loss of vision due to suspected SRMH is depicted in Figure 2.

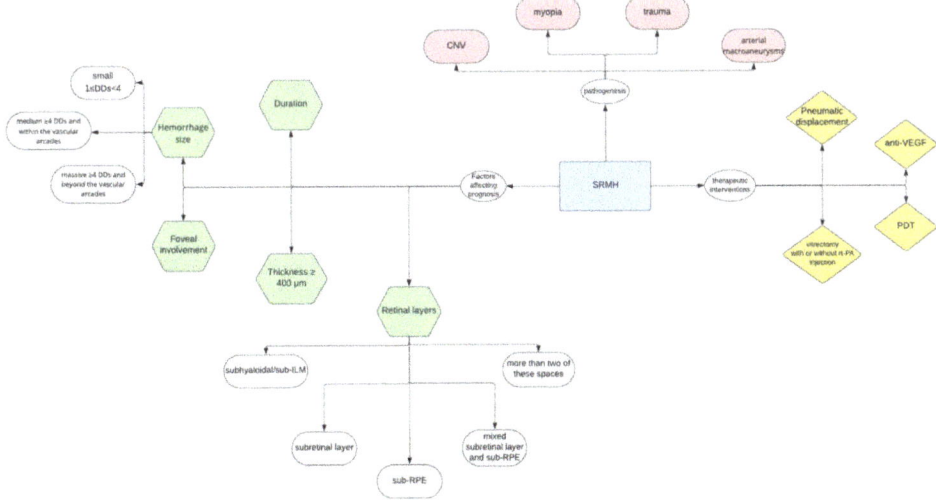

**Figure 2.** Flow chart on the clinical diagnostics, management, and treatment of patients with acute loss of vision due to suspected SRMH. Disc diameter (DD); photodynamic therapy (PDT).

As research continues to evolve, new treatment modalities and refinements to existing approaches may emerge, offering hope for improved outcomes and quality of life for individuals affected by SRMH. The optimal approach to managing this condition will depend on the specific characteristics and needs of each patient, and ongoing clinical trials and research will help shape the future of SRMH treatment.

## 5. Conclusions

In conclusion, the management of subretinal macular hemorrhage presents a complex and challenging clinical scenario. Various treatment modalities have been explored, each with its own set of pros and cons. The choice of treatment should be tailored to the individual patient, taking into consideration the specific characteristics of the hemorrhage, the patient's overall health, and their visual acuity goals.

Intravitreal injection of anti-VEGF agents has emerged as a promising non-invasive option for some patients. Its advantages include rapid resolution of hemorrhage, minimal invasiveness, and a potential for improved visual outcomes. However, it may not be effective in all cases, especially in instances of massive hemorrhage or when fibrotic changes have already occurred. Additionally, the need for multiple injections and the long-term safety profile of these drugs require ongoing research.

Surgical interventions, such as pneumatic displacement and vitrectomy, offer the advantage of direct visualization and removal of the hemorrhage. These procedures can be effective in a wider range of cases and may yield significant improvements in vision. Nevertheless, they come with the risk of surgical complications, prolonged recovery periods, and potential long-term anatomical changes. The choice of surgery should be made carefully, considering the individual patient's surgical risk profile and the likelihood of postoperative complications.

The use of subretinal tPA and gas injection, while it may achieve faster resolution compared to observation alone, it is still an invasive procedure like traditional vitrectomy. This technique is, however, not suitable for all cases and requires experienced surgical hands to minimize risks.

Ultimately, the decision on the most appropriate treatment modality for subretinal macular hemorrhage should be made through a multidisciplinary approach involving the ophthalmologist, the patient, and other healthcare providers. It is imperative to weigh the potential benefits against the risks and limitations of each approach while considering the patient's individual circumstances and preferences. Ongoing research and clinical trials will continue to refine our understanding of these treatment modalities and potentially lead to further advancements in the management of this challenging condition. As we move forward, it is crucial that clinicians remain vigilant in their pursuit of improved therapies, with the goal of optimizing visual outcomes and enhancing the quality of life for patients with subretinal macular hemorrhage.

**Author Contributions:** Conceptualization, F.C.; methodology, F.C., G.B., X.L. and G.P.; software, V.F., G.B., G.P. and F.C.; validation, G.B., F.C., V.F., A.D.M., B.É.P., J.L.V.G., P.V., A.R. and G.P.; formal analysis, G.B.; investigation, F.C., V.F., A.D.M., G.B., X.L. and G.P.; resources, F.C., X.L., G.P., A.D.M. and G.B.; data curation, F.C., V.F., A.D.M., G.B. and G.P.; writing—original draft preparation, A.D.M., G.B. and F.C.; writing—review and editing, all authors; supervision, X.L., G.P. and F.C.; project administration, G.P. and F.C.; funding acquisition, F.C., V.F., A.D.M., G.B., X.L. and G.P. All authors have read and agreed to the published version of the manuscript.

**Funding:** This research received no external funding.

**Institutional Review Board Statement:** Not applicable.

**Informed Consent Statement:** Not applicable.

**Data Availability Statement:** Data are available on reasonable request to the corresponding authors.

**Conflicts of Interest:** The authors declare no conflicts of interest.

## Appendix A

Documentation on the literature search for:
Subretinal haemorrhage

Search date: 14 June 2022
The following databases were searched:

| Database | Number of Retrieved References |
|---|---|
| Ovid Medline | 1312 |
| Embase | 1411 |
| Cochrane Central Register of Controlled Trials | 22 |
| Cochrane Database of Systematic Reviews | 0 |
| Number of references before deduplication: | 2745 |
| Number of references after deduplication: | 1654 |

Search syntax:

| / | After an index term indicates a subject heading was selected |
|---|---|
| .ti,ab,kf. | Search for a term in title, abstract, and author keywords |
| * | At the end of a term indicates that this term has been truncated; hemorrhag* retrieves haemorrhage, haemorrhages |
| Adj2 | ADJ = adjacent operator in the Ovid databases. Adj2: search for two terms next to each other, in any order, up to 2 words in between. |
| NEAR/3 | NEAR = proximity operator in the Cochrane Database of Systematic Reviews. NEAR/3: search for two terms next to each other, in any order, up to 2 words in between. |

Search strategies:
Ovid MEDLINE(R) ALL 1946 to 8 June 2022

| # | Searches | Results |
|---|---|---|
| 1 | ((subretin* or sub-retin* or submacula* or sub-macula*) adj2 (hemorrhag* or haemorrhag* or bleed*)).ti,ab,kf. | 1346 |
| 2 | Retinal Haemorrhage/ | 5523 |
| 3 | (subretin* or sub-retin* or submacula* or sub-macula*).ti,ab,kf. | 11,699 |
| 4 | 1 or (2 and 3) | 1509 |
| 5 | limit 4 to english language | 1312 |

Embase Classic + Embase 1947 to 8 June 2022

| # | Searches | Results |
|---|---|---|
| 1 | ((subretin* or sub-retin* or submacula* or sub-macula*) adj2 (hemorrhag* or haemorrhag* or bleed*)).ti,ab,kf. | 1672 |
| 2 | retina haemorrhage/ or retina macula haemorrhage/ | 10,977 |
| 3 | (subretin* or sub-retin* or submacula* or sub-macula*).ti,ab,kf. | 16,004 |
| 4 | 1 or (2 and 3) | 2098 |
| 5 | limit 4 to conference abstracts | 234 |
| 6 | 4 not 5 | 1864 |
| 7 | limit 6 to (article or review) | 1725 |
| 8 | limit 7 to english language | 1411 |

Cochrane Central Register of Controlled Trials

| | | |
|---|---|---|
| 1 | ((subretin* or sub-retin* or submacula* or sub-macula*) AND (hemorrhag* or haemorrhag* or bleed*)): in Record Title | 22 |

Cochrane Database of Systematic Reviews

| | | |
|---|---|---|
| 1 | ((subretin* or sub-retin* or submacula* or sub-macula*) NEAR/3 (hemorrhag* or haemorrhag* or bleed*)): in ti,ab,kw. | 0 |

**Appendix B**

Summary of the 155 records screened for inclusion/exclusion and the determining reasons behind each choice.

| | Title | Included (N. of Eyes) | Excluded | Explanation for Exclusion (or Comments) |
|---|---|---|---|---|
| 1 | Olivier S, Chow DR, Packo KH, MacCumber MW, Awh CC. Subretinal recombinant tissue plasminogen activator injection and pneumatic displacement of thick submacular haemorrhage in Age-Related macular degeneration. Ophthalmology. 2004 Jun;111(6):1201–8. doi: 10.1016/j.ophtha.2003.10.020. Erratum in: Ophthalmology. 2004 Sep;111(9):1640. PMID: 15177972. | 1 included (29 eyes) | | |
| 2 | Woo, J. John M.D.; Lou, Peter L. M.D.; Ryan, Edward A. M.D.; Kroll, Arnold J. M.D. Surgical Treatment of Submacular Haemorrhage in Age-Related Macular Degeneration. International Ophthalmology Clinics: Winter 2004-Volume 44-Issue 1-p 43–50 | | Excluded | Review |
| 3 | Chan, W.-M., Liu, D.T., Lai, T.Y., Li, H., Tong, J.-P. and Lam, D.S. (2005), Extensive submacular haemorrhage in polypoidal choroidal vasculopathy managed by sequential gas displacement and photodynamic therapy: a pilot study of one-year follow up. Clinical & Experimental Ophthalmology, 33: 611–618. https://doi-org.ezproxy.uio.no/10.1111/j.1442-9071.2005.01105.x | | Excluded | Pilot study, 6 eyes |
| 4 | Puchta, Koch, F., & Hattenbach, L. (2005). Prospektive, randomisierte Studie zur intravitrealen Gabe von rt-PA mit SF6-Gas vs. SF6-Gas in der Behandlung von submakulären Blutungen bei AMD. Klinische Monatsblätter für Augenheilkunde. https://doi.org/10.1055/s-2005-922145 | | Excluded | Languages other than English |
| 5 | Ratanasukon, M., Kittantong, A. Results of intravitreal tissue plasminogen activator and expansile gas injection for submacular haemorrhage in Thais. Eye 19, 1328–1332 (2005). https://doi.org/10.1038/sj.eye.6701769 | 2 included (24 eyes) | | |
| 6 | Thompson JT, Sjaarda RN. Vitrectomy for the treatment of submacular haemorrhages from macular degeneration: a comparison of submacular haemorrhage/membrane removal and submacular tissue plasminogen activator-assisted pneumatic displacement. Trans Am Ophthalmol Soc. 2005;103:98–107; discussion 107. PMID: 17057793; PMCID: PMC1447564. | 3 included (42 eyes) | | |

| | | | |
|---|---|---|---|
| 7 | Wu TT, Sheu SJ. Intravitreal tissue plasminogen activator and pneumatic displacement of submacular haemorrhage secondary to retinal artery macroaneurysm. J Ocul Pharmacol Ther. 2005 Feb;21(1):62–7. doi: 10.1089/jop.2005.21.62. PMID: 15718829. | Excluded | Case series of only 6 eyes |
| 8 | Yang PM, Kuo HK, Kao ML, Chen YJ, Tsai HH. Pneumatic displacement of a dense submacular haemorrhage with or without tissue plasminogen activator. Chang Gung Med J. 2005 Dec;28(12):852–9. PMID: 16515019. | 4 included (24 eyes) | |
| 9 | Mozaffarieh M, Heinzl H, Sacu S, Wedrich A. In-patient management and treatment satisfaction after intravitreous plasminogen activator injection. Graefes Arch Clin Exp Ophthalmol. 2006 Nov;244(11):1421–8. doi: 10.1007/s00417-005-0232-z. Epub 2006 Apr 5. PMID: 16596407. | 5 included (101 eyes) | (No anatomical parameters) |
| 10 | Oie Y, Emi K. Surgical excision of retinal macroaneurysms with submacular haemorrhage. Jpn J Ophthalmol. 2006 Nov-Dec;50(6):550–553. doi: 10.1007/s10384-006-0369-2. Epub 2006 Dec 18. PMID: 17180532. | Excluded | Only 2 patients |
| 11 | Singh RP, Patel C, Sears JE. Management of subretinal macular haemorrhage by direct administration of tissue plasminogen activator. Br J Ophthalmol. 2006 Apr;90(4):429–31. doi: 10.1136/bjo.2005.085001. PMID: 16547320; PMCID: PMC1856980. | 6 included (17 eyes) | |
| 12 | Chen CY, Hooper C, Chiu D, Chamberlain M, Karia N, Heriot WJ. Management of submacular haemorrhage with intravitreal injection of tissue plasminogen activator and expansile gas. Retina. 2007 Mar;27(3):321–8. doi: 10.1097/01.iae.0000237586.48231.75. PMID: 17460587. | 7 included (104 eyes) | |
| 13 | Gopalakrishan M, Giridhar A, Bhat S, Saikumar SJ, Elias A, N S. Pneumatic displacement of submacular haemorrhage: safety, efficacy, and patient selection. Retina. 2007 Mar;27(3):329–34. doi: 10.1097/01.iae.0000231544.43093.40. PMID: 17460588. | 8 included (20 eyes) | |
| 14 | Hasler PW, la Cour M, Villumsen J. Pneumatic displacement and intravitreal bevacizumab in the management of subretinal haemorrhage caused by choroidal neovascularization. Acta Ophthalmol Scand. 2007 Aug;85(5):577–9. doi: 10.1111/j.1600-0420.2007.00914.x. Epub 2007 Jun 8. PMID: 17559558. | Excluded | Case report |
| 15 | Oshima Y, Ohji M, Tano Y. Pars plana vitrectomy with peripheral retinotomy after injection of preoperative intravitreal tissue plasminogen activator: a modified procedure to drain massive subretinal haemorrhage. Br J Ophthalmol. 2007 Feb;91(2):193–8. doi: 10.1136/bjo.2006.101444. Epub 2006 Aug 17. PMID: 16916872; PMCID: PMC1857597. | Excluded | Surgical technique |
| 16 | Ron Y, Ehrlich R, Axer-Siegel R, Rosenblatt I, Weinberger D. Pneumatic displacement of submacular haemorrhage due to age-related macular degeneration. Ophthalmologica. 2007;221(1):57–61. doi: 10.1159/000096524. PMID: 17183203. | 9 included (24 eyes) | |

| | | | |
|---|---|---|---|
| 17 | Stifter E, Michels S, Prager F, Georgopoulos M, Polak K, Hirn C, Schmidt-Erfurth U. Intravitreal bevacizumab therapy for neovascular age-related macular degeneration with large submacular haemorrhage. Am J Ophthalmol. 2007 Dec;144(6):886–892. doi: 10.1016/j.ajo.2007.07.034. Epub 2007 Oct 4. PMID: 17916314. | 10 included (21 eyes) | |
| 18 | Liu, W. Current management of submacular haemorrhage in age-related macular degeneration. International Journal of Ophthalmology-Volume 8, Issue 0, pp. 867–870-published 2008-01-01 | Excluded | Review |
| 19 | Meyer CH, Scholl HP, Eter N, Helb HM, Holz FG. Combined treatment of acute subretinal haemorrhages with intravitreal recombined tissue plasminogen activator, expansile gas and bevacizumab: a retrospective pilot study. Acta Ophthalmol. 2008 Aug;86(5):490–4. doi: 10.1111/j.1600-0420.2007.01125.x. Epub 2008 Jan 24. PMID: 18221499. | 11 included (19 eyes) | |
| 20 | Nakamura H, Hayakawa K, Sawaguchi S, Gaja T, Nagamine N, Medoruma K. Visual outcome after vitreous, sub-internal limiting membrane, and/or submacular haemorrhage removal associated with ruptured retinal arterial macroaneurysms. Graefes Arch Clin Exp Ophthalmol. 2008 May;246(5):661–9. doi: 10.1007/s00417-007-0724-0. Epub 2007 Dec 11. PMID: 18071732. | Excluded | SRMH secondary to RAM |
| 21 | Chawla S, Misra V, Khemchandani M. Pneumatic displacement and intravitreal bevacizumab: a new approach for management of submacular haemorrhage in choroidal neovascular membrane. Indian J Ophthalmol. 2009 Mar-Apr;57(2):155–7. doi: 10.4103/0301-4738.45511. PMID: 19237795; PMCID: PMC2684421. | Excluded | Only 4 cases |
| 22 | Fang IM, Lin YC, Yang CH, Yang CM, Chen MS. Effects of intravitreal gas with or without tissue plasminogen activator on submacular haemorrhage in age-related macular degeneration. Eye (Lond). 2009 Feb;23(2):397–406. doi: 10.1038/sj.eye.6703017. Epub 2007 Nov 2. PMID: 17975562. | 12 included (53 eyes) | |
| 23 | Gibran SK, Romano MR, Wong D. Surgical management of massive submacular haemorrhage associated with age-related macular degeneration. Retin Cases Brief Rep. 2009 Fall;3(4):391–4. doi: 10.1097/ICB.0b013e31818a470e. PMID: 25389857. | Excluded | 6 eyes |
| 24 | Kamei M, Tano Y. Tissue plasminogen activator-assisted vitrectomy: surgical drainage of submacular haemorrhage. Dev Ophthalmol. 2009;44:82–88. doi: 10.1159/000223948. Epub 2009 Jun 3. PMID: 19494655. | Excluded | 12 eyes |
| 25 | Arias L, Monés J. Transconjunctival sutureless vitrectomy with tissue plasminogen activator, gas and intravitreal bevacizumab in the management of predominantly hemorrhagic age-related macular degeneration. Clin Ophthalmol. 2010 Feb 18;4:67–72. doi: 10.2147/opth.s8635. PMID: 20186279; PMCID: PMC2827187. | 13 included (15 eyes) | |

| | | | |
|---|---|---|---|
| 26 | Cakir M, Cekiç O, Yilmaz OF. Pneumatic displacement of acute submacular haemorrhage with and without the use of tissue plasminogen activator. Eur J Ophthalmol. 2010 May-Jun;20(3):565–71. doi: 10.1177/112067211002000305. PMID: 20037915. | 14 included (21 eyes) | |
| 27 | Fine HF, Iranmanesh R, Del Priore LV, Barile GR, Chang LK, Chang S, Schiff WM. Surgical outcomes after massive subretinal haemorrhage secondary to age-related macular degeneration. Retina. 2010 Nov-Dec;30(10):1588–94. doi: 10.1097/IAE.0b013e3181e2263c. PMID: 20856172. | 15 included (15 eyes) | |
| 28 | Hillenkamp J, Surguch V, Framme C, Gabel VP, Sachs HG. Management of submacular haemorrhage with intravitreal versus subretinal injection of recombinant tissue plasminogen activator. Graefes Arch Clin Exp Ophthalmol. 2010 Jan;248(1):5–11. doi: 10.1007/s00417-009-1158-7. Epub 2009 Aug 11. PMID: 19669780. | 16 included (18 + 29 eyes) | |
| 29 | Höhn F, Mirshahi A, Hattenbach LO. Kombinierte intravitreale Injektion von Bevacizumab und SF(6)-Gas bei AMD-assoziierter, submakulärer Hämorrhagie [Combined intravitreal injection of bevacizumab and SF6 gas for treatment of submacular haemorrhage secondary to age-related macular degeneration]. Ophthalmologe. 2010 Apr;107(4):328–32. German. doi: 10.1007/s00347-009-2004-3. PMID: 19669150. | Excluded | Language other than English |
| 30 | Kung YH, Wu TT, Hong MC, Sheu SJ. Intravitreal tissue plasminogen activator and pneumatic displacement of submacular haemorrhage. J Ocul Pharmacol Ther. 2010 Oct;26(5):469–74. doi: 10.1089/jop.2010.0066. PMID: 20925578. | 17 included (46 eyes) | |
| 31 | McAllister IL, Chen SD, Patel JI, Fleming BL, Yu DY. Management of submacular haemorrhage in age-related macular degeneration with intravitreal tenecteplase. Br J Ophthalmol. 2010 Feb;94(2):260–1. doi: 10.1136/bjo.2009.158170. PMID: 20139293. | Excluded | 8 eyes |
| 32 | McKibbin M, Papastefanou V, Matthews B, Cook H, Downey L. Ranibizumab monotherapy for sub-foveal haemorrhage secondary to choroidal neovascularisation in age-related macular degeneration. Eye (Lond). 2010 Jun;24(6):994–8. doi: 10.1038/eye.2009.271. Epub 2009 Nov 13. PMID: 19911016. | Excluded | 12 eyes |
| 33 | Sandhu SS, Manvikar S, Steel DH. Displacement of submacular haemorrhage associated with age-related macular degeneration using vitrectomy and submacular rt-PA injection followed by intravitreal ranibizumab. Clin Ophthalmol. 2010 Jul 21;4:637–42. doi: 10.2147/opth.s10060. PMID: 20668667; PMCID: PMC2909894. | 18 included (16 eyes) | |
| 34 | Treumer F, Klatt C, Roider J, Hillenkamp J. Subretinal coapplication of recombinant tissue plasminogen activator and bevacizumab for neovascular age-related macular degeneration with submacular haemorrhage. Br J Ophthalmol. 2010 Jan;94(1):48–53. doi: 10.1136/bjo.2009.164707. Epub 2009 Nov 27. PMID: 19946027. | Excluded | 12 eyes |
| 35 | Georgalas I, Papaconstantinou D, Karagiannis D, Ladas I. Pneumatic displacement of acute submacular haemorrhage with and without the use of rt-PA. Eur J Ophthalmol. 2011 Mar-Apr;21(2):220; author reply 221. doi: 10.5301/ejo.2010.5685. PMID: 20853260. | Excluded | Comment to the editor |

| | | | | |
|---|---|---|---|---|
| 36 | Guthoff R, Guthoff T, Meigen T, Goebel W. Intravitreous injection of bevacizumab, tissue plasminogen activator, and gas in the treatment of submacular haemorrhage in age-related macular degeneration. Retina. 2011 Jan;31(1):36–40. doi: 10.1097/IAE.0b013e3181e37884. PMID: 20921929. | 19 included (38 eyes) | | |
| 37 | Mizutani T, Yasukawa T, Ito Y, Takase A, Hirano Y, Yoshida M, Ogura Y. Pneumatic displacement of submacular haemorrhage with or without tissue plasminogen activator. Graefes Arch Clin Exp Ophthalmol. 2011 Aug;249(8):1153–7. doi: 10.1007/s00417-011-1649-1. Epub 2011 Mar 29. PMID: 21445629. | 20 included (53 eyes) | | |
| 38 | Moriyama M, Ohno-Matsui K, Shimada N, Hayashi K, Kojima A, Yoshida T, Tokoro T, Mochizuki M. Correlation between visual prognosis and fundus autofluorescence and optical coherence tomographic findings in highly myopic eyes with submacular haemorrhage and without choroidal neovascularization. Retina. 2011 Jan;31(1):74–80. doi: 10.1097/IAE.0b013e3181e91148. PMID: 21187733. | | Excluded | Macular hemorrhage secondary to pathologic myopia |
| 39 | Shultz RW, Bakri SJ. Treatment for submacular haemorrhage associated with neovascular age-related macular degeneration. Semin Ophthalmol. 2011 Nov;26(6):361–71. doi: 10.3109/08820538.2011.585368. PMID: 22044334. | | Excluded | Review |
| 40 | Steel DH, Sandhu SS. Submacular haemorrhages associated with neovascular age-related macular degeneration. Br J Ophthalmol. 2011 Aug;95(8):1051–7. doi: 10.1136/bjo.2010.182253. Epub 2010 Sep 2. PMID: 20813746. | | Excluded | Review |
| 41 | Tognetto D, Skiadaresi E, Cecchini P, Ravalico G. Subretinal recombinant tissue plasminogen activator and pneumatic displacement for the management of subretinal haemorrhage occurring after anti-VEGF injections for wet AMD. Clin Ophthalmol. 2011;5:459–63. doi: 10.2147/OPTH.S15864. Epub 2011 Apr 13. PMID: 21573092; PMCID: PMC3090299. | | Excluded | 3 cases |
| 42 | Treumer F, Roider J, Hillenkamp J. Long-term outcome of subretinal coapplication of rt-PA and bevacizumab followed by repeated intravitreal anti-VEGF injections for neovascular AMD with submacular haemorrhage. Br J Ophthalmol. 2012 May;96(5):708–13. doi: 10.1136/bjophthalmol-2011-300655. Epub 2011 Dec 15. PMID: 22174095. | 21 included (41 eyes) | | |
| 43 | Wu TT, Kung YH, Hong MC. Vitreous haemorrhage complicating intravitreal tissue plasminogen activator and pneumatic displacement of submacular haemorrhage. Retina. 2011 Nov;31(10):2071–7. doi: 10.1097/IAE.0b013e31822528c8. PMID: 21817964. | | Excluded | Aim out of the scope: to evaluate the clinical factors associated with vitreous hemorrhage |
| 44 | Hesgaard HB, Torkashvand M, la Cour M. Failure to detect an effect of pneumatic displacement in the management of submacular haemorrhage secondary to age-related macular degeneration: a retrospective case series. Acta Ophthalmol. 2012 Sep;90(6):e498–500. doi: 10.1111/j.1755-3768.2011.02352.x. Epub 2012 Jan 23. PMID: 22268661. | | Excluded | Letter to the editor |
| 45 | Hesse, L. Intravitreale Injektionen. Ophthalmologe 109, 644–647 (2012). https://doi.org/10.1007/s00347-012-2565-4 | | Excluded | Language other than English |

| | | | |
|---|---|---|---|
| 46 | Hillenkamp J, Klettner A, Puls S, Treumer F, Roider J. Subretinale Koapplikation von rt-PA und Bevacizumab bei exsudativer altersbedingter Makuladegeneration mit submakulärer Blutung. Kompatibilität der Wirkstoffe und klinische Langzeitergebnisse [Subretinal co-application of rt-PA and bevacizumab for exudative AMD with submacular haemorrhage. Compatibility and clinical long-term results]. Ophthalmologe. 2012 Jul;109(7):648–56. German. doi: 10.1007/s00347-012-2564-5. PMID: 22752624. | Excluded | Language other than English |
| 47 | Cochrane Central Register of Controlled Trials Intravitreal versus submacular injection of rt-PA for acute submacular haemorrhages NTR3359 https://trialsearch.who.int/Trial2.aspx?TrialID=NTR3359, 2012 \| added to CENTRAL: 31 March 2019 \| 2019 Issue 3 accessed on 1 July 2023. | Excluded | Trial protocol |
| 48 | Sonmez K, Ozturk F, Ozcan PY. Treatment of multilevel macular haemorrhage secondary to retinal arterial macroaneurysm with submacular tissue plasminogen activator. Eur J Ophthalmol. 2012 Nov-Dec;22(6):1026–31. doi: 10.5301/ejo.5000140. Epub 2012 Mar 20. PMID: 22467586. | Excluded | SRMH secondary to RAM |
| 49 | Szurman P. Subretinale Chirurgie bei Massenblutung [Subretinal surgery for massive haemorrhage]. Ophthalmologe. 2012 Jul;109(7):657–64. German. doi: 10.1007/s00347-012-2566-3. PMID: 22814924. | Excluded | Language other than English |
| 50 | Tsymanava A, Uhlig CE. Intravitreal recombinant tissue plasminogen activator without and with additional gas injection in patients with submacular haemorrhage associated with age-related macular degeneration. Acta Ophthalmol. 2012 Nov;90(7):633–8. doi: 10.1111/j.1755-3768.2011.02115.x. Epub 2011 Feb 18. PMID: 21332673. | 22 included (110 eyes) | |
| 51 | Ueda-Arakawa N, Tsujikawa A, Yamashiro K, Ooto S, Tamura H, Yoshimura N. Visual prognosis of eyes with submacular haemorrhage associated with exudative age-related macular degeneration. Jpn J Ophthalmol. 2012 Nov;56(6):589–98. doi: 10.1007/s10384-012-0191-y. Epub 2012 Oct 4. PMID: 23053632. | 23 included (31 eyes) | |
| 52 | Injection of Lucentis (Ranibizumab) in the vitreous body of the eye after eye surgery and application of recombinant tissue plasminogen activator (rt-PA) in patients with submacular bleeding complications suffering from wet age-related macular degeneration (AMD) EUCTR2010-018637-21-DE https://trialsearch.who.int/Trial2.aspx?TrialID=EUCTR2010-018637-21-DE, 2013 \| added to CENTRAL: 31 March 2019 \| 2019 Issue 3 | Excluded | Protocol clinical trial |
| 53 | Intravitreal rt-PA and $C_3F_8$ for the Treatment of Submacular Haemorrhage as a Complication of Neovascular Age-related Macular Degeneration NCT01835067 https://clinicaltrials.gov/show/NCT01835067, 2013 \| added to CENTRAL: 31 May 2018 \| 2018 Issue 5 | Excluded | Protocol clinical trial |

| | | | |
|---|---|---|---|
| 54 | Cheung CM, Bhargava M, Xiang L, Mathur R, Mun CC, Wong D, Wong TY. Six-month visual prognosis in eyes with submacular haemorrhage secondary to age related macular degeneration or polypoidal choroidal vasculopathy. Graefes Arch Clin Exp Ophthalmol. 2013 Jan;251(1):19–25. doi: 10.1007/s00417-012-2029-1. Epub 2012 May 26. PMID: 22638617. | Excluded | |
| 55 | Cho HJ, Koh KM, Kim HS, Lee TG, Kim CG, Kim JW. Anti-vascular endothelial growth factor monotherapy in the treatment of submacular haemorrhage secondary to polypoidal choroidal vasculopathy. Am J Ophthalmol. 2013 Sep;156(3):524–531.e1. doi: 10.1016/j.ajo.2013.04.029. Epub 2013 Jun 13. PMID: 23769197. | 24 included (27 eyes) | |
| 56 | Cho HJ, Koh KM, Kim HS, Lee TG, Kim CG, Kim JW. Anti-vascular endothelial growth factor monotherapy in the treatment of submacular haemorrhage secondary to polypoidal choroidal vasculopathy. Am J Ophthalmol. 2013 Sep;156(3):524–531.e1. doi: 10.1016/j.ajo.2013.04.029. Epub 2013 Jun 13. PMID: 23769197. | 25 included (17 eyes) | |
| 57 | Han L, Ma Z, Wang C, Dou H, Hu Y, Feng X, Xu Y, Yin Z, Wang X. Autologous transplantation of simple retinal pigment epithelium sheet for massive submacular haemorrhage associated with pigment epithelium detachment. Invest Ophthalmol Vis Sci. 2013 Jul 24;54(7):4956–63. doi: 10.1167/iovs.13-11957. PMID: 23744996. | 26 included (14 eyes) | |
| 58 | Jain S, Kishore K, Sharma YR. Intravitreal anti-VEGF monotherapy for thick submacular haemorrhage of less than 1 week duration secondary to neovascular age-related macular degeneration. Indian J Ophthalmol. 2013 Sep;61(9):490–6. doi: 10.4103/0301-4738.119432. PMID: 24104707; PMCID: PMC3831764. | 27 included (14 eyes) | |
| 59 | Kapran Z, Ozkaya A, Uyar OM. Hemorrhagic age-related macular degeneration managed with vitrectomy, subretinal injection of tissue plasminogen activator, gas tamponade, and upright positioning. Ophthalmic Surg Lasers Imaging Retina. 2013 Sep-Oct;44(5):471–6. doi: 10.3928/23258160-20130909-09. PMID: 24044710. | Excluded | 10 eyes |
| 60 | Lumi X, Sulak M. Treatment of submacular haemorrhage in patients with neovascular age related macular degeneration. Coll Antropol. 2013 Apr;37 Suppl 1:223–6. PMID: 23837248. | Excluded | 9 patients |
| 61 | Martel JN, Mahmoud TH. Subretinal pneumatic displacement of subretinal haemorrhage. JAMA Ophthalmol. 2013 Dec;131(12):1632–5. doi: 10.1001/jamaophthalmol.2013.5464. PMID: 24337559. | Excluded | Surgical technique |
| 62 | Mayer WJ, Hakim I, Haritoglou C, Gandorfer A, Ulbig M, Kampik A, Wolf A. Efficacy and safety of recombinant tissue plasminogen activator and gas versus bevacizumab and gas for subretinal haemorrhage. Acta Ophthalmol. 2013 May;91(3):274–8. doi: 10.1111/j.1755-3768.2011.02264.x. Epub 2011 Sep 22. PMID: 21952010. | 28 included (45 eyes) | |

| | | | |
|---|---|---|---|
| 63 | Papavasileiou E, Steel DH, Liazos E, McHugh D, Jackson TL. Intravitreal tissue plasminogen activator, perfluoropropane ($C_3F_8$), and ranibizumab or photodynamic therapy for submacular haemorrhage secondary to wet age-related macular degeneration. Retina. 2013 Apr;33(4):846–53. doi: 10.1097/IAE.0b013e318271f278. PMID: 23400079. | Excluded | 7 eyes |
| 64 | Rishi E, Gopal L, Rishi P, Sengupta S, Sharma T. Submacular haemorrhage: a study amongst Indian eyes. Indian J Ophthalmol. 2012 Nov-Dec;60(6):521–5. doi: 10.4103/0301-4738.103779. PMID: 23202390; PMCID: PMC3545128. | 29 included (46 eyes) | |
| 65 | Mark Sherman, Charles Barr, Shlomit Schaal; Functional and Anatomical Outcomes of Tissue Plasminogen Activator (rt-PA) Treatment for Submacular Haemorrhage Associated with Exudative Macular Degeneration (ExAMD): A Comparative Analysis Between Intra-vitreal and Sub-retinal rt-PA injected Patients. Invest. Ophthalmol. Vis. Sci. 2013;54(15):3304. | Excluded | Meeting abstract |
| 66 | Shienbaum G, Garcia Filho CA, Flynn HW Jr, Nunes RP, Smiddy WE, Rosenfeld PJ. Management of submacular haemorrhage secondary to neovascular age-related macular degeneration with anti-vascular endothelial growth factor monotherapy. Am J Ophthalmol. 2013 Jun;155(6):1009–13. doi: 10.1016/j.ajo.2013.01.012. Epub 2013 Mar 7. PMID: 23465269. | 30 included (19 eyes) | |
| 67 | van Zeeburg EJ, Cereda MG, van Meurs JC. Recombinant tissue plasminogen activator, vitrectomy, and gas for recent submacular haemorrhage displacement due to retinal macroaneurysm. Graefes Arch Clin Exp Ophthalmol. 2013 Mar;251(3):733–40. doi: 10.1007/s00417-012-2116-3. Epub 2012 Aug 4. PMID: 22865261. | Excluded | SRMH secondary to RAM |
| 68 | van Zeeburg EJ, van Meurs JC. Literature review of recombinant tissue plasminogen activator used for recent-onset submacular haemorrhage displacement in age-related macular degeneration. Ophthalmologica. 2013;229(1):1–14. doi: 10.1159/000343066. Epub 2012 Oct 12. PMID: 23075629. | Excluded | Review |
| 69 | Chang W, Garg SJ, Maturi R, Hsu J, Sivalingam A, Gupta SA, Regillo CD, Ho AC. Management of thick submacular haemorrhage with subretinal tissue plasminogen activator and pneumatic displacement for age-related macular degeneration. Am J Ophthalmol. 2014 Jun;157(6):1250–7. doi: 10.1016/j.ajo.2014.02.007. Epub 2014 Feb 13. PMID: 24531021. | 31 included (101 eyes) | |
| 70 | Dewilde E, Delaere L, Vaninbroukx I, Van Calster J, Stalmans P. Subretinal tissue plasminogen activator injection to treat submacular haemorrhage during age-related macular degeneration. Acta Ophthalmol. 2014 Sep;92(6):e497–8. doi: 10.1111/aos.12458. Epub 2014 Jun 18. PMID: 24943231. | Excluded | Letter to the editor |
| 71 | Iacono P, Parodi MB, Introini U, La Spina C, Varano M, Bandello F. Intravitreal ranibizumab for choroidal neovascularization with large submacular haemorrhage in age-related macular degeneration. Retina. 2014 Feb;34(2):281–7. doi: 10.1097/IAE.0b013e3182979e33. PMID: 23851632. | 32 included (23 eyes) | |

| | | | |
|---|---|---|---|
| 72 | Kitahashi M, Baba T, Sakurai M, Yokouchi H, Kubota-Taniai M, Mitamura Y, Yamamoto S. Pneumatic displacement with intravitreal bevacizumab for massive submacular haemorrhage due to polypoidal choroidal vasculopathy. Clin Ophthalmol. 2014 Mar 3;8:485–92. doi: 10.2147/OPTH.S55413. PMID: 24623972; PMCID: PMC3949732. | 33 included (32 eyes) | |
| 73 | Gerard F McGowan, David Steel, David Yorston; AMD with submacular haemorrhage: new insights from a population-based study. Invest. Ophthalmol. Vis. Sci. 2014;55(13):662. | Excluded | Meeting abstract |
| 74 | Moisseiev E, Ben Ami T, Barak A. Vitrectomy and subretinal injection of tissue plasminogen activator for large submacular haemorrhage secondary to AMD. Eur J Ophthalmol. 2014 Nov-Dec;24(6):925–31. doi: 10.5301/ejo.5000500. Epub 2014 Jun 12. PMID: 24966031. | 34 included (31 eyes) | |
| 75 | Dimopoulos S, Leitritz MA, Ziemssen F, Voykov B, Bartz-Schmidt KU, Gelisken F. Submacular predominantly hemorrhagic choroidal neovascularization: resolution of bleedings under anti-VEGF therapy. Clin Ophthalmol. 2015 Aug 24;9:1537–41. doi: 10.2147/OPTH.S87919. PMID: 26346691; PMCID: PMC4554429. | 35 included (46 eyes) | |
| 76 | Hirashima T, Moriya T, Bun T, Utsumi T, Hirose M, Oh H. Optical coherence tomography findings and surgical outcomes of tissue plasminogen activator-assisted vitrectomy for submacular haemorrhage secondary to age-related macular degeneration. Retina. 2015 Oct;35(10):1969–78. doi: 10.1097/IAE.0000000000000574. PMID: 26079475. | Excluded | 9 eyes |
| 77 | Inoue M, Shiraga F, Shirakata Y, Morizane Y, Kimura S, Hirakata A. Subretinal injection of recombinant tissue plasminogen activator for submacular haemorrhage associated with ruptured retinal arterial macroaneurysm. Graefes Arch Clin Exp Ophthalmol. 2015 Oct;253(10):1663–9. doi: 10.1007/s00417-014-2861-6. Epub 2014 Nov 25. PMID: 25418034. | Excluded | RAM |
| 78 | Prospective intervention study for drainage of subretinal haemorrhage using tissue plasminogen activator Authors: Jprn, Umin; Journal: https://trialsearch.who.int/Trial2.aspx?TrialID=JPRN-UMIN000019668 | Excluded | Clinical trial protocol |
| 79 | Kadonosono K, Arakawa A, Yamane S, Inoue M, Yamakawa T, Uchio E, Yanagi Y. Displacement of submacular haemorrhages in age-related macular degeneration with subretinal tissue plasminogen activator and air. Ophthalmology. 2015 Jan;122(1):123–8. doi: 10.1016/j.ophtha.2014.07.027. Epub 2014 Sep 4. PMID: 25200400. | 36 included (13 eyes) | |
| 80 | Kim HS, Cho HJ, Yoo SG, Kim JH, Han JI, Lee TG, Kim JW. Intravitreal anti-vascular endothelial growth factor monotherapy for large submacular haemorrhage secondary to neovascular age-related macular degeneration. Eye (Lond). 2015 Sep;29(9):1141–51. doi: 10.1038/eye.2015.131. Epub 2015 Aug 14. PMID: 26272443; PMCID: PMC4565949. | 37 included (49 eyes) | |

| | | | |
|---|---|---|---|
| 81 | Kimura S, Morizane Y, Hosokawa M, Shiode Y, Kawata T, Doi S, Matoba R, Hosogi M, Fujiwara A, Inoue Y, Shiraga F. Submacular haemorrhage in polypoidal choroidal vasculopathy treated by vitrectomy and subretinal tissue plasminogen activator. Am J Ophthalmol. 2015 Apr;159(4):683–9. doi: 10.1016/j.ajo.2014.12.020. Epub 2014 Dec 30. PMID: 25555798. | 38 included (15 eyes) | |
| 82 | Nayak S, Padhi TR, Basu S, Das T. Pneumatic displacement and intra-vitreal bevacizumab in management of sub-retinal and sub-retinal pigment epithelial haemorrhage at macula in polypoidal choroidal vasculopathy (PCV): rationale and outcome. Semin Ophthalmol. 2015 Jan;30(1):53–5. doi: 10.3109/08820538.2013.807849. Epub 2013 Aug 15. PMID: 23947424. | Excluded | 3 eyes |
| 83 | Schaal, S.; Apenbrinck, E.; Barr, C. C.; Management of thick submacular haemorrhage with subretinal tissue plasminogen activator and pneumatic displacement for age-related macular degeneration. February 2015American Journal of Ophthalmology 159(2) DOI: 10.1016/j.ajo.2014.10.024 | Excluded | Correspondence article |
| 84 | Shin JY, Lee JM, Byeon SH. Anti-vascular endothelial growth factor with or without pneumatic displacement for submacular haemorrhage. Am J Ophthalmol. 2015 May;159(5):904–14.e1. doi: 10.1016/j.ajo.2015.01.024. Epub 2015 Jan 28. PMID: 25637179. | 39 included (82 eyes) | |
| 85 | Wei Y, Zhang Z, Jiang X, Li F, Zhang T, Qiu S, Yang Y, Zhang S. A surgical approach to large subretinal haemorrhage using pars plana vitrectomy and 360° retinotomy. Retina. 2015 Aug;35(8):1631–9. doi: 10.1097/IAE.0000000000000501. PMID: 26214315. | 40 included (21 eyes) | |
| 86 | Abdelkader E, Yip KP, Cornish KS. Pneumatic displacement of submacular haemorrhage. Saudi J Ophthalmol. 2016 Oct-Dec;30(4):221–226. doi: 10.1016/j.sjopt.2016.10.002. Epub 2016 Oct 13. PMID: 28003779; PMCID: PMC5161816. | Excluded | 12 eyes, 9 with SRMH secondary to AMD |
| 87 | Araújo J, Sousa C, Faria PA, Carneiro Â, Rocha-Sousa A, Falcão-Reis F. Intravitreal injection of recombinant tissue plasminogen activator in submacular haemorrhage: case series. Eur J Ophthalmol. 2016 Apr 12;26(3):e49–51. doi: 10.5301/ejo.5000682. PMID: 26428222. | Excluded | 6 eyes |
| 88 | Bae K, Cho GE, Yoon JM, Kang SW. Optical Coherence Tomographic Features and Prognosis of Pneumatic Displacement for Submacular Haemorrhage. PLoS One. 2016 Dec 19;11(12):e0168474. doi: 10.1371/journal.pone.0168474. PMID: 27992524; PMCID: PMC5167395. | 41 included (37 eyes) | |
| 89 | de Jong JH, van Zeeburg EJ, Cereda MG, van Velthoven ME, Faridpooya K, Vermeer KA, van Meurs JC. Intravitreal versus subretinal administration of recombinant tissue plasminogen activator combined with gas for acute submacular haemorrhages due to age-related macular degeneration: An Exploratory Prospective Study. Retina. 2016 May;36(5):914–25. doi: 10.1097/IAE.0000000000000954. PMID: 26807631. | 42 included (24 eyes) | |

| | | | |
|---|---|---|---|
| 90 | de Silva SR, Bindra MS. Early treatment of acute submacular haemorrhage secondary to wet AMD using intravitreal tissue plasminogen activator, C3F8, and an anti-VEGF agent. Eye (Lond). 2016 Jul;30(7):952–7. doi: 10.1038/eye.2016.67. Epub 2016 Apr 15. PMID: 27080482; PMCID: PMC4941069. | Excluded | 8 eyes |
| 91 | Dhawan, B.; Vig, V.; Singh, P.; Singh, R.; Management of sub macular haemorrhage with intravitreal injection of tissue plasminogen activator and sulfur hexafluoride. Journal Retina-Vitreus | Excluded | Not retrievable |
| 92 | Fassbender JM, Sherman MP, Barr CC, Schaal S. Tissue plasminogen activator for subfoveal haemorrhage due to age-related macular degeneration: Comparison of 3 Treatment Modalities. Retina. 2016 Oct;36(10):1860–5. doi: 10.1097/IAE.0000000000001030. PMID: 26945238. | 43 included (39 eyes) | |
| 93 | González-López JJ, McGowan G, Chapman E, Yorston D. Vitrectomy with subretinal tissue plasminogen activator and ranibizumab for submacular haemorrhages secondary to age-related macular degeneration: retrospective case series of 45 consecutive cases. Eye (Lond). 2016 Jul;30(7):929–35. doi: 10.1038/eye.2016.65. Epub 2016 Apr 8. PMID: 27055681; PMCID: PMC4941067. | 44 included (45 eyes) | |
| 94 | Isizaki E, Morishita S, Sato T, Fukumoto M, Suzuki H, Kida T, Ueki M, Ikeda T. Treatment of massive subretinal hematoma associated with age-related macular degeneration using vitrectomy with intentional giant tear. Int Ophthalmol. 2016 Apr;36(2):199–206. doi: 10.1007/s10792-015-0102-6. Epub 2015 Jul 28. PMID: 26216161. | Excluded | 12 eyes |
| 95 | Kitagawa Y, Shimada H, Mori R, Tanaka K, Yuzawa M. Intravitreal Tissue Plasminogen Activator, Ranibizumab, and Gas Injection for Submacular Haemorrhage in Polypoidal Choroidal Vasculopathy. Ophthalmology. 2016 Jun;123(6):1278–86. doi: 10.1016/j.ophtha.2016.01.035. Epub 2016 Mar 2. PMID: 26949121. | 45 included (20 eyes) | |
| 96 | Kumar A, Roy S, Bansal M, Tinwala S, Aron N, Temkar S, Pujari A. Modified Approach in Management of Submacular Haemorrhage Secondary to Wet Age-Related Macular Degeneration. Asia Pac J Ophthalmol (Phila). 2016 Mar-Apr;5(2):143–6. doi: 10.1097/APO.0000000000000130. PMID: 26302314. | Excluded | 10 eyes |
| 97 | Lee JP, Park JS, Kwon OW, You YS, Kim SH. Management of Acute Submacular Haemorrhage with Intravitreal Injection of Tenecteplase, Anti-vascular Endothelial Growth Factor and Gas. Korean J Ophthalmol. 2016 Jun;30(3):192–7. doi: 10.3341/kjo.2016.30.3.192. Epub 2016 May 18. PMID: 27247518; PMCID: PMC4878979. | 46 included (25 eyes) | |
| 98 | Lin TC, Hwang DK, Lee FL, Chen SJ. Visual prognosis of massive submacular haemorrhage in polypoidal choroidal vasculopathy with or without combination treatment. J Chin Med Assoc. 2016 Mar;79(3):159–65. doi: 10.1016/j.jcma.2015.11.004. Epub 2016 Jan 8. PMID: 26775600. | 47 included (20 eyes) | |

| | | | |
|---|---|---|---|
| 99 | Liu H, Zhang LY, Li XX, Wu MQ. 23-Gauge vitrectomy with external drainage therapy as a novel procedure to displace massive submacular haemorrhage secondary to polypoidal choroidal vasculopathy. Medicine (Baltimore). 2016 Aug;95(32):e4192. doi: 10.1097/MD.0000000000004192. PMID: 27512837; PMCID: PMC4985292. | Excluded | 4 eyes |
| 100 | Sadeghi Y, Elalouf M, Mantel I, Pournaras JA. Vitrectomy with Gas Tamponade and anti-VEGF Injections for the Management of Submacular Haemorrhage. Klin Monbl Augenheilkd. 2016 Apr;233(4):500–2. English. doi: 10.1055/s-0042-102567. Epub 2016 Apr 26. PMID: 27116519. | Excluded | Case report |
| 101 | Stanescu-Segall D, Balta F, Jackson TL. Submacular haemorrhage in neovascular age-related macular degeneration: A synthesis of the literature. Surv Ophthalmol. 2016 Jan-Feb;61(1):18–32. doi: 10.1016/j.survophthal.2015.04.004. Epub 2015 Jul 23. PMID: 26212151. | Excluded | Review |
| 102 | Waizel M, Todorova MG, Kazerounian S, Rickmann A, Blanke BR, Szurman P. Efficacy of Vitrectomy Combined with Subretinal Recombinant Tissue Plasminogen Activator for Subretinal versus Subpigment Epithelial versus Combined Haemorrhages. Ophthalmologica. 2016;236(3):123–132. doi: 10.1159/000449172. Epub 2016 Sep 16. PMID: 27631507. | 48 included (19 eyes) | |
| 103 | Bell JE, Shulman JP, Swan RJ, Teske MP, Bernstein PS. Intravitreal Versus Subretinal Tissue Plasminogen Activator Injection for Submacular Haemorrhage. Ophthalmic Surg Lasers Imaging Retina. 2017 Jan 1;48(1):26–32. doi: 10.3928/23258160-20161219-04. PMID: 28060391. | 49 included (18 eyes) | |
| 104 | Fleissig E, Barak A, Goldstein M, Loewenstein A, Schwartz S. Massive subretinal and subretinal pigment epithelial haemorrhage displacement with perfluorocarbon liquid using a two-step vitrectomy technique. Graefes Arch Clin Exp Ophthalmol. 2017 Jul;255(7):1341–1347. doi: 10.1007/s00417-017-3648-3. Epub 2017 Apr 15. PMID: 28412773. | Excluded | 7 eyes |
| 105 | Fotis K, Garcia-Cabrera R, Ohn M, Chandra A. Anatomical and Functional Outcome of Pars Plana Vitrectomy and Subretinal Recombinant Tissue Plasminogen Activator for a Macular Subpigment Epithelial Haemorrhage. Ophthalmologica. 2017;238(1–2):106–108. doi: 10.1159/000475891. Epub 2017 May 24. PMID: 28535542. | Excluded | Case report |
| 106 | Gok M, Karabaş VL, Aslan MS, Kara Ö, Karaman S, Yenihayat F. Tissue plasminogen activator-assisted vitrectomy for submacular haemorrhage due to age-related macular degeneration. Indian J Ophthalmol. 2017 Jun;65(6):482–487. doi: 10.4103/ijo.IJO_129_16. PMID: 28643713; PMCID: PMC5508459. | 50 included (17 eyes) | |
| 107 | Kimura S, Morizane Y, Matoba R, Hosokawa M, Shiode Y, Hirano M, Doi S, Toshima S, Takahashi K, Hosogi M, Fujiwara A, Shiraga F. Retinal sensitivity after displacement of submacular haemorrhage due to polypoidal choroidal vasculopathy: effectiveness and safety of subretinal tissue plasminogen activator. Jpn J Ophthalmol. 2017 Nov;61(6):472–478. doi: 10.1007/s10384-017-0530-0. Epub 2017 Aug 23. PMID: 28836011. | Excluded | 11 eyes |

| | | | |
|---|---|---|---|
| 108 | Amy Q. Lu, Jay G. Prensky, Paul S. Baker, Ingrid U. Scott, Tamer H. Mahmoud, Bozho Todorich. (2020) Update on medical and surgical management of submacular haemorrhage. Expert Review of Ophthalmology 15:1, pages 43–57. | Excluded | Review |
| 109 | Tan, C.S., Lim, L.W. & Ngo, W.K. Treatment of massive subretinal haemorrhage from polypoidal choroidal vasculopathy and age-related macular degeneration. Int Ophthalmol 37, 779–780 (2017). https://doi.org/10.1007/s10792-016-0351-z | Excluded | Letter to the editor |
| 110 | Waizel M, Todorova MG, Rickmann A, Blanke BR, Szurman P. Efficacy of Vitrectomy Combined with Subretinal rt-PA Injection with Gas or Air Tamponade. Klin Monbl Augenheilkd. 2017 Apr;234(4):487–492. English. doi: 10.1055/s-0042-121575. Epub 2017 Jan 31. PMID: 28142164. | 51 included (85 eyes) | |
| 111 | Waizel M, Todorova MG, Rickmann A, Blanke BR, Szurman P. Structural and Functional Outcome of Vitrectomy Combined with Subretinal Recombinant Tissue Plasminogen Activator for Isolated Subpigment Epithelial Haemorrhages. Ophthalmologica. 2017;238(1–2):109. doi: 10.1159/000475892. Epub 2017 May 24. PMID: 28535505. | Excluded | Letter to the editor |
| 112 | Cochrane Central Register of Controlled Trials Impacts of pneumatic displacement of submacular haemorrhage secondary to age-related macular degeneration on retinal pigment epithelial detachment UMIN000031065 https://trialsearch.who.int/Trial2.aspx?TrialID=JPRN-UMIN000031065, 2018 | added to CENTRAL: 31 March 2019 | 2019 Issue 3 Sourced from: ICTRP Links: WHO ICTRP | Excluded | Trial registration |
| 113 | Bardak H, Bardak Y, Erçalık Y, Erdem B, Arslan G, Timlioglu S. Sequential tissue plasminogen activator, pneumatic displacement, and anti-VEGF treatment for submacular haemorrhage. Eur J Ophthalmol. 2018 May;28(3):306–310. doi: 10.5301/ejo.5001074. PMID: 29148027. | 52 included (16 eyes) | |
| 114 | Juncal VR, Hanout M, Altomare F, Chow DR, Giavedoni LR, Muni RH, Wong DT, Berger AR. Surgical management of submacular haemorrhage: experience at an academic Canadian centre. Can J Ophthalmol. 2018 Aug;53(4):408–414. doi: 10.1016/j.jcjo.2017.10.010. Epub 2017 Dec 23. PMID: 30119797. | 53 included (99 eyes) | |
| 115 | Kim JH, Chang YS, Lee DW, Kim CG, Kim JW. Quantification of retinal changes after resolution of submacular haemorrhage secondary to polypoidal choroidal vasculopathy. Jpn J Ophthalmol. 2018 Jan;62(1):54–62. doi: 10.1007/s10384-017-0549-2. Epub 2017 Nov 29. PMID: 29188462. | 54 included (21 eyes) | |
| 116 | Management of Submacular Haemorrhage in Age-Related Macular Degeneration Authors: Kim, L. A.; Eliott, D.; Journal: Ophthalmology Retina-Volume 2, Issue 3, pp. 177–179-published 2018-01-01 | Excluded | Review |

| | | | |
|---|---|---|---|
| 117 | Kimura M, Yasukawa T, Shibata Y, Kato A, Hirano Y, Uemura A, Yoshida M, Ogura Y. Flattening of retinal pigment epithelial detachments after pneumatic displacement of submacular haemorrhages secondary to age-related macular degeneration. Graefes Arch Clin Exp Ophthalmol. 2018 Oct;256(10):1823–1829. doi: 10.1007/s00417-018-4059-9. Epub 2018 Jul 1. PMID: 29961921. | 55 included (33 eyes) | |
| 118 | Ozkaya A, Erdogan G, Tarakcioglu HN. Submacular haemorrhage secondary to age-related macular degeneration managed with vitrectomy, subretinal injection of tissue plasminogen activator, haemorrhage displacement with liquid perfluorocarbon, gas tamponade, and face-down positioning. Saudi J Ophthalmol. 2018 Oct-Dec;32(4):269–274. doi: 10.1016/j.sjopt.2018.08.002. Epub 2018 Aug 15. PMID: 30581295; PMCID: PMC6300785. | Excluded | 9 eyes |
| 119 | Sharma S, Kumar JB, Kim JE, Thordsen J, Dayani P, Ober M, Mahmoud TH. Pneumatic Displacement of Submacular Haemorrhage with Subretinal Air and Tissue Plasminogen Activator: Initial United States Experience. Ophthalmol Retina. 2018 Mar;2(3):180–186. doi: 10.1016/j.oret.2017.07.012. Epub 2017 Sep 28. PMID: 31047581. | 56 included (24 eyes) | |
| 120 | Adrean SD, Chaili S, Pirouz A, Grant S. Rapid displacement of subretinal haemorrhage from a choroidal neovascular membrane with intravitreal $C_3F_8$ gas and face-down positioning. Am J Ophthalmol Case Rep. 2019 Mar 14;14:79–82. doi: 10.1016/j.ajoc.2019.03.003. PMID: 30949612; PMCID: PMC6428934. | Excluded | Case report |
| 121 | Balughatta P, Kadri V, Braganza S, Jayadev C, Mehta RA, Nakhate V, Yadav NK, Shetty R. Pneumatic displacement of limited traumatic submacular haemorrhage without tissue plasminogen activator: a case series. Retin Cases Brief Rep. 2019 Winter;13(1):34–38. doi: 10.1097/ICB.0000000000000525. PMID: 28079650. | Excluded | Case report |
| 122 | Gujral GS, Agarwal M, Mayor R, Shroff D, Chhablani J, Shanmugam MP. Clinical profile and management outcomes of traumatic submacular haemorrhage. J Curr Ophthalmol. 2019 Oct 22;31(4):411–415. doi: 10.1016/j.joco.2019.09.001. PMID: 31844792; PMCID: PMC6896465. | Excluded | Traumatic SRMH |
| 123 | Li ZX, Hu YJ, Atik A, Lu L, Hu J. Long-term observation of vitrectomy without subretinal haemorrhage management for massive vitreous haemorrhage secondary to polypoidal choroidal vasculopathy. Int J Ophthalmol. 2019 Dec 18;12(12):1859–1864. doi: 10.18240/ijo.2019.12.07. PMID: 31850169; PMCID: PMC6901888. | Excluded | Vitreous hemorrhage without SRMH |
| 124 | Plemel DJA, Lapere SRJ, Rudnisky CJ, Tennant MTS. VITRECTOMY WITH SUBRETINAL TISSUE PLASMINOGEN ACTIVATOR AND GAS TAMPONADE FOR SUBFOVEAL HAEMORRHAGE: Prognostic Factors and Clinical Outcomes. Retina. 2019 Jan;39(1):172–179. doi: 10.1097/IAE.0000000000001931. PMID: 29135798. | 57 included (78 eyes) | |

| | | | |
|---|---|---|---|
| 125 | Erdogan G, Kirmaci A, Perente I, Artunay O. Gravitational displacement of submacular haemorrhage in patients with age-related macular disease. Eye (Lond). 2020 Jun;34(6):1136–1141. doi: 10.1038/s41433-019-0720-8. Epub 2019 Dec 2. PMID: 31792350; PMCID: PMC7253466. | Excluded | 9 eyes |
| 126 | Helaiwa K, Paez LR, Szurman P, Januschowski K. Combined Administration of Preoperative Intravitreal and Intraoperative Subretinal Recombinant Tissue Plasminogen Activator in Acute Hemorrhagic Age-related Macular Degeneration. Cureus. 2020 Mar 10;12(3):e7229. doi: 10.7759/cureus.7229. PMID: 32190528; PMCID: PMC7065728. | 58 included (14 eyes) | |
| 127 | Jeong S, Park DG, Sagong M. Management of a Submacular Haemorrhage Secondary to Age-Related Macular Degeneration: A Comparison of Three Treatment Modalities. J Clin Med. 2020 Sep 24;9(10):3088. doi: 10.3390/jcm9103088. PMID: 32987903; PMCID: PMC7601376. | 59 included (77 eyes) | |
| 128 | Karamitsos A, Papastavrou V, Ivanova T, Cottrell D, Stannard K, Karachrysafi S, Cheristanidis S, Ziakas N, Papamitsou T, Hillier R. Management of acute submacular haemorrhage using intravitreal injection of tissue plasminogen activator and gas: A case series. SAGE Open Med Case Rep. 2020 Nov 13;8:2050313X20970337. doi: 10.1177/2050313X20970337. PMID: 33240500; PMCID: PMC7675899. | 60 included (28 eyes) | |
| 129 | Kim JH, Kim CG, Lee DW, Yoo SJ, Lew YJ, Cho HJ, Kim JY, Lee SH, Kim JW. Intravitreal aflibercept for submacular haemorrhage secondary to neovascular age-related macular degeneration and polypoidal choroidal vasculopathy. Graefes Arch Clin Exp Ophthalmol. 2020 Jan;258(1):107–116. doi: 10.1007/s00417-019-04474-0. Epub 2019 Nov 18. PMID: 31741044. | 61 included (29 eyes) | |
| 130 | Lee K, Park YG, Park YH. Visual prognosis after pneumatic displacement of submacular haemorrhage according to age-related macular degeneration subtypes. Retina. 2020 Dec;40(12):2304–2311. doi: 10.1097/IAE.0000000000002762. PMID: 31985556. | 62 included (67 eyes) | |
| 131 | Amy Q. Lu, Jay G. Prensky, Paul S. Baker, Ingrid U. Scott, Tamer H. Mahmoud & Bozho Todorich (2020) Update on medical and surgical management of submacular haemorrhage, Expert Review of Ophthalmology, 15:1, 43–57, DOI: 10.1080/17469899.2020.1725474 | Excluded | Review |
| 132 | Maggio E, Peroglio Deiro A, Mete M, Sartore M, Polito A, Prigione G, Guerriero M, Pertile G. Intravitreal Recombinant Tissue Plasminogen Activator and Sulphur Hexafluoride Gas for Submacular Haemorrhage Displacement in Age-Related Macular Degeneration: Looking behind the Blood. Ophthalmologica. 2020;243(3):224–235. doi: 10.1159/000505752. Epub 2020 Jan 7. PMID: 31905361. | 63 included (96) | |
| 133 | Onder Tokuc, E.; Levent Karabas, V.; Surgical management of subretinal haemorrhage. Journal: Retina-Vitreus-Volume 29, Issue 0, pp. 1–9-published 2020-01-01 | Excluded | Review |

| | | | |
|---|---|---|---|
| 134 | Sun, T.; Wan, Z.; Gao, Y.; Zhang, L.; Peng, Q. Fundus imaging features of massive hemorrhaging in polypoidal choroidal vasculopathy after treatment. International Journal of Clinical and Experimental Medicine-Volume 13, Issue 0, pp. 5736–5744-published 2020-01-01 | Excluded | Case series of 9 eyes |
| 135 | Wilkins CS, Mehta N, Wu CY, Barash A, Deobhakta AA, Rosen RB. Outcomes of pars plana vitrectomy with subretinal tissue plasminogen activator injection and pneumatic displacement of fovea-involving submacular haemorrhage. BMJ Open Ophthalmol. 2020 Mar 16;5(1):e000394. doi: 10.1136/bmjophth-2019-000394. PMID: 32201733; PMCID: PMC7076260. | 64 included (37 eyes) | |
| 136 | Ali Said Y, Dewilde E, Stalmans P. Visual Outcome after Vitrectomy with Subretinal rt-PA Injection to Treat Submacular Haemorrhage Secondary to Age-Related Macular Degeneration or Macroaneurysm. J Ophthalmol. 2021 Dec 30;2021:3160963. doi: 10.1155/2021/3160963. PMID: 35003789; PMCID: PMC8736698. | 65 included (93 eyes) | |
| 137 | Avcı R, Mavi Yıldız A, Çınar E, Yılmaz S, Küçükerdönmez C, Akalp FD, Avcı E. Subretinal Coapplication of Tissue Plasminogen Activator and Bevacizumab with Concurrent Pneumatic Displacement for Submacular Haemorrhages Secondary to Neovascular Age-Related Macular Degeneration. Turk J Ophthalmol. 2021 Feb 25;51(1):38–44. doi: 10.4274/tjo.galenos.2020.72540. PMID: 33631914; PMCID: PMC7931654. | 66 included (30 patients) | |
| 138 | Caporossi T, Bacherini D, Governatori L, Oliverio L, Di Leo L, Tartaro R, Rizzo S. Management of submacular massive haemorrhage in age-related macular degeneration: comparison between subretinal transplant of human amniotic membrane and subretinal injection of tissue plasminogen activator. Acta Ophthalmol. 2022 Aug;100(5):e1143–e1152. doi: 10.1111/aos.15045. Epub 2021 Oct 5. PMID: 34609787. | 67 included (44 eyes) | |
| 139 | Iannetta D, De Maria M, Bolletta E, Mastrofilippo V, Moramarco A, Fontana L. Subretinal Injection of Recombinant Tissue Plasminogen Activator and Gas Tamponade to Displace Acute Submacular Haemorrhages Secondary to Age-Related Macular Degeneration. Clin Ophthalmol. 2021;15:3649–3659 https://doi.org/10.2147/OPTH.S324091 | 68 included (25 eyes) | |
| 140 | Iyer PG, Brooks HL Jr, Flynn HW Jr. Long-Term Favorable Visual Outcomes in Patients with Large Submacular Haemorrhage. Clin Ophthalmol. 2021;15:1189–1192 https://doi.org/10.2147/OPTH.S300662 | Excluded | Case series (2 eyes) |
| 141 | Aslı Kırmacı Kabakcı, Gürkan Erdoğan, Burcu Kemer Atik, İrfan Perente. Outcomes of Surgical Treatment in Cases with Submacular Haemorrhage. | 69 included (54 eyes) | |
| 142 | Kawakami S, Wakabayashi Y, Umazume K, Usui Y, Muramatsu D, Agawa T, Yamamoto K, Goto H. Long-Term Outcome of Eyes with Vitrectomy for Submacular and/or Vitreous Haemorrhage in Neovascular Age-Related Macular Degeneration. J Ophthalmol. 2021 Nov 2;2021:2963822. doi: 10.1155/2021/2963822. PMID: 34765261; PMCID: PMC8577947. | 70 included (25 eyes) | |

| | | | |
|---|---|---|---|
| 143 | Kishikova L, Saad AAA, Vaideanu-Collins D, Isac M, Hamada D, El-Haig WM. Comparison between different techniques for treatment of submacular haemorrhage due to Age-Related Macular Degeneration. Eur J Ophthalmol. 2021 Sep;31(5):2621–2624. doi: 10.1177/1120672120959551. Epub 2020 Sep 29. PMID: 32993349. | 71 included (29 eyes) | |
| 144 | Pierre M, Mainguy A, Chatziralli I, Pakzad-Vaezi K, Ruiz-Medrano J, Bodaghi B, Loewenstein A, Ambati J, de Smet MD, Tadayoni R, Touhami S. Macular Haemorrhage Due to Age-Related Macular Degeneration or Retinal Arterial Macroaneurysm: Predictive Factors of Surgical Outcome. J Clin Med. 2021 Dec 10;10(24):5787. doi: 10.3390/jcm10245787. PMID: 34945083; PMCID: PMC8703651. | 72 included (65 eyes) | |
| 145 | Matsuo Y, Haruta M, Ishibashi Y, Ishibashi K, Furushima K, Kato N, Murotani K, Yoshida S. Visual Outcomes and Prognostic Factors of Large Submacular Haemorrhages Secondary to Polypoidal Choroidal Vasculopathy. Clin Ophthalmol. 2021 Aug 24;15:3557–3562. doi: 10.2147/OPTH.S327138. PMID: 34465976; PMCID: PMC8403222. | 73 included (30 eyes) | |
| 146 | Rickmann A, Paez LR, Della Volpe Waizel M, Bisorca-Gassendorf L, Schulz A, Vandebroek AC, Szurman P, Januschowski K. Functional and structural outcome after vitrectomy combined with subretinal rt-PA Injection with or without additional intravitreal Bevacizumab injection for submacular haemorrhages. PLoS ONE. 2021 Apr 30;16(4):e0250587. doi: 10.1371/journal.pone.0250587. PMID: 33930041; PMCID: PMC8087026. | 74 included (31 eyes) | |
| 147 | Saito-Uchida S, Inoue M, Koto T, Kato Y, Hirakata A. Vitrectomy combined with subretinal injection of tissue plasminogen activator for successful treatment of massive subretinal haemorrhage. Eur J Ophthalmol. 2021 Sep;31(5):2588–2595. doi: 10.1177/1120672120970404. Epub 2020 Nov 4. PMID: 33148019. | Excluded | 11 eyes |
| 148 | Sniatecki JJ, Ho-Yen G, Clarke B, Barbara R, Lash S, Papathomas T, Antonakis S, Gupta B. Treatment of submacular haemorrhage with tissue plasminogen activator and pneumatic displacement in age-related macular degeneration. Eur J Ophthalmol. 2021 Mar;31(2):643–648. doi: 10.1177/1120672119891625. Epub 2019 Dec 9. PMID: 31813290. | 75 included (54 eyes) | |
| 149 | Tranos P, Tsiropoulos GN, Koronis S, Vakalis A, Asteriadis S, Stavrakas P. Comparison of subretinal versus intravitreal injection of recombinant tissue plasminogen activator with gas for submacular haemorrhage secondary to wet age-related macular degeneration: treatment outcomes and brief literature review. Int Ophthalmol. 2021 Dec;41(12):4037–4046. doi: 10.1007/s10792-021-01976-x. Epub 2021 Jul 30. PMID: 34331185. | 76 included (25 eyes) | |

| | | | |
|---|---|---|---|
| 150 | Fukuda Y, Nakao S, Kohno RI, Ishikawa K, Shimokawa S, Shiose S, Takeda A, Morizane Y, Sonoda KH. Postoperative follow-up of submacular haemorrhage displacement treated with vitrectomy and subretinal injection of tissue plasminogen activator: ultrawide-field fundus autofluorescence imaging in gas-filled eyes. Jpn J Ophthalmol. 2022 May;66(3):264–270. doi: 10.1007/s10384-022-00910-7. Epub 2022 Mar 9. PMID: 35260984. | 77 included (24 eyes) | |
| 151 | Jackson, T.L., Bunce, C., Desai, R. et al. Vitrectomy, subretinal Tissue plasminogen activator and Intravitreal Gas for submacular haemorrhage secondary to Exudative Age-Related macular degeneration (TIGER): study protocol for a phase 3, pan-European, two-group, non-commercial, active-control, observer-masked, superiority, randomised controlled surgical trial. Trials 23, 99 (2022). https://doi.org/10.1186/s13063-021-05966-3 | Excluded | Study protocol |
| 152 | Kitagawa Y, Shimada H, Mori R, Tanaka K, Wakatsuki Y, Onoe H, Kaneko H, Machida Y, Nakashizuka H. One-Year Outcome of Intravitreal Tissue Plasminogen Activator, Ranibizumab, and Gas Injections for Submacular Haemorrhage in Polypoidal Choroidal Vasculopathy. J Clin Med. 2022 Apr 13;11(8):2175. doi: 10.3390/jcm11082175. PMID: 35456268; PMCID: PMC9032067. | 78 included (64 eyes) | |
| 153 | Mehta A, Steel DH, Muldrew A, Peto T, Reeves BC, Evans R, Chakravarthy U; IVAN Study Investigators. Associations and Outcomes of Patients with Submacular Haemorrhage Secondary to Age-related Macular Degeneration in the IVAN Trial. Am J Ophthalmol. 2022 Apr;236:89–98. doi: 10.1016/j.ajo.2021.09.033. Epub 2021 Oct 6. PMID: 34626573. | 79 included (535 eyes) | |
| 154 | Tiosano A, Gal-Or O, Fradkin M, Elul R, Dotan A, Hadayer A, Brody J, Ehrlich R. Visual acuity outcome in patients with subretinal haemorrhage-office procedure vs. surgical treatment. Eur J Ophthalmol. 2022 May 9:11206721221098208. doi: 10.1177/11206721221098208. Epub ahead of print. PMID: 35532042. | 80 included (107 eyes) | |
| 155 | Ura S, Miyata M, Ooto S, Yasuhara S, Tamura H, Ueda-Arakawa N, Muraoka Y, Miyake M, Takahashi A, Wakazono T, Uji A, Yamashiro K, Tsujikawa A. Contrast-to-noise ratio is a useful predictor of early displacement of large submacular haemorrhage by intravitreal sf6 gas injection. Retina. 2022 Apr 1;42(4):661–668. doi: 10.1097/IAE.0000000000003360. PMID: 35350046. | 81 included (16 eyes) | |

## Appendix C

| Author (et al.) | Year | Study Design | Study Sample (Eyes) | Type of Surgery | Mean Size of the Bleeding | Outcome Final BCVA | Mean Days from Onset | Complications | GRADE [1] |
|---|---|---|---|---|---|---|---|---|---|
| Olivier [85] | 2004 | Retrospective, noncomparative, interventional case series | 29 | PPV + subretinal rt-PA + air | N/A | 17 eyes (59%) gained more than 2 lines; 3 eyes (10%) lost more than 2 lines at 3 months | 23 | 2 vitreous hemorrhages and 1 relapse | Very low |
| Ratanasukon [56] | 2005 | Retrospective, noncomparative, interventional case series | 19 | Intravitreal rt-PA + expansile gas | More than 3 disc diameters | BCVA improved 2 lines or greater in 12 eyes (63.2%), stabilized in 6 eyes (31.6%), and worsened in 1 (5.2%) (at 13 months) | 13.1 | 3 vitreous hemorrhages, 3 cataracts, and 2 retinal detachments | Very low |
| Thompson [90] | 2005 | Retrospective, comparative, interventional case series | 42 | PPV + removal of subretinal hemorrhage versus PPV + subretinal rt-PA | 12 disc diameters or less | From 20/1000-1 to 20/640-2 at 3 months | N/A | 1 RD, 1 hyphema, 2 VH | Low |
| Yang [58] | 2005 | Retrospective, comparative, interventional case series | 24 | Intravitreal injection of expansile gas, with or without adjunctive commercial rt-PA solution | N/A | BCVA improved two or more lines in 11 (45.8%) of the 24 eyes, and measured 20/100 or better in 10 (41.7%) of the 11 eyes | N/A | 2 recurrent SRMH, 7 VH, 1 massive VH | Very low |
| Mozafarieh [27] | 2006 | Longitudinal prospective study | 101 | Intravitreous plasminogen activator injection | At least one disc diameter | - | Less than 4 weeks | None | Moderate |
| Singh [57] | 2006 | Retrospective, noncomparative, interventional case series | 17 | PPV + subretinal rt-PA + air | N/A | Improvement was made in all but five patients | Mean duration before surgery was 11.9 days | 3 rebleeds, 1 RD | Very low |

| Chen [58] | 2007 | Retrospective, noncomparative, interventional case series | 85 | PPV + subretinal rt-PA + gas | N/A | 52 eyes (64%) achieved 2 Snellen acuity lines or better improvement at 3 months | Mean duration of symptoms before surgery was 9.3 days | Vitreous hemorrhage in 8 eyes (8%) and retinal detachment in 3 eyes | Low |
|---|---|---|---|---|---|---|---|---|---|
| Gopalakrishan [28] | 2007 | Prospective, consecutive, single-center, noncomparative, interventional case series | 20 | Intravitreal $C_3F_8$ injection without rt-PA | N/A | Mean BCVA improved from 1.6 to 0.72 LogMAR | Range from 1 to 30 days | 4 VH | Moderate |
| Ron [91] | 2007 | Retrospective, noncomparative, interventional case series | 24 | PPV + subretinal rt-PA + gas (SF 6 and $C_3F_8$) | At least 3 disc diameters | SF6 used in 13 patients (54.2%). Seven (53.8%) showed improvement of 2 lines on the Snellen chart. $C_3F_8$ was injected in 11 patients (45.8%). Four of them (36.3%) showed an improvement of 2 lines on the Snellen chart | Range from 1 to 30 days | No complications | Low |
| Stifter [59] | 2007 | Retrospective, noncomparative, interventional case series | 21 | Intravitreal bevacizumab | At least 3 disc diameters | VA improved in 48% (10/21) of the treated eyes with a mean VA gain of 0.2 0.16, was stable in 9% (2/21), and decreased in 43% (9/21) of the treated eyes with a mean VA loss of 0.1 0.06 | The mean period between symptomatic onset of submacular hemorrhage and the time of initial presentation was 12.9 days | N/A | Very low |

| Meyer [92] | 2008 | Retrospective, noncomparative, interventional case series | 19 | Intravitreal injections of recombined tissue plasminogen activator (rt-PA), expansile gas and bevacizumab | 1–3 disc diameters | VA improved two or more lines in 19% of the surgery group compared to 17% of the observation group at 3 months | Onset < 3 months | 5 High IOP > 30 mmHg | Very low |
| --- | --- | --- | --- | --- | --- | --- | --- | --- | --- |
| Fang [93] | 2009 | Retrospective, noncomparative, interventional case series | 53 | PPV with or without subretinal rt-PA + Gas | N/A | Best visual acuity improvement was significantly higher in the rt-PA and gas group than in the gas-alone group (60.7 vs. 32.0%; $p$ = 0.037) | Duration < 14 days or > 14 days | VH and endophthalmitis | Low |
| Arias [60] | 2010 | Retrospective, noncomparative, interventional case series | 15 | PPV with intravitreal or subretinal rt-PA + Gas SF6 + intravitreal bevacizumab | 1–3 disc diameters | The mean VA (ETDRS) improved from 9.4 letters to 28.2 letters with a mean change of +18.7 letters | Within 5 days from symptoms' onset | 3 VH and 1 RPE tear | Very low |
| Cakir [61] | 2010 | Retrospective, noncomparative, interventional case series | 21 | $C_3F_8$ gas-assisted pneumatic displacement, with and without intravitreal rt-PA | N/A | Visual acuity in all patients either improved at least one Snellen line ($n$ = 13) or remained the same ($n$ = 8) | Up to 10 days | 2 recurrences | Very low |
| Fine [94] | 2010 | Retrospective, noncomparative, interventional case series | 15 | Subretinal injection of rt-PA (15 of 15) + gas tamponade (12 of 15), oil tamponade (3 of 15) | At least two quadrants | LogMAR 2.77 at baseline vs. 1.95 at 12 months follow-up | Less than 3 weeks after the onset | 6 vitreous hemorrhages, 2 RD, 1 glaucoma, 1 cataract, 1 aphakia | Very low |

| | | | | | | | | |
|---|---|---|---|---|---|---|---|---|
| Hillenkamp [35] | 2010 | Nonrandomized, retrospective, interventional, comparative consecutive series | 47 | PPV with intravitreal injection of rt-PA and SF6 (Group A) versus PPV with subretinal injection of rt-PA and intravitreal injection of SF6 (Group B) | N/A | The difference in BCVA change between Group A and Group B was not statistically significant | 6.6 days (Group A), 5.9 days (Group B) | Group A: 1 vitreous hemorrhage and 1 recurrence; Group B: 3 RD, 2 vitreous hemorrhages | Low |
| Kung [62] | 2010 | Retrospective, interventional case series | 46 | rt-PA + $C_3F_8$ | From 0.5 to 35 disc areas (median, 8 disc areas) | Postoperative BCVA improved by 2 Snellen lines or greater in 21 of 45 eyes (46.67%) | 10 | 9 vitreous hemorrhages | Low |
| Sandhu [63] | 2010 | Retrospective, interventional case series | 16 | PPV + submacular rt-PA injection + pneumatic displacement with air followed by postoperative intravitreal ranibizumab (RZB) (12 patients) | 6 disc diameters (range 3–12) | At 6 months, 10 of 16 patients had improved by 2 lines; 10 of the 12 patients treated with RZB improved by 2, and all improved by at least 1 line. The mean number of lines of improvement was 3.4 | 12.5 | 2 recurrences (treated with another RZB injection) | Very low |
| Guthoff [36] | 2011 | Nonrandomized, retrospective, interventional, comparative consecutive series | 38 | Group A: intravitreal rt-PA + SF6 (26 patients) vs. Group B: intravitreal bevacizumab + rt-PA + SF6 (12 patients) | More than 1 disc diameter | After 7 months, BCVA was significantly higher in the bevacizumab/rt-PA/gas group (B) | 1–31 days | No complications | Low |

| Mizutani [95] | 2011 | Nonrandomized, retrospective, interventional, comparative consecutive series | 53 | Intravitreal injection SF6 with/without rt-PA | N/A | Intravitreal SF6 + rt-PA have good visual outcomes and no remarkable complications for treating submacular hemorrhage secondary to AMD. rt-PA is not recommended for ruptured retinal arterial macroaneurysms, because of a higher incidence of subsequent vitreous hemorrhage | N/A | All eyes with macroaneurysms have recurrence. 5 postoperative transient ocular hypertensions | Low |
|---|---|---|---|---|---|---|---|---|---|
| Treumer [64] | 2011 | Retrospective, consecutive, interventional case series | 41 | PPV + subretinal rt-PA and bevacizumab + SF6 | Mean 4.5 disc diameters (range 1.5–12) | LogMAR BCVA improved significantly from the preoperative value 1.7 (3.0–0.5) to 0.8 (1.6–0.2) | Maximum 2 weeks | 8 recurrences | Low |
| Tsymanava [37] | 2012 | Retrospective, non-randomized, comparative case study | 110 | rt-PA injection without gas injection (group A1: 50 μg of rt-PA; A2: 100 μg; A3: 200 μg) and with gas injection (group B1: 50 μg of rt-PA; B2: 100 μg; B3: 200 μg) | 12.5 (1–38) | BCVA was better in B1 and B2 groups | 10.0 (0.5–180.0) | 2 endophthalmitis, 10 vitreous hemorrhages, 3 increased intraocular pressure | Low |

| Ueda-Arakawa [103] | 2012 | Nonrandomized, retrospective, comparative consecutive series | 31 | None, the study valued the retinal structural changes associated with submacular hemorrhage and their relationships with visual prognosis | $6.0 \pm 3.1$ disc areas | The initial OCT detection of the IS/OS just beneath the fovea may predict good visual outcomes | $3.7 \pm 2.3$ months | N/A | Low |
|---|---|---|---|---|---|---|---|---|---|
| Cho [65] | 2013 | Retrospective, interventional case series | 27 | Anti-VEGF injection with an initial 3 loading injections by month, followed by an as-needed reinjection in patients with PCV | $18.2 \pm 13.8$ mm² | LogMAR visual acuity at baseline was $1.02 \pm 0.51$ and improved significantly to $0.76 \pm 0.48$ at 12 months | $9.8 \pm 7.5$ days | 3 vitreous hemorrhages | Very low |
| Han [96] | 2013 | Retrospective, interventional case series | 14 | 180° peripheral temporal retinotomy, choroidal neovascular membrane (CNVM) excision, and transplantation of an autologous simple RPE sheet developed from the PED region outside the CNVM lesion | Massive submacular hemorrhage (extending to at least one temporal vessel arch) | Mean ETDRS score increased from $14.0 \pm 23.4$ preoperatively to $31.9 \pm 23.8$ at 18 months | Less than 6 months | 1 RD, 1 delayed recurrent submacular hemorrhage | Very low |

| Jain [66] | 2013 | Retrospective chart review | 14 | Anti-VEGF monotherapy | More than 2 disc areas | Mean change in VA from baseline at final follow-up was −0.58 LogMAR (range −1.6 to +1, Snellen range 20/30–20/400, median 20/60; $p = 0.0022$) | 4 (range 1–7) | N/A | Very low |
| --- | --- | --- | --- | --- | --- | --- | --- | --- | --- |
| Mayer [38] | 2013 | Nonrandomized, retrospective, interventional, comparative consecutive series | 45 | Group A: rt-PA (50 µg/0.05 mL) + SF6. Group B: bevacizumab (1.25 mg/0.05 mL) + SF6. Thereafter, all patients received bevacizumab | From 1 to 5 disc areas | Better VA in the rt-PA and gas group (14 letters improvement) compared with VA increase in the bevacizumab and gas group (8 letters improvement) from baseline to 12 months follow-up ($p < 0.03$) | N/A | 10 vitreous hemorrhages | Low |
| Rishi [39] | 2012 | Retrospective, single-center study | 46 | PPV + subretinal rt-PA (group 1); pneumatic displacement with intravitreal rt-PA and gas (group 2); pneumatic displacement with intraocular gas (group 3) | 5.6 ± 3.4 disc areas | No statistically significant difference amongst groups | 10 | 4 cataracts, 4 RD, 2 secondary glaucoma, 2 vitreous hemorrhages | Low |

| Shienbaum [97] | 2013 | Retrospective, interventional, consecutive case series | 19 | Anti-VEGF monotherapy | 39.0 mm² (range 4.3–170.2 mm²) | The mean change in approximate ETDRS letter score from baseline was +12 letters at 3 months ($p < 0.003$), +18 letters at 6 months ($p < 0.001$), and +17 letters at 12 months follow-up ($p < 0.02$) | N/A | No adverse ocular or systemic events | Very low |
|---|---|---|---|---|---|---|---|---|---|
| Chang [98] | 2014 | Retrospective, comparative, interventional case series | 101 | PPV + subretinal rt-PA + gas tamponade with and without postsurgical antiVEGF injection | N/A | BCVA of the group that received post-operative anti-VEGF injection showed greater visual acuity improvement 6 months postoperatively compared to the group that did not receive post-operative anti-VEGF | N/A | 6 recurrences, 4 RD, 2 vitreous hemorrhages | Low |
| Iacono [29] | 2014 | Prospective interventional case series | 23 | Intravitreal ranibizumab | Occult choroidal neovascularization with flat large submacular hemorrhage > 50% of the entire lesion | At 12-months mean visual acuity improved significantly to $0.68 \pm 0.41$ ($p = 0.04$) | N/A | None | Very low |

| Kitahashi [40] | 2014 | Retrospective, comparative, interventional case series | 32 | Pneumatic displacement (SF6) + intravitreal bevacizumab vs. pneumatic displacement (SF6) alone | More than 2 disc areas | Mean BCVA in the SF6 + IVB group was significantly better than that in the SF6 group at 1, 3, and 6 months postoperatively ($p$ 0.001, $p$ 0.001 and $p$ 0.001, respectively) | Less than 10 days | 1 RD | Low |
|---|---|---|---|---|---|---|---|---|---|
| Moisseiev [67] | 2014 | Retrospective, noncomparative, interventional case series | 31 | PPV + subretinal rt-PA | N/A | Patients who improved by at least one line in VA (change in LogMAR $-0.41 \pm 0.17$) had worse VA at presentation and better final VA than those who did not improve (change in LogMAR $0.37 \pm 0.18$) | $13.4 \pm 12.4$ (range 1–60) days | 6 RD, 2 recurrences, 2 elevated IOP following surgery | Low |
| Dimopoulos [41] | 2015 | Retrospective, noncomparative, interventional case series | 46 | Intravitreal bevacizumab in group A (from 1 to 4 disc area), group B (from 4 to 9 DA), group C (more than 9 DA) | 6 DA | The mean BCVA increased from 0.81 LogMAR (Snellen 20/125) at baseline to 0.75 LogMAR (20/125) after 1 year. Amongst the three groups, improvement of the BCVA was found in 57% (13/23), 53% (8/15), and 38% (3/8) of eyes, respectively. | $11.5 \pm 19$ days (range: 1–45 days) | None | Low |

| Author | Year | Study design | N | Intervention | Size | Outcome | Duration | Complications | Quality |
|---|---|---|---|---|---|---|---|---|---|
| Kadonosono [86] | 2015 | Prospective, consecutive, interventional case series | 13 | 25-gauge vitrectomy and submacular injection of rt-PA and air | N/A | Mean ETDRS score improvement was 19.4 letters at 1 month and 23.3 letters at 3 months | 19 days (range 7–40) | 1 FTMH, 1 VH | Moderate |
| Kim [68] | 2015 | Retrospective, noncomparative, interventional case series | 49 | Intravitreal anti-VEGF injection | 13.9 ± 8.8 disc areas | Mean BCVA improved from 1.14 ± 0.61 LogMAR (20/276, Snellen equivalent) to 0.82 ± 0.53 LogMAR (20/132) at 12 months | 7.25 ± 5.9 days | 10 VH | Low |
| Kimura [69] | 2015 | Prospective, noncomparative, interventional case series | 15 | PPV + subretinal rt-PA injection + air tamponade, followed by intravitreal antiVEGF injection | 5.6 ± 4.7 disc diameters (range, 1.5–20 disc diameters) | Mean BCVA at baseline (0.98 ± 0.44) had improved significantly both 1 month after surgery (0.41 ± 0.25) and at final visit (0.23 ± 0.25) | 9.5 ± 4.5 (range 5–21) days | None | Moderate |
| Shin [42] | 2015 | Retrospective, comparative, interventional case series | 82 | Pneumatic displacement (SF6 or $C_3F_8$) + intravitreal anti-VEGF vs. anti-VEGF monotherapy | N/A | Improvement in BCVA was not significantly different between the 2 groups at baseline, 3 months, or 6 months after initial treatment, but the combination therapy group showed better visual acuity at 1 month after initial treatment compared with the monotherapy group | 11.4 ± 10.4 days in the combination therapy group and 13.8 ± 11.5 days in the monotherapy group | 6 recurrences, 12 RPE tears, 5 VH, 2 RRD, 1 HRD with choroidal hemorrhage | Low |

| Wei [30] | 2015 | Prospective, nonrandomized, and noncomparative case series study | 21 | PPV + 360° retinotomy + silicon oil (Oxane 5700) tamponade | N/A | The mean BCVA in LogMAR (Snellen equivalent) significantly improved from preoperatively 2.64 (hand movement) to 1.73 (7/400), 1.50 (6/200), 1.51 (6/200), and 1.45 (7/200) at 1 month, 3 months, 6 months after the initial surgery, and final follow-up | N/A | 10 mild subretinal fibrosis | Moderate |
|---|---|---|---|---|---|---|---|---|---|
| Bae [105] | 2016 | Retrospective, interventional case series | 37 | Pneumatic displacement + laser or anti-VEGF | $12.9 \pm 8.3$ DA | The mean BCVA was $1.08 \pm 0.55$ at baseline, $0.74 \pm 0.57$ at 3 months, and $0.63 \pm 0.58$ at 6 months. The mean BCVA of PCV patients was significantly better than that of typical exudative AMD patients | $16.1 \pm 12.5$ | None | Low |
| De Jong [31] | 2016 | Prospective, noncomparative, interventional case series | 24 | Group A: PPV + gas + subretinal rt-PA; Group B: intravitreal rt-PA + gas | Group A: 11.1 DA (range 0.5–31.0); Group B: 9.7 DA (range 2.9–20.2) | Median visual acuity improvement in ETDRS lines at Week 4, 6, and 12 shows no significant differences between groups | Group A: 5 (range 1–11), Group B: 6 (range 1–14 | Group A: 3 increased IOP > 50 mmHg, 2 VH, 1 RD, 1 recurrence. Group B: 2 RD, 2 recurrences | Very low |

| | | | | | | | | |
|---|---|---|---|---|---|---|---|---|
| Fassbender [43] | 2016 | Retrospective case series | 39 | Group A: PPV + subretinal (rt-PA) injection; Group B: pneumatic displacement (PD) + intravitreal rt-PA; Group C: PD without rt-PA | Group A: 9.1 mm$^2$; Group B: 8.1 mm$^2$; Group C: 9.1 mm$^2$ | Final visual acuity improved significantly in both the vitrectomy and subretinal rt-PA injection group and the intravitreal rt-PA injection group, but not with PD alone | Group A: 5 ± 4.6; Group B: 6 ± 4.2; Group C: 6 ± 2.2 | None | Low |
| González-López [70] | 2016 | Retrospective, nonrandomized, and noncomparative case series study | 45 | Small gauge PPV + subretinal rt-PA + ranibizumab | 40.64 ± 20.20 mm$^2$ | Visual acuity improved −0.59 ± 0.61 LogMAR between presentation and last follow-up | 6.98 ± 5.70 | N/A | Low |
| Kitagawa [32] | 2016 | Prospective, interventional, consecutive case series | 20 | Intravitreal rt-PA + ranibizumab + gas without vitrectomy | 11.1 ± 8.7 disc diameters (range, 2–31 disc diameters) | Mean change in ETDRS score from baseline was +13 letters | 9.9 ± 9.8 days (range 2–30 days) | 3 VH, 1 RD | Very low |
| Lee [71] | 2016 | Retrospective clinical case series | 25 | Intravitreal injections of tenecteplase, antiVEGF, and expansile gas | 7.5 ± 5.0 disc areas (range, 1.5 to 19) | BCVA improved from 1.09 ± 0.77 LogMAR at baseline to 0.52 ± 0.60 LogMAR at 12 months | 7.2 ± 8.2 days (range, 1 to 30 days) | 1 VH, 1 RPE tear | Very low |

| | | | | | | | | |
|---|---|---|---|---|---|---|---|---|
| Lin [44] | 2016 | Retrospective, comparative, interventional case series | 20 | Group A: subretinal rt-PA + PPV; Group B: or intravitreal rt-PA + gas to achieve pneumatic displacement. Additionally, combination treatment with either (PDT) or intravitreal injection of anti-VEGF was performed | 17.8 ± 19.2 disc diameter (DD) compared (2.64 DD) | Combination treatment with PDT showed significant efficacy in the improvement of BCVA | 14.3 ± 16.6 days | 2 VH | Very low |
| Waizel [72] | 2016 | Observational analysis | 83 | PPV + rt-PA + gas for subretinal hemorrhages (SRH), subpigment epithelial hemorrhages (SPH), and combined subretinal and subpigment epithelial hemorrhages (CH). 68.7% received additional anti-VEGF | N/A | Vitrectomy combined with subretinal rt-PA injection and gas or air tamponade has a strong functional and anatomical effect on both SRH and CH and also seems to slightly improve the anatomical outcome in SPH | 13.4 ± 13.4 in CH; 8.3 ± 10.3 in SRH; 4.9 ± 8.0 in SPH | 1 FTMH, 1 RD, 3 recurrences | Low |
| Bell [45] | 2017 | Retrospective chart review | 18 | Pneumatic displacement followed by intravitreal rt-PA if needed vs. PPV with subretinal rt-PA | N/A | The percentage of patients achieving three lines or greater improvement at 1 year was 46% and 18% in these groups; the difference was not statistically significant | N/A | 1 recurrence | Very low |

| Author | Year | Study Design | N | Intervention | Size of SMH | Visual Acuity Outcome | Follow-up | Complications | Quality |
|---|---|---|---|---|---|---|---|---|---|
| Gok [73] | 2017 | Retrospective, nonrandomized, consecutive case series | 17 | PPV + subretinal rt-PA + SF6 | 8.6 ± 5.3 disc areas | Improvement from initial VA (mean LogMAR, 1.8 ± 0.3) and the final BCVA (mean LogMAR, 0.97 ± 0.52) | 12.8 ± 18.2 days | 1 recurrence, 1 RRD | Very low |
| Waizel [74] | 2017 | Retrospective observational study | 85 | PPV with rt-PA combined with gas or air tamponade | N/A | In air tamponade group, mean VA improved from LogMAR 1.42 ± 0.52 to LogMAR 1.25 ± 0.51 (20/530 to 20/355 Snellen equivalent, average gain in visual acuity of 1.7 lines). In gas tamponade group, VA improved from LogMAR 1.37 ± 0.42 to LogMAR 1.29 ± 0.39 (20/471 to 20/394 Snellen equivalent, average gain in visual acuity of 0.8 lines) | 13.5 ± 12.3 days in gas tamponade; 10.9 ± 15.2 days in air tamponade | 1 FTMH, 3 recurrences | Low |
| Bardak [75] | 2018 | Retrospective pilot study | 16 | Intravitreal rt-PA + pneumatic displacement + anti-VEGF | N/A | Mean BCVA was 2.08 ± 0.79 LogMAR at baseline, 1.09 ± 0.73 LogMAR at the last follow up | 7.9 ± 3.6 days | 1 retinal pigment epithelium tear | Very low |

| Juncal [84] | 2018 | Retrospective case series | 99 | PPV + subretinal rt-PA + pneumatic displacement | 15.7% 1–5 DA; 18.6% 6–10 DA; 65.7% > 10 DA | Mean LogMAR BCVA improved from 2.03 ± 0.81 (Snellen 20/2143) at baseline to 1.80 ± 1.00 (Snellen 20/1262) at final follow-up | 19.6 ± 29.1 (2–160) | 13 VH, 8 RD, 4 RPE tears, 2 expulsive choroidal hemorrhages, 12 recurrences | Low |
| --- | --- | --- | --- | --- | --- | --- | --- | --- | --- |
| Kim [87] | 2017 | Retrospective observational study | 21 | Anti-VEGF monotherapy | 19.3 ± 9.1 mm² (range: 5.6 to 32.3 mm²) | From 0.86 ± 0.39 LogMAR at baseline to 0.53 ± 0.43 LogMAR after resolution of the hemorrhage | 16.0 ± 10.1 | N/A | Very low |
| Kimura [99] | 2018 | Retrospective analysis | 33 | Pneumatic displacement with SF6 with or without rt-PA | N/A | The BCVAs improved significantly in eyes with PCV compared with eyes with typical AMD | N/A | 4 persistent PED | Low |
| Sharma [76] | 2017 | Retrospective, noncomparative, interventional case series | 24 | PPV + subretinal air injection in combination with rt-PA + partial fluid-gas exchange and preoperative, intraoperative, or postoperative anti-VEGF | Small (does not reach arcades) in 6 patients (25%), large (extending to the arcades) in 9 patients (37.5%), and massive (extending to 2 quadrants, past the equator, or both) in 7 patients (29.2%) | Mean preoperative VA was 1.95 (Snellen equivalent, 20/1783), mean postoperative VA was 0.85 LogMAR (Snellen equivalent, 20/141) | 11.3 days (range, 1–59 days; median, 9 days) | 5 recurrences, 3 VH, 2 RD, 1 FTMH | Very low |

| Study | Year | Study type | N | Treatment | Size/Groups | Outcome | Follow-up | Complications | Evidence level |
|---|---|---|---|---|---|---|---|---|---|
| Plemel [100] | 2019 | Retrospective, noncomparative, interventional case series | 78 | PPV + subretinal rt-PA + gas tamponade | 13.6 DA | Visual acuity improved from 20/1449 preoperatively to 20/390 after a mean follow-up time of 6.3 months, corresponding to approximately 5 lines of Snellen acuity improvement | N/A | 9 recurrences | Low |
| Helaiwa [101] | 2020 | Single-center, case series report | 14 | Intravitreal rt-PA + (next day) PPV + subretinal rt-PA + air tamponade | $21.6 \pm 17.8$ mm$^2$ | Significant ($p = 0.01$) overall improvement in the visual acuity post-treatment (from $1.4 \pm 0.5$ log MAR to $0.9 \pm 0.4$) | N/A | None | Very low |
| Jeong [46] | 2020 | Retrospective chart review | 77 | Group A: anti-VEGF monotherapy; Group B: PD + anti-VEGF; Group C: PPV + subretinal rt-PA and gas tamponade | Three groups according to the dimensions: small-sized (optic disc diameter (ODD) $\geq 1$ to $<4$), medium-sized (ODD $\geq 4$ within the temporal arcade) and large-sized (ODD $\geq 4$, exceeding the temporal arcade) | In the small-sized group, all treatment modalities showed a gradual BCVA improvement. In the medium-sized group, PD and surgery were associated with better BCVA than anti-VEGF monotherapy (67% and 83%, respectively, vs. 33%). In the large-sized group, surgery showed a better visual improvement with a higher displacement rate than PD (86% vs. 25%) | $14.3 \pm 25.8$ | 1 recurrence, 1 RPE rip, 1 FTMH | Low |

| Karamitsos [77] | 2020 | Retrospective case series | 28 | Intravitreal rt-PA + gas ± anti-VEGF | 4.9 mm in patients with no anatomical displacement; 4.5 ± 1.4 mm in patients with anatomical displacement | The mean improvement of all patients with anatomical displacement of the hemorrhage in visual acuity was 0.7 ± 0.5 (LogMAR) in 1 month | 3.5 ± 2.1 days in patients with no anatomical displacement and 3.4 ± 3.6 days in patients with anatomical displacement | 2 VH, 1 RD | Very low |
|---|---|---|---|---|---|---|---|---|---|
| Kim [104] | 2019 | Retrospective, nonrandomized, and noncomparative case series study | 29 | Intravitreal aflibercept | 6.2 ± 4.8 DA | BCVA significantly improved from 52.9 ± 17.8 ETDRS letters at week 0 to 71.8 ± 16.1 letters at week 56 | ≤7 days in 18 patients (62.1%), >7 days but ≤1 month in 7 patients (24.1%), and >1 month but <3 months in 4 patients (13.8%) | 8 reactivations | Very low |
| Lee [78] | 2020 | Retrospective, comparative, interventional case series | 67 | Pneumatic displacement among patients with different subtypes of age-related macular degeneration (AMD): typical AMD, polypoidal choroidal vasculopathy (PCV), and retinal angiomatous proliferation (RAP) | 6.63 ± 4.66 DA in typical AMD; 5.95 ± 4.58 DA in PCV; 8.35 ± 4.00 DA in RAP | The proportion of eyes with improved visual acuity was highest in the PCV subtype and lowest in the RAP subtype | 7.85 ± 6.89 | N/A | Low |

| | | | | | | | | |
|---|---|---|---|---|---|---|---|---|
| Maggio [47] | 2020 | Retrospective, noncomparative, interventional case series | 96 | Intravitreal rt-PA + SF6 for guiding the selection of additional treatments (anti-VEGF, PDT, or submacular surgery) or observation (CNV) | At least 3 DA involving the fovea | BCVA improved from 1.8 (SD = 0.96) LogMAR to BCVA significantly improved to 1.29 (SD = 0.78) LogMAR at 3 months | Less than 14 days | 7 recurrences, 2 VH | Low |
| Wilkins [102] | 2020 | Retrospective, interventional case series | 37 | PPV + subretinal rt-PA + pneumatic displacement | N/A | Median preoperative VA was 20/2000, at postoperative month 3 was 20/152 | N/A | 5 VH, 4 recurrent H, 3 RD, 1 blood stained cornea, 1 glaucoma, 1 phthisis | Low |
| Ali Said [79] | 2021 | Retrospective analysis | 93 | PPV + subretinal rt-PA + air | N/A | Mean BCVA at baseline was 0.06 Snellen; after the surgery, BCVA improved to 0.16 Snellen; at 8 months, decreased to 0.08 Snellen | The majority of eyes were operated within two days after the onset of the hemorrhage (60, 2%), 90.3% of eyes within one week, and all 93 eyes within 14 days | 2 RPE tears, 7 VH, 4 hyphema, 6 RD, 2 sub-choroidal hemorrhages | Low |
| Avci [80] | 2021 | Retrospective study | 30 | PPV + $C_3F_8$ 5% + subretinal rt-PA + anti-VEGF | $61.95 \pm 43.47$ (range: 10.75–176.42) $mm^2$ | Mean VA improved from LogMAR $2.11 \pm 0.84$ at baseline to LogMAR $1.32 \pm 0.91$, $0.94 \pm 0.66$, $1.13 \pm 0.84$, and $1.00 \pm 0.70$ at postoperative month 1, 2, 3, and 6, respectively | $13.70 \pm 8.05$ (range: 2–30) days | 2 recurrences | Low |

| Caporossi [88] | 2022 | Retrospective, consecutive, comparative, non-randomized interventional study | 44 | Group A: PPV + massive submacular hemorrhage and neovascular membrane removal + hAM subretinal implant + silicone oil; Group B: PPV + subretinal rt-PA + SF6 20% | N/A | Mean preoperative BCVA was 1.9 LogMAR in the amniotic membrane group and 2 LogMAR in the rt-PA group. The mean final BCVA values were 1.25 and 1.4 LogMAR, respectively, with a statistically significant difference | 25.9 ± 36 days (range, 1–150 days) | 2 VH, 2 RD | Low |
| Iannetta [81] | 2021 | Single-center, retrospective, case series | 25 | PPV + subretinal rt-PA + SF6 20% | 68.34 ± 42.42 mm$^2$ | BCVA significantly improved from 1.81 ± 0.33 to 1.37 ± 0.52 LogMAR at 12 months from surgery | 9.24 (±3.37) | 2 recurrences, 1 RD | Very low |
| Asli [48] | | Retrospective case series | 54 | - 21 eyes PPV + submacular rt-PA + 20% SF6 or 14% C$_3$F$_8$; - 14 eyes PPV + submacular rt-PA + 20% SF6 or 14% C$_3$F$_8$ + antiVEGF; - 10 eyes PPV + subretinal rt-PA without gas; - 4 eyes intravitreal gas + rt-PA; - 3 eyes PPV + subretinal rt-PA + drainage; - 2 eyes intravitreal gas + intravitreal antiVEGF | 31.5 ± 26.5 (2.8–145.3) mm$^2$ | BCVA improved from 2.0 ± 0.8 (0.3–3) at presentation to 1.67 ± 0.87 (0.22–3) LogMAR on postoperative month 1, 1.65 ± 0.79 (0.40–3) LogMAR on month 3, 1.76 ± 0.88 (0.22–3) LogMAR on month 6, 1.71 ± 0.85 (0.30–3) LogMAR at year 1, and 1.76 ± 0.81 (0.22–3) LogMAR at final visit | 13.7 ± 16.3 (1–95) days | 6 RD, 3 VH, 2 FTMH, 4 recurrences | Low |

| | | | | | | | | |
|---|---|---|---|---|---|---|---|---|
| Kawakami [82] | 2021 | Retrospective case series | 25 | PPV ± anti-VEGF (2 eyes in SMH group) | 4.0 ± 1.6 (range 2.0–6.7) disc diameters | BCVA improved in eyes with SMH at 6 and 12 months after PPV, and the BCVA was maintained until the end of the study (24 months) | 9.3 ± 4.6 (range 4–17) | 2 FTMH | Very low |
| Kishikova [49] | 2020 | Retrospective analysis | 29 | Group 1: intravitreal rt-PA + SF6 Group 2: PPV + subretinal rt-PA + SF6 with (2A) or without (2B) subretinal air | 9.45 DD ± 2.34 in Group 1 and 9.72 DD ± 2.02 in Group 2 | The mean BCVA at presentation was 0.0068 in Group 1 and 0.0067 in Group 2. The mean postoperative BCVA at 6 months was 0.31 in Group 1 and 0.58 in Group 2. Subgroup analysis of Group 2 did not show statistically significant difference in outcome when adding subretinal air to the vitrectomy procedure | N/A | 3 high IOP, 2 RD, 3 cataracts | Very low |
| Pierre [13] | 2021 | Multicentric retrospective case series | 65 | PPV + subretinal rt-PA + gas | 5441.3 ± 1323.1 microns in AMD group; 5085.2 ± 3012.3 microns in RAM group | BCVA improved from 20/500 to 20/125 at month 1 and month 6 | 7.1 ± 6.7 days (range 0–30 days) | 7 VH, 5 RRD, 7 recurrences | Low |

| Matsuo [50] | 2021 | Retrospective study | 30 | 13 eyes underwent pneumatic displacement, 22 eyes received anti-VEGF therapy, and four eyes underwent PPV | 17.0 ± 4.8 disc areas | The mean BCVA at the development, 1 month, and 1 year after the development of large SMHs, and at the final visit were LogMAR 0.88 ± 0.61 (Snellen equivalent 20/151), LogMAR 1.12 ± 0.82 (Snellen equivalent 20/263), LogMAR 0.84 ± 0.72 (Snellen equivalent 20/138), and LogMAR 0.88 ± 0.75 (Snellen equivalent 20/152), respectively | N/A | 2 VH, 1 RRD | Low |
|---|---|---|---|---|---|---|---|---|---|
| Rickmann [51] | 2021 | Retrospective, consecutive case series | 31 | PPV + subretinal rt-PA + air displacement with (group +B) or without Group − B) intravitreal bevacizumab | 11.78 ± 3.04 mm² in +B; 14.75 ± 3.98 mm² in −B | The mean visual acuity improved significantly in both groups, from 1.37 ± 0.39 to 1.03 ± 0.57 LogMAR in +B and from 1.48 ± 0.48 to 1.01 ± 0.38 LogMAR in group B | 3.3 ± 1.6 in +B; 3.4 ± 1.5 in −B | 1 FTMH, 2 RD, 1 recurrence | Low |

| Sniatecki [52] | 2019 | Retrospective study | 54 | PPV + subretinal rt-PA + pneumatic displacement vs. antiVEGF monotherapy | In rt-PA group, 5.0 DA; in anti-VEGF group, 4.2 DA | Mean LogMAR in rt-PA group at baseline was 1.56, and it was improved at 1 year to 1.07. Mean BCVA in anti-VEGF group at baseline was 1.22 LogMAR with no significant improvement (1.36 at 1 year) | 5 days (range 1–13) | 2 RD, 3 VH, 7 cataracts | Low |
| Tranos [53] | 2021 | Retrospective, comparative, interventional case series | 25 | Group A: PPV + subretinal rt-PA + gas; Group B: intravitreal rt-PA + gas | 4.604 ± 2079 μm | BCVA improved significantly but did not differ between the 2 groups | 8.2 (±7.3) days | N/A | Very low |
| Fukuda [83] | 2022 | Retrospective, consecutive case series | 24 | PPV + subretinal rt-PA | N/A | BCVAs at baseline (1.16 ± 0.52) had improved significantly at the final visit (0.52 ± 0.39) | 11.5 ± 6.6 days | N/A | Very low |
| Kitagawa [33] | 2022 | Extended study of a previous prospective study | 64 | Intravitreal rt-PA + ranibizumab + gas injection | 8 ± 6 (range, 2–27) disc diameters | Mean ETDRS score increased from 58 at baseline to 64 letters | 7 ± 7 (range, 1–30) days | 46 recurrences | Low |

| Author | Year | Study Type | N | Purpose/Method | Results | Follow-up | Complications | Grade |
|---|---|---|---|---|---|---|---|---|
| Mehta [34] | 2021 | Secondary analyses of a randomized, controlled trial of image and clinical data | 535 | Randomly divided into monthly ranibizumab, as-needed ranibizumab, monthly bevacizumab or as-needed bevacizumab | 89% were smaller than 1 standard disc area | SMH at baseline was associated with worse baseline BCVA compared with eyes with no SMH (median letters, 62 vs. 68; $p < 0.001$; estimate of difference 6 letters, 95% CI, 4–8 letters). By month 12, the BCVA had improved in both groups (median letters 71 vs. 75) and was not significantly associated with the presence of baseline SMH ($p = 0.570$) | N/A | 1 RPE tear, 28 fibrosis, 10 atrophic scars, 6 geographic atrophies, 7 epiretinal membranes | Moderate |
| Tiosano [54] | 2022 | Retrospective study | 107 | Group A: intravitreal injection of rt-PA + gas; Group B: PPV | 767 microns in Group A and 962.5 microns in Group B | Visual acuity (in LogMAR) was similar in the two groups prior to the diagnosis of subretinal hemorrhage but better in the rt-PA and gas group at the end of follow-up | N/A | N/A | Low |
| Ura [89] | 2022 | Retrospective study | 16 | Investigate predictors of early displacement of submacular hemorrhage by simple intravitreal SF6 gas injections before inception of subretinal rt-PA | $33.10 \pm 13.98$ mm$^2$ | LogMAR BCVA at 1 week after the injection showed no statistically significant association with any of the measured parameters | $20.6 \pm 44.2$ days | N/A | Very low |

[1] Grading of Recommendations Assessment, Development and Evaluation (GRADE) system [25,26].

## References

1. Kanukollu, V.M.; Ahmad, S.S. *Retinal Haemorrhage*; StatPearls Publishing: Treasure Island, FL, USA, 2022.
2. Shukla, U.V.; Kaufman, E.J. *Intraocular Haemorrhage*; StatPearls Publishing: Treasure Island, FL, USA, 2022.
3. Ohji, M.; Saito, Y.; Hayashi, A.; Lewis, J.M.; Tano, Y. Pneumatic Displacement of Subretinal Haemorrhage without Tissue Plasminogen Activator. *Arch. Ophthalmol.* **1998**, *116*, 1326–1332. [CrossRef]
4. Nayak, S.; Padhi, T.R.; Basu, S.; Das, T. Pneumatic Displacement and Intra-Vitreal Bevacizumab in Management of Sub-Retinal and Sub-Retinal Pigment Epithelial Haemorrhage at Macula in Polypoidal Choroidal Vasculopathy (PCV): Rationale and Outcome. *Semin. Ophthalmol.* **2015**, *30*, 53–55. [CrossRef]
5. Thuruthumaly, C.; Yee, D.C.; Rao, P.K. Presumed Ocular Histoplasmosis. *Curr. Opin. Ophthalmol.* **2014**, *25*, 508–512. [CrossRef]
6. Moriyama, M.; Ohno-Matsui, K.; Shimada, N.; Hayashi, K.; Kojima, A.; Yoshida, T.; Tokoro, T.; Mochizuki, M. Correlation between Visual Prognosis and Fundus Autofluorescence and Optical Coherence Tomographic Findings in Highly Myopic Eyes with Submacular Haemorrhage and without Choroidal Neovascularization. *Retina* **2011**, *31*, 74–80. [CrossRef]
7. Nakamura, H.; Hayakawa, K.; Sawaguchi, S.; Gaja, T.; Nagamine, N.; Medoruma, K. Visual Outcome after Vitreous, Sub-Internal Limiting Membrane, and/or Submacular Haemorrhage Removal Associated with Ruptured Retinal Arterial Macroaneurysms. *Graefes Arch. Clin. Exp. Ophthalmol.* **2008**, *246*, 661–669. [CrossRef]
8. Avery, R.L.; Fekrat, S.; Hawkins, B.S.; Bressler, N.M. Natural History of Subfoveal Subretinal Haemorrhage in Age-Related Macular Degeneration. *Retina* **1996**, *16*, 183–189. [CrossRef]
9. Stevens, T.S.; Bressler, N.M.; Maguire, M.G.; Bressler, S.B.; Fine, S.L.; Alexander, J.; Phillips, D.A.; Margherio, R.R.; Murphy, P.L.; Schachat, A.P. Occult Choroidal Neovascularization in Age-Related Macular Degeneration. A Natural History Study. *Arch. Ophthalmol.* **1997**, *115*, 345–350. [CrossRef]
10. Bressler, N.M.; Bressler, S.B.; Childs, A.L.; Haller, J.A.; Hawkins, B.S.; Lewis, H.; MacCumber, M.W.; Marsh, M.J.; Redford, M.; Sternberg, P.; et al. Surgery for Hemorrhagic Choroidal Neovascular Lesions of Age-Related Macular Degeneration: Ophthalmic Findings: SST Report No. 13. *Ophthalmology* **2004**, *111*, 1993–2006. [CrossRef]
11. Fleckenstein, M.; Keenan, T.D.L.; Guymer, R.H.; Chakravarthy, U.; Schmitz-Valckenberg, S.; Klaver, C.C.; Wong, W.T.; Chew, E.Y. Age-Related Macular Degeneration. *Nat. Rev. Dis. Primer* **2021**, *7*, 31. [CrossRef]
12. Steel, D.H.W.; Sandhu, S.S. Submacular Haemorrhages Associated with Neovascular Age-Related Macular Degeneration. *Br. J. Ophthalmol.* **2011**, *95*, 1051–1057. [CrossRef]
13. Pierre, M.; Mainguy, A.; Chatziralli, I.; Pakzad-Vaezi, K.; Ruiz-Medrano, J.; Bodaghi, B.; Loewenstein, A.; Ambati, J.; de Smet, M.D.; Tadayoni, R.; et al. Macular Haemorrhage Due to Age-Related Macular Degeneration or Retinal Arterial Macroaneurysm: Predictive Factors of Surgical Outcome. *J. Clin. Med.* **2021**, *10*, 5787. [CrossRef]
14. Al-Hity, A.; Steel, D.H.; Yorston, D.; Gilmour, D.; Koshy, Z.; Young, D.; Hillenkamp, J.; McGowan, G. Incidence of Submacular Haemorrhage (SMH) in Scotland: A Scottish Ophthalmic Surveillance Unit (SOSU) Study. *Eye* **2019**, *33*, 486–491. [CrossRef]
15. McGowan, G.F.; Steel, D.; Yorston, D. AMD with Submacular Haemorrhage: New Insights from a Population-Based Study. *Investig. Ophthalmol. Vis. Sci.* **2014**, *55*, 662.
16. A Historic Shift: More Elderly than Children and Teenagers. Available online: https://www.ssb.no/en/befolkning/artikler-og-publikasjoner/a-historic-shift-more-elderly-than-children-and-teenagers (accessed on 16 August 2022).
17. Scupola, A.; Coscas, G.; Soubrane, G.; Balestrazzi, E. Natural History of Macular Subretinal Haemorrhage in Age-Related Macular Degeneration. *Ophthalmologica* **1999**, *213*, 97–102. [CrossRef]
18. Glatt, H.; Machemer, R. Experimental Subretinal Haemorrhage in Rabbits. *Am. J. Ophthalmol.* **1982**, *94*, 762–773. [CrossRef]
19. Papanikolaou, G.; Pantopoulos, K. Iron Metabolism and Toxicity. *Toxicol. Appl. Pharmacol.* **2005**, *202*, 199–211. [CrossRef]
20. Imam, M.U.; Zhang, S.; Ma, J.; Wang, H.; Wang, F. Antioxidants Mediate Both Iron Homeostasis and Oxidative Stress. *Nutrients* **2017**, *9*, 671. [CrossRef]
21. Hochman, M.A.; Seery, C.M.; Zarbin, M.A. Pathophysiology and Management of Subretinal Haemorrhage. *Surv. Ophthalmol.* **1997**, *42*, 195–213. [CrossRef]
22. Hassan, A.S.; Johnson, M.W.; Schneiderman, T.E.; Regillo, C.D.; Tornambe, P.E.; Poliner, L.S.; Blodi, B.A.; Elner, S.G. Management of Submacular Haemorrhage with Intravitreous Tissue Plasminogen Activator Injection and Pneumatic Displacement. *Ophthalmology* **1999**, *106*, 1900–1906; discussion 1906–1907. [CrossRef]
23. Balughatta, P.; Kadri, V.; Braganza, S.; Jayadev, C.; Mehta, R.A.; Nakhate, V.; Yadav, N.K.; Shetty, R. Pneumatic displacement of limited traumatic submacular haemorrhage without tissue plasminogen activator: A case series. *Retin. Cases Brief Rep.* **2019**, *13*, 34–38. [CrossRef]
24. Moher, D.; Liberati, A.; Tetzlaff, J.; Altman, D.G. Preferred Reporting Items for Systematic Reviews and Meta-Analyses: The PRISMA Statement. *Ann. Intern. Med.* **2009**, *151*, 264–269. [CrossRef]
25. Howick, J.; Glasziou, P.; Aronson, J.K. Evidence-Based Mechanistic Reasoning. *J. R. Soc. Med.* **2010**, *103*, 433–441. [CrossRef]
26. Guyatt, G.; Oxman, A.D.; Akl, E.A.; Kunz, R.; Vist, G.; Brozek, J.; Norris, S.; Falck-Ytter, Y.; Glasziou, P.; deBeer, H.; et al. GRADE Guidelines: 1. Introduction—GRADE Evidence Profiles and Summary of Findings Tables. *J. Clin. Epidemiol.* **2011**, *64*, 383–394. [CrossRef]
27. Mozaffarieh, M.; Heinzl, H.; Sacu, S.; Wedrich, A. In-Patient Management and Treatment Satisfaction after Intravitreous Plasminogen Activator Injection. *Graefes Arch. Clin. Exp. Ophthalmol.* **2006**, *244*, 1421–1428. [CrossRef]

28. Gopalakrishan, M.; Giridhar, A.; Bhat, S.; Saikumar, S.J.; Elias, A.; Sandhya, N. Pneumatic Displacement of Submacular Haemorrhage: Safety, Efficacy, and Patient Selection. *Retina* **2007**, *27*, 329–334. [CrossRef]
29. Iacono, P.; Parodi, M.B.; Introini, U.; La Spina, C.; Varano, M.; Bandello, F. Intravitreal Ranibizumab for Choroidal Neovascularization with Large Submacular Haemorrhage in Age-Related Macular Degeneration. *Retina* **2014**, *34*, 281–287. [CrossRef]
30. Wei, Y.; Zhang, Z.; Jiang, X.; Li, F.; Zhang, T.; Qiu, S.; Yang, Y.; Zhang, S. A surgical approach to large subretinal haemorrhage using pars plana vitrectomy and 360° retinotomy. *Retina* **2015**, *35*, 1631–1639. [CrossRef]
31. De Jong, J.H.; van Zeeburg, E.J.; Cereda, M.G.; van Velthoven, M.E.; Faridpooya, K.; Vermeer, K.A.; van Meurs, J.C. Intravitreal versus subretinal administration of recombinant tissue plasminogen activator combined with gas for acute submacular haemorrhages due to age-related macular degeneration: An Exploratory Prospective Study. *Retina* **2016**, *36*, 914–925. [CrossRef]
32. Kitagawa, Y.; Shimada, H.; Mori, R.; Tanaka, K.; Yuzawa, M. Intravitreal Tissue Plasminogen Activator, Ranibizumab, and Gas Injection for Submacular Haemorrhage in Polypoidal Choroidal Vasculopathy. *Ophthalmology* **2016**, *123*, 1278–1286. [CrossRef]
33. Kitagawa, Y.; Shimada, H.; Mori, R.; Tanaka, K.; Wakatsuki, Y.; Onoe, H.; Kaneko, H.; Machida, Y.; Nakashizuka, H. One-Year Outcome of Intravitreal Tissue Plasminogen Activator, Ranibizumab, and Gas Injections for Submacular Haemorrhage in Polypoidal Choroidal Vasculopathy. *J. Clin. Med.* **2022**, *11*, 2175. [CrossRef]
34. Mehta, A.; Steel, D.H.; Muldrew, A.; Peto, T.; Reeves, B.C.; Evans, R.; Chakravarthy, U.; IVAN Study Investigators. Associations and Outcomes of Patients with Submacular Haemorrhage Secondary to Age-Related Macular Degeneration in the IVAN Trial. *Am. J. Ophthalmol.* **2022**, *236*, 89–98. [CrossRef]
35. Hillenkamp, J.; Surguch, V.; Framme, C.; Gabel, V.P.; Sachs, H.G. Management of Submacular Haemorrhage with Intravitreal versus Subretinal Injection of Recombinant Tissue Plasminogen Activator. *Graefes Arch. Clin. Exp. Ophthalmol.* **2010**, *248*, 5–11. [CrossRef]
36. Guthoff, R.; Guthoff, T.; Meigen, T.; Goebel, W. Intravitreous Injection of Bevacizumab, Tissue Plasminogen Activator, and Gas in the Treatment of Submacular Haemorrhage in Age-Related Macular Degeneration. *Retina* **2011**, *31*, 36–40. [CrossRef]
37. Tsymanava, A.; Uhlig, C.E. Intravitreal Recombinant Tissue Plasminogen Activator without and with Additional Gas Injection in Patients with Submacular Haemorrhage Associated with Age-Related Macular Degeneration. *Acta Ophthalmol.* **2012**, *90*, 633–638. [CrossRef]
38. Mayer, W.J.; Hakim, I.; Haritoglou, C.; Gandorfer, A.; Ulbig, M.; Kampik, A.; Wolf, A. Efficacy and Safety of Recombinant Tissue Plasminogen Activator and Gas versus Bevacizumab and Gas for Subretinal Haemorrhage. *Acta Ophthalmol.* **2013**, *91*, 274–278. [CrossRef]
39. Rishi, E.; Gopal, L.; Rishi, P.; Sengupta, S.; Sharma, T. Submacular Haemorrhage: A Study amongst Indian Eyes. *Indian J Ophthalmol.* **2012**, *60*, 521–525. [CrossRef]
40. Kitahashi, M.; Baba, T.; Sakurai, M.; Yokouchi, H.; Kubota-Taniai, M.; Mitamura, Y.; Yamamoto, S. Pneumatic Displacement with Intravitreal Bevacizumab for Massive Submacular Haemorrhage Due to Polypoidal Choroidal Vasculopathy. *Clin. Ophthalmol.* **2014**, *8*, 485–492. [CrossRef]
41. Dimopoulos, S.; Leitritz, M.A.; Ziemssen, F.; Voykov, B.; Bartz-Schmidt, K.U.; Gelisken, F. Submacular Predominantly Hemorrhagic Choroidal Neovascularization: Resolution of Bleedings under Anti-VEGF Therapy. *Clin. Ophthalmol.* **2015**, *9*, 1537–1541. [CrossRef]
42. Shin, J.Y.; Lee, J.M.; Byeon, S.H. Anti-Vascular Endothelial Growth Factor with or without Pneumatic Displacement for Submacular Haemorrhage. *Am. J. Ophthalmol.* **2015**, *159*, 904–914.E1. [CrossRef]
43. Fassbender, J.M.; Sherman, M.P.; Barr, C.C.; Schaal, S. Tissue plasminogen activator for subfoveal haemorrhage due to age-related macular degeneration: Comparison of 3 Treatment Modalities. *Retina* **2016**, *36*, 1860–1865. [CrossRef]
44. Lin, T.C.; Hwang, D.K.; Lee, F.L.; Chen, S.J. Visual Prognosis of Massive Submacular Haemorrhage in Polypoidal Choroidal Vasculopathy with or without Combination Treatment. *J. Chin. Med. Assoc.* **2016**, *79*, 159–165. [CrossRef]
45. Bell, J.E.; Shulman, J.P.; Swan, R.J.; Teske, M.P.; Bernstein, P.S. Intravitreal Versus Subretinal Tissue Plasminogen Activator Injection for Submacular Haemorrhage. *Ophthalmic Surg. Lasers Imaging Retina* **2017**, *48*, 26–32. [CrossRef]
46. Jeong, S.; Park, D.G.; Sagong, M. Management of a Submacular Haemorrhage Secondary to Age-Related Macular Degeneration: A Comparison of Three Treatment Modalities. *J. Clin. Med.* **2020**, *9*, 3088. [CrossRef]
47. Maggio, E.; Peroglio Deiro, A.; Mete, M.; Sartore, M.; Polito, A.; Prigione, G.; Guerriero, M.; Pertile, G. Intravitreal Recombinant Tissue Plasminogen Activator and Sulphur Hexafluoride Gas for Submacular Haemorrhage Displacement in Age-Related Macular Degeneration: Looking behind the Blood. *Ophthalmologica* **2020**, *243*, 224–235. [CrossRef]
48. Kabakcı, A.K.; Erdoğan, B.; Atik, B.K.; Perente, İ. Outcomes of Surgical Treatment in Cases with Submacular Haemorrhage. *Retin.-Vitr. J. Retin.-Vitr.* **2021**, *30*, 2.
49. Kishikova, L.; Saad, A.A.A.; Vaideanu-Collins, D.; Isac, M.; Hamada, D.; El-Haig, W.M. Comparison between Different Techniques for Treatment of Submacular Haemorrhage Due to Age-Related Macular Degeneration. *Eur. J. Ophthalmol.* **2021**, *31*, 2621–2624. [CrossRef]
50. Matsuo, Y.; Haruta, M.; Ishibashi, Y.; Ishibashi, K.; Furushima, K.; Kato, N.; Murotani, K.; Yoshida, S. Visual Outcomes and Prognostic Factors of Large Submacular Haemorrhages Secondary to Polypoidal Choroidal Vasculopathy. *Clin. Ophthalmol.* **2021**, *15*, 3557–3562. [CrossRef]

51. Rickmann, A.; Paez, L.R.; Della Volpe Waizel, M.; Bisorca-Gassendorf, L.; Schulz, A.; Vandebroek, A.C.; Szurman, P.; Januschowski, K. Functional and Structural Outcome after Vitrectomy Combined with Subretinal Rt-PA Injection with or without Additional Intravitreal Bevacizumab Injection for Submacular Haemorrhages. *PLoS ONE* **2021**, *16*, E0250587. [CrossRef]
52. Sniatecki, J.J.; Ho-Yen, G.; Clarke, B.; Barbara, R.; Lash, S.; Papathomas, T.; Antonakis, S.; Gupta, B. Treatment of Submacular Haemorrhage with Tissue Plasminogen Activator and Pneumatic Displacement in Age-Related Macular Degeneration. *Eur. J. Ophthalmol.* **2021**, *31*, 643–648. [CrossRef]
53. Tranos, P.; Tsiropoulos, G.N.; Koronis, S.; Vakalis, A.; Asteriadis, S.; Stavrakas, P. Comparison of Subretinal versus Intravitreal Injection of Recombinant Tissue Plasminogen Activator with Gas for Submacular Haemorrhage Secondary to Wet Age-Related Macular Degeneration: Treatment Outcomes and Brief Literature Review. *Int. Ophthalmol.* **2021**, *41*, 4037–4046. [CrossRef]
54. Tiosano, A.; Gal-Or, O.; Fradkin, M.; Elul, R.; Dotan, A.; Hadayer, A.; Brody, J.; Ehrlich, R. Visual Acuity Outcome in Patients with Subretinal Haemorrhage—Office Procedure vs. Surgical Treatment. *Eur. J. Ophthalmol.* **2022**, *33*, 506–513. [CrossRef]
55. Confalonieri, F.; Stene-Johansen, I.; Lumi, X.; Petrovski, G. Intravitreal RT-PA Injection and Pneumatic Displacement for Submacular Retinal Haemorrhage: A Case Series. *Case Rep. Ophthalmol.* **2022**, *13*, 630–637. [CrossRef]
56. Ratanasukon, M.; Kittantong, A. Results of Intravitreal Tissue Plasminogen Activator and Expansile Gas Injection for Submacular Haemorrhage in Thais. *Eye* **2005**, *19*, 1328–1332. [CrossRef]
57. Singh, R.P.; Patel, C.; Sears, J.E. Management of Subretinal Macular Haemorrhage by Direct Administration of Tissue Plasminogen Activator. *Br. J. Ophthalmol.* **2006**, *90*, 429–431. [CrossRef]
58. Yang, P.-M.; Kuo, H.-K.; Kao, M.-L.; Chen, Y.-J.; Tsai, H.-H. Pneumatic Displacement of a Dense Submacular Haemorrhage with or without Tissue Plasminogen Activator. *Chang. Gung Med. J.* **2005**, *28*, 852–859.
59. Stifter, E.; Michels, S.; Prager, F.; Georgopoulos, M.; Polak, K.; Hirn, C.; Schmidt-Erfurth, U. Intravitreal Bevacizumab Therapy for Neovascular Age-Related Macular Degeneration with Large Submacular Haemorrhage. *Am. J. Ophthalmol.* **2007**, *144*, 886–892.e2. [CrossRef]
60. Arias, L.; Monés, J. Transconjunctival Sutureless Vitrectomy with Tissue Plasminogen Activator, Gas and Intravitreal Bevacizumab in the Management of Predominantly Hemorrhagic Age-Related Macular Degeneration. *Clin. Ophthalmol.* **2010**, *4*, 67–72.
61. Cakir, M.; Cekiç, O.; Yilmaz, O.F. Pneumatic Displacement of Acute Submacular Haemorrhage with and without the Use of Tissue Plasminogen Activator. *Eur. J. Ophthalmol.* **2010**, *20*, 565–571. [CrossRef]
62. Kung, Y.H.; Wu, T.T.; Hong, M.C.; Sheu, S.J. Intravitreal Tissue Plasminogen Activator and Pneumatic Displacement of Submacular Haemorrhage. *J. Ocul. Pharmacol Ther.* **2010**, *26*, 469–474. [CrossRef]
63. Sandhu, S.S.; Manvikar, S.; Steel, D.H. Displacement of Submacular Haemorrhage Associated with Age-Related Macular Degeneration Using Vitrectomy and Submacular RT-PA Injection Followed by Intravitreal Ranibizumab. *Clin. Ophthalmol.* **2010**, *4*, 637–642. [CrossRef]
64. Treumer, F.; Roider, J.; Hillenkamp, J. Long-Term Outcome of Subretinal Coapplication of Rt-PA and Bevacizumab Followed by Repeated Intravitreal Anti-VEGF Injections for Neovascular AMD with Submacular Haemorrhage. *Br. J. Ophthalmol.* **2012**, *96*, 708–713. [CrossRef]
65. Cho, H.J.; Koh, K.M.; Kim, H.S.; Lee, T.G.; Kim, C.G.; Kim, J.W. Anti-Vascular Endothelial Growth Factor Monotherapy in the Treatment of Submacular Haemorrhage Secondary to Polypoidal Choroidal Vasculopathy. *Am. J. Ophthalmol.* **2013**, *156*, 524–531.E1. [CrossRef]
66. Jain, S.; Kishore, K.; Sharma, Y.R. Intravitreal Anti-VEGF Monotherapy for Thick Submacular Haemorrhage of Less than 1 Week Duration Secondary to Neovascular Age-Related Macular Degeneration. *Indian J. Ophthalmol.* **2013**, *61*, 490–496. [CrossRef]
67. Moisseiev, E.; Ben Ami, T.; Barak, A. Vitrectomy and Subretinal Injection of Tissue Plasminogen Activator for Large Submacular Haemorrhage Secondary to AMD. *Eur. J. Ophthalmol.* **2014**, *24*, 925–931. [CrossRef]
68. Kim, H.S.; Cho, H.J.; Yoo, S.G.; Kim, J.H.; Han, J.I.; Lee, T.G.; Kim, J.W. Intravitreal Anti-Vascular Endothelial Growth Factor Monotherapy for Large Submacular Haemorrhage Secondary to Neovascular Age-Related Macular Degeneration. *Eye* **2015**, *29*, 1141–1151. [CrossRef]
69. Kimura, S.; Morizane, Y.; Hosokawa, M.; Shiode, Y.; Kawata, T.; Doi, S.; Matoba, R.; Hosogi, M.; Fujiwara, A.; Inoue, Y.; et al. Submacular Haemorrhage in Polypoidal Choroidal Vasculopathy Treated by Vitrectomy and Subretinal Tissue Plasminogen Activator. *Am. J. Ophthalmol.* **2015**, *159*, 683–689. [CrossRef]
70. González-López, J.J.; McGowan, G.; Chapman, E.; Yorston, D. Vitrectomy with Subretinal Tissue Plasminogen Activator and Ranibizumab for Submacular Haemorrhages Secondary to Age-Related Macular Degeneration: Retrospective Case Series of 45 Consecutive Cases. *Eye* **2016**, *30*, 929–935. [CrossRef]
71. Lee, J.P.; Park, J.S.; Kwon, O.W.; You, Y.S.; Kim, S.H. Management of Acute Submacular Haemorrhage with Intravitreal Injection of Tenecteplase, Anti-Vascular Endothelial Growth Factor and Gas. *Korean J. Ophthalmol.* **2016**, *30*, 192–197. [CrossRef]
72. Waizel, M.; Todorova, M.G.; Kazerounian, S.; Rickmann, A.; Blanke, B.R.; Szurman, P. Efficacy of Vitrectomy Combined with Subretinal Recombinant Tissue Plasminogen Activator for Subretinal versus Subpigment Epithelial versus Combined Haemorrhages. *Ophthalmologica* **2016**, *236*, 123–132. [CrossRef]
73. Gok, M.; Karabaş, V.L.; Aslan, M.S.; Kara, Ö.; Karaman, S.; Yenihayat, F. Tissue Plasminogen Activator-Assisted Vitrectomy for Submacular Haemorrhage Due to Age-Related Macular Degeneration. *Indian J. Ophthalmol.* **2017**, *65*, 482–487. [CrossRef]
74. Waizel, M.; Todorova, M.G.; Rickmann, A.; Blanke, B.R.; Szurman, P. Efficacy of Vitrectomy Combined with Subretinal Rt-PA Injection with Gas or Air Tamponade. *Klin. Monbl. Augenheilkd.* **2017**, *234*, 487–492. (In English) [CrossRef]

75. Bardak, H.; Bardak, Y.; Erçalık, Y.; Erdem, B.; Arslan, G.; Tımlıoglu, S. Sequential Tissue Plasminogen Activator, Pneumatic Displacement, and Anti-VEGF Treatment for Submacular Haemorrhage. *Eur. J. Ophthalmol.* **2018**, *28*, 306–310. [CrossRef]
76. Sharma, S.; Kumar, J.B.; Kim, J.E.; Thordsen, J.; Dayani, P.; Ober, M.; Mahmoud, T.H. Pneumatic Displacement of Submacular Haemorrhage with Subretinal Air and Tissue Plasminogen Activator: Initial United States Experience. *Ophthalmol. Retina* **2018**, *2*, 180–186. [CrossRef]
77. Karamitsos, A.; Papastavrou, V.; Ivanova, T.; Cottrell, D.; Stannard, K.; Karachrysafi, S.; Cheristanidis, S.; Ziakas, N.; Papamitsou, T.; Hillier, R. Management of Acute Submacular Haemorrhage Using Intravitreal Injection of Tissue Plasminogen Activator and Gas: A Case Series. *SAGE Open Med. Case Rep.* **2020**, *8*, 2050313X20970337. [CrossRef]
78. Lee, K.; Park, Y.G.; Park, Y.H. Visual prognosis after pneumatic displacement of submacular haemorrhage according to age-related macular degeneration subtypes. *Retina* **2020**, *40*, 2304–2311. [CrossRef]
79. Ali Said, Y.; Dewilde, E.; Stalmans, P. Visual Outcome after Vitrectomy with Subretinal RT-PA Injection to Treat Submacular Haemorrhage Secondary to Age-Related Macular Degeneration or Macroaneurysm. *J. Ophthalmol.* **2021**, *2021*, 3160963. [CrossRef]
80. Avcı, R.; Mavi Yıldız, A.; Çınar, E.; Yılmaz, S.; Küçükerdönmez, C.; Akalp, F.D.; Avcı, E. Subretinal Coapplication of Tissue Plasminogen Activator and Bevacizumab with Concurrent Pneumatic Displacement for Submacular Haemorrhages Secondary to Neovascular Age-Related Macular Degeneration. *Turk. J. Ophthalmol.* **2021**, *51*, 38–44. [CrossRef]
81. Iannetta, D.; De Maria, M.; Bolletta, E.; Mastrofilippo, V.; Moramarco, A.; Fontana, L. Subretinal Injection of Recombinant Tissue Plasminogen Activator and Gas Tamponade to Displace Acute Submacular Haemorrhages Secondary to Age-Related Macular Degeneration. *Clin. Ophthalmol.* **2021**, *15*, 3649–3659. [CrossRef]
82. Kawakami, S.; Wakabayashi, Y.; Umazume, K.; Usui, Y.; Muramatsu, D.; Agawa, T.; Yamamoto, K.; Goto, H. Long-Term Outcome of Eyes with Vitrectomy for Submacular and/or Vitreous Haemorrhage in Neovascular Age-Related Macular Degeneration. *J. Ophthalmol.* **2021**, *2021*, 2963822. [CrossRef]
83. Fukuda, Y.; Nakao, S.; Kohno, R.I.; Ishikawa, K.; Shimokawa, S.; Shiose, S.; Takeda, A.; Morizane, Y.; Sonoda, K.H. Postoperative Follow-up of Submacular Haemorrhage Displacement Treated with Vitrectomy and Subretinal Injection of Tissue Plasminogen Activator: Ultrawide-Field Fundus Autofluorescence Imaging in Gas-Filled Eyes. *Jpn. J. Ophthalmol.* **2022**, *66*, 264–270. [CrossRef]
84. Juncal, V.R.; Hanout, M.; Altomare, F.; Chow, D.R.; Giavedoni, L.R.; Muni, R.H.; Wong, D.T.; Berger, A.R. Surgical Management of Submacular Haemorrhage: Experience at an Academic Canadian Centre. *Can. J. Ophthalmol.* **2018**, *53*, 408–414. [CrossRef]
85. Olivier, S.; Chow, D.R.; Packo, K.H.; MacCumber, M.W.; Awh, C.C. Subretinal Recombinant Tissue Plasminogen Activator Injection and Pneumatic Displacement of Thick Submacular Haemorrhage in Age-Related Macular Degeneration. *Ophthalmology* **2004**, *111*, 1201–1208. [CrossRef]
86. Kadonosono, K.; Arakawa, A.; Yamane, S.; Inoue, M.; Yamakawa, T.; Uchio, E.; Yanagi, Y. Displacement of Submacular Haemorrhages in Age-Related Macular Degeneration with Subretinal Tissue Plasminogen Activator and Air. *Ophthalmology* **2015**, *122*, 123–128. [CrossRef]
87. Kim, J.H.; Chang, Y.S.; Lee, D.W.; Kim, C.G.; Kim, J.W. Quantification of Retinal Changes after Resolution of Submacular Haemorrhage Secondary to Polypoidal Choroidal Vasculopathy. *Jpn. J. Ophthalmol.* **2018**, *62*, 54–62. [CrossRef]
88. Caporossi, T.; Bacherini, D.; Governatori, L.; Oliverio, L.; Di Leo, L.; Tartaro, R.; Rizzo, S. Management of Submacular Massive Haemorrhage in Age-Related Macular Degeneration: Comparison between Subretinal Transplant of Human Amniotic Membrane and Subretinal Injection of Tissue Plasminogen Activator. *Acta Ophthalmol.* **2022**, *100*, E1143–E1152. [CrossRef]
89. Ura, S.; Miyata, M.; Ooto, S.; Yasuhara, S.; Tamura, H.; Ueda-Arakawa, N.; Muraoka, Y.; Miyake, M.; Takahashi, A.; Wakazono, T.; et al. Contrast-to-noise ratio is a useful predictor of early displacement of large submacular haemorrhage by intravitreal sf6 gas injection. *Retina* **2022**, *42*, 661–668. [CrossRef]
90. Thompson, J.T.; Sjaarda, R.N. Vitrectomy for the treatment of submacular haemorrhages from macular degeneration: A comparison of submacular haemorrhage/membrane removal and submacular tissue plasminogen activator–assisted pneumatic displacement. *Trans. Am. Ophthalmol. Soc.* **2005**, *103*, 98–107.
91. Ron, Y.; Ehrlich, R.; Axer-Siegel, R.; Rosenblatt, I.; Weinberger, D. Pneumatic Displacement of Submacular Haemorrhage Due to Age-Related Macular Degeneration. *Ophthalmologica* **2006**, *221*, 57–61. [CrossRef]
92. Meyer, C.H.; Scholl, H.P.; Eter, N.; Helb, H.-M.; Holz, F.G. Combined Treatment of Acute Subretinal Haemorrhages with Intravitreal Recombined Tissue Plasminogen Activator, Expansile Gas and Bevacizumab: A Retrospective Pilot Study. *Acta Ophthalmol.* **2008**, *86*, 490–494. [CrossRef]
93. Fang, I.-M.; Lin, Y.-C.; Yang, C.-H.; Yang, C.-M.; Chen, M.-S. Effects of Intravitreal Gas with or without Tissue Plasminogen Activator on Submacular Haemorrhage in Age-Related Macular Degeneration. *Eye* **2009**, *23*, 397–406. [CrossRef]
94. Fine, H.F.; Iranmanesh, R.; Del Priore, L.V.; Barile, G.R.; Chang, L.K.; Chang, S.; Schiff, W.M. Surgical Outcomes after Massive Subretinal Haemorrhage Secondary to Age-Related Macular Degeneration. *Retina* **2010**, *30*, 1588–1594. [CrossRef]
95. Mizutani, T.; Yasukawa, T.; Ito, Y.; Takase, A.; Hirano, Y.; Yoshida, M.; Ogura, Y. Pneumatic Displacement of Submacular Haemorrhage with or without Tissue Plasminogen Activator. *Graefes Arch. Clin. Exp. Ophthalmol.* **2011**, *249*, 1153–1157. [CrossRef]
96. Han, L.; Ma, Z.; Wang, C.; Dou, H.; Hu, Y.; Feng, X.; Xu, Y.; Yin, Z.; Wang, X. Autologous Transplantation of Simple Retinal Pigment Epithelium Sheet for Massive Submacular Haemorrhage Associated with Pigment Epithelium Detachment. *Investig. Ophthalmol. Vis. Sci.* **2013**, *54*, 4956–4963. [CrossRef]

97. Shienbaum, G.; Garcia Filho, C.A.; Flynn, H.W., Jr.; Nunes, F.; Smiddy, W.E.; Rosenfeld, P.J. Management of Submacular Haemorrhage Secondary to Neovascular Age-Related Macular Degeneration with Anti-Vascular Endothelial Growth Factor Monotherapy. *Am. J. Ophthalmol.* **2013**, *155*, 1009–1013. [CrossRef]
98. Chang, W.; Garg, S.J.; Maturi, R.; Hsu, J.; Sivalingam, A.; Gupta, S.A.; Regillo, C.D.; Ho, A.C. Management of Thick Submacular Haemorrhage with Subretinal Tissue Plasminogen Activator and Pneumatic Displacement for Age-Related Macular Degeneration. *Am. J. Ophthalmol.* **2014**, *157*, 1250–1257. [CrossRef]
99. Kimura, M.; Yasukawa, T.; Shibata, Y.; Kato, A.; Hirano, Y.; Uemura, A.; Yoshida, M.; Ogura, Y. Flattening of Retinal Pigment Epithelial Detachments after Pneumatic Displacement of Submacular Haemorrhages Secondary to Age-Related Macular Degeneration. *Graefes Arch. Clin. Exp. Ophthalmol.* **2018**, *256*, 1823–1829. [CrossRef]
100. Plemel, D.J.A.; Lapere, S.R.J.; Rudnisky, C.J.; Tennant, M.T.S. Vitrectomy with subretinal tissue plasminogen activator and gas tamponade for subfoveal haemorrhage: Prognostic Factors and Clinical Outcomes. *Retina* **2019**, *39*, 172–179. [CrossRef]
101. Helaiwa, K.; Paez, L.R.; Szurman, P.; Januschowski, K. Combined Administration of Preoperative Intravitreal and Intraoperative Subretinal Recombinant Tissue Plasminogen Activator in Acute Hemorrhagic Age-Related Macular Degeneration. *Cureus* **2020**, *12*, E7229. [CrossRef]
102. Wilkins, C.S.; Mehta, N.; Wu, C.Y.; Barash, A.; Deobhakta, A.A.; Rosen, R.B. Outcomes of Pars Plana Vitrectomy with Subretinal Tissue Plasminogen Activator Injection and Pneumatic Displacement of Fovea-Involving Submacular Haemorrhage. *BMJ Open Ophthalmol.* **2020**, *5*, E000394. [CrossRef]
103. Ueda-Arakawa, N.; Tsujikawa, A.; Yamashiro, K.; Ooto, S.; Tamura, H.; Yoshimura, N. Visual Prognosis of Eyes with Submacular Haemorrhage Associated with Exudative Age-Related Macular Degeneration. *Jpn. J. Ophthalmol.* **2012**, *56*, 589–598. [CrossRef]
104. Kim, J.H.; Kim, C.G.; Lee, D.W.; Yoo, S.J.; Lew, Y.J.; Cho, H.J.; Kim, J.Y.; Lee, S.H.; Kim, J.W. Intravitreal Aflibercept for Submacular Haemorrhage Secondary to Neovascular Age-Related Macular Degeneration and Polypoidal Choroidal Vasculopathy. *Graefes Arch. Clin. Exp. Ophthalmol.* **2020**, *258*, 107–116. [CrossRef]
105. Bae, K.; Cho, G.E.; Yoon, J.M.; Kang, S.W. Optical Coherence Tomographic Features and Prognosis of Pneumatic Displacement for Submacular Haemorrhage. *PLoS ONE* **2016**, *11*, E0168474. [CrossRef]

**Disclaimer/Publisher's Note:** The statements, opinions and data contained in all publications are solely those of the individual author(s) and contributor(s) and not of MDPI and/or the editor(s). MDPI and/or the editor(s) disclaim responsibility for any injury to people or property resulting from any ideas, methods, instructions or products referred to in the content.

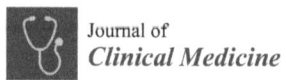 

*Article*

# Intraoperative Iridectomy in Femto-Laser Assisted Smaller-Incision New Generation Implantable Miniature Telescope

Rodolfo Mastropasqua [1], Matteo Gironi [1], Rossella D'Aloisio [1,*], Valentina Pastore [2], Giacomo Boscia [2], Luca Vecchiarino [1], Fabiana Perna [1,3], Katia Clemente [1], Ilaria Palladinetti [1], Michela Calandra [1], Marina Piepoli [2], Annamaria Porreca [4], Marta Di Nicola [4] and Francesco Boscia [2]

[1] Ophthalmology Clinic, Department of Medicine and Science of Ageing, University "G. d'Annunzio" of Chieti-Pescara, Via dei Vestini 31, 66100 Chieti, Italy; rodolfo.mastropasqua@gmail.com (R.M.); matteo.gironi@hotmail.it (M.G.); l.vecchiarino@unich.it (L.V.); fabiana975@hotmail.com (F.P.); katiaclem90@hotmail.it (K.C.); ilaria.palladinetti@libero.it (I.P.); michela.calandra1@gmail.com (M.C.)

[2] Eye Clinic, Department of Medical Science, Neuroscience and Sense Organs, University of Bari, 70121 Bari, Italy; valentinapastore@hotmail.it (V.P.); bosciagiacomo@gmail.com (G.B.); marinapiepoli93@gmail.com (M.P.); francescoboscia@hotmail.com (F.B.)

[3] International Agency of Prevention of Blindness, 00185 Rome, Italy

[4] Laboratory of Biostatistics, Department of Medical, Oral and Biotechnological Sciences, University "G. d'Annunzio" of Chieti-Pescara, Via dei Vestini 31, 66100 Chieti, Italy; annamaria.porreca@unich.it (A.P.); marta.dinicola@unich.it (M.D.N.)

* Correspondence: ross.daloisio@gmail.com; Tel.: +39-0871358410; Fax: +39-087135794

**Abstract:** Background: In this study, we aimed to report the short-term (6 months) effects on visual functionality and safety of femto-laser assisted smaller-incision new-generation implantable miniature telescope (SING-IMT™) implanting, particularly related to postsurgical intraocular pressure increase, in patients suffering from end-stage age-related macular degeneration (AMD) and cataract. This device, designed for monocular use, aims to minimise the impact of the central scotoma by projecting the images onto a larger area of the photoreceptors surrounding the macula. Methods: In this prospective multicentric observational case series study, 6 eyes of 6 patients who underwent SING-IMT™ implantations were enrolled. At baseline and 6 months follow-up, best corrected distance visual acuity (BCDV) and best corrected near visual acuity (BCNVA), intraocular pressure (IOP), anterior chamber depth, endothelial cells count were assessed. In addition, IOP was also measured at 7, 15, 30, 45 days, and at 3 months follow-up. Finally, the incidence of complications was evaluated. Results: At final follow-up, in the study eyes, mean BCDVA improved by +10.0 letters (6.25; 13.8) letters and mean BCNVA improved by −0.30 logMAR (−0.55; −0.20). At postoperative month 6, we reported a mean IOP decrease of 4.50 mmHg (−5.75; −0.25). Interestingly, 83.3% of patients had an increased IOP value in at least one of the first two postoperative follow-ups (7 days and 15 days). In patients in whom intraoperative mechanical iridotomy was not performed, it was necessary to perform a postoperative YAG laser iridotomy to improve IOP management. Compared to the baseline, ECD loss at 6 months follow-up was 12.6%. Conclusions: The SING IMT™ device was found to be effective in the distance and near vision improvement, without serious postoperative complications. We recommend intraoperative mechanical iridectomy in order to easily manage post-operative IOP and to avoid sudden IOP rise with its possible consequences. These good results can be a hope to partially improve the quality of life of patients suffering from severe end stage macular atrophy.

**Keywords:** small-incision new-generation implantable miniature telescope; age-related macular degeneration; maculopathy; geographic atrophy; visual prosthesis; visual impairment; implantable ophthalmic micro telescope; SING IMT; iridectomy

## 1. Introduction

Age-related macular degeneration (AMD) is still a leading cause of central vision loss in developed countries [1]. As one of the main reasons for legal blindness in Western countries, late AMD has a remarkable impact on public health [2,3], affecting 10–13% of over 65 year-old people and with an estimated prevalence of 13.1% and 0.1–0.3% after the age of 85 in European Caucasian and in Asiatic population respectively [4–6].

Ageing has a key role as a risk factor for dry-AMD, thus explaining the geographic distribution of disease prevalence [7].

Nowadays, no medical treatment has proven its efficacy for end-stage AMD, which dramatically impacts daily activities and quality of life [8,9].

Extraocular low vision aids have been used for many years in visual rehabilitation settings to enlarge the retinal image of individuals with low vision, including hand/stand magnifiers, handheld telescopes, contact lenses and other tools. However, they showed several limitations in daily life application [10].

Different intraocular implants have been developed as alternative devices for improving quality of life and visual acuity (VA) in AMD as better described in the Supplementary Materials [11–16]. The IMT™ works projecting the images onto a larger area of the photoreceptors surrounding the macula.

Based on the positive results of these devices, Samsara SING IMT™ has recently introduced a new IMT™ model, the Smaller-Incision New Generation Implantable Miniature Telescope (SING-IMT™). SING-IMT™ is an in the capsular bag implantable Galilean telescope after lens extraction, providing 2.7× magnification of central VF. It has an ultra-precision wide-angle glass micro-optics mounted on a silicon carrying device, which should be implanted in the capsular bag after removing the natural lenses through a 6.5–7.5 mm clear cut or limbal incision tunnel to extend through the pupil and acquire vertical positioning. It is provided by a preloaded delivery system and a new foldable haptic design to enhance stability and centration.

Recently a large retrospective case series study was published to describe the safety and efficacy outcomes at 3 months follow-up of the SING IMT™ prosthesis [17].

The purpose of this study was to report the short-term effects on visual functionality and safety, at 6 months follow-up, of femto-laser assisted SING-IMT™ implanting in patients suffering from end-stage AMD and cataract.

## 2. Materials and Methods

This prospective multicentric observational case series study was conducted at the Ophthalmology Clinic, University of Chieti-Pescara, Italy and the Ophthalmology Clinic, University of Bari, Italy. This work was approved by the Institutional Review Board, following the principles of the Declaration of Helsinki. The informed consent form was obtained from all patients.

The cases (n = 6) selection was accomplished in May 2022, and patients underwent surgery implantation between June 2022 and March 2023. Inclusion criteria for the enrollment were irreversible late-stage AMD, resulting from dry-type AMD or wet AMD that has been considered stable for at least 6 months, best corrected distance visual acuity (BCDVA) from 20/80 to 20/800 bilaterally, an expectation five-letter improvement using an external telescope, age of 55 years or older with a visual cataract, anterior chamber depth of ≥2.5 mm and axial length > 21 mm. In addition, good peripheral vision in the eye, not receiving an implant, was required. Exclusion criteria for the study were a history of other retinal or retinal vascular diseases, myopia > 6.0 D or hyperopia > 4.0 D in the planned operative eye, unilateral involvement of macular degeneration, uncontrolled glaucoma or IOP > 22 mmHg, steroid-responsive rise in IOP, endothelial cell density (ECD) ≤ 1600 cells/mm², cornea stromal or endothelial dystrophies, including guttae, poor compliance during the preoperative rehabilitation process.

Patients who met the inclusion criteria received additional pre-operative screening by undergoing simulation of the post-operative expected field of view and scotoma reduction effect on visual acuity tested with an external telescope simulator (ETS). Fellow eye is occluded during the test, and it is requested at least a 5 letter improvement in the selected eye, to meet the criteria for implantation.

*2.1. Preoperative Evaluation*

Patients included in the study underwent a complete ophthalmic examination for both eyes, including BCDVA and best corrected near visual acuity (BCNVA), intraocular pressure, axial length, anterior chamber depth, endothelial cells count, corneal thickness, slit-lamp biomicroscopy, fundoscopy, optical coherence tomography biometry, anterior-segment optical coherence tomography (AS-OCT), corneal topography, spectral domain-optical coherence tomography (SD-OCT) and optical coherence tomography angiography OCTA, along with complete medical history. BCVA was measured by the Early Treatment of Diabetic Retinopathy Study (ETDRS) chart from 2 m. Near vision acuity was evaluated using the ETDRS near chart for 40 cm distance. Goldmann applanation tonometer was used for Intraocular pressure (IOP) measurement. Endothelial cells count was obtained with CEM-530 specular microscope (Nidek Co., Ltd., Gamagori, Japan) IOL Master 700 (Carl Zeiss Meditec AG, Jena, Germany) was used for the biometry, axial length and anterior chamber depth. AS-OCT and corneal topography were realized using MS-39 device (CSO, Phoenix software, v.4.1.1.5, Italy) OCT and OCTA examinations were performed using Spectralis® HRA+ OCT (Heidelberg Engineering, Heidelberg, Germany).

*2.2. Surgical Technique*

Topical mydriatic agents were preoperatively administered in order to obtain iris dilation (>5.70 mm). All patients included in the study underwent femtosecond laser-assisted cataract surgery (FLACS) with LenSx®Laser System (Alcon, Fort Worth, TX, USA), for anterior capsulotomy, but assisted corneal incision and nuclear fragmentation was not performed. FLACS allows improved precision during corneal incisions and anterior capsulotomy (>5.5 mm diameter). A conjunctival peritomy was performed at the 12 o'clock position, and a 2.75 mm triplanar corneal incision was subsequently created in the upper quadrant. Standard cataract surgery procedure was completed using Alcon Costellation System (Alcon, Fort Worth, TX, USA). After phacoemulsification, the corneal incision was enlarged to 7.5 mm and a cohesive ophthalmic viscosurgical device (OVD) was injected in the anterior chamber (AC) in order to maintain the AC depth stable. Thereafter, we performed the in-the-bag SING-IMT™ implantation using preloaded injector. The parameters of the device are 4.4 mm long, 3.6 mm in diameter and an overall haptic-to-haptic diameter of 10.8 mm. Intraoperative peripheral surgical iridectomy was realized in 3 patients (50%), and no iridectomy was performed in the 3 remaining patients intraoperatively. 10/0 Nylon interrupted sutures were placed to close the corneal incision. Cefuroxime was injected into the anterior chamber. Antibiotic, steroid and cycloplegic eye drops were prescribed to be administered post-operatively. Antibiotic and steroid eye drops were applied for around 1 month postoperatively.

*2.3. Postoperative Evaluation*

Patients underwent complete ophthalmologic examination, including slit-lamp biomicroscopy, fundoscopy and intraocular pressure, at 7, 15, 30, 45 days, and at 3 months. Additional evaluations were performed when necessary. At 6 months all parameters were recorded, by an extensive ophthalmologic examination, as described in the preoperative evaluation. Corneal sutures were removed at the discretion of the examiner. Eventually significant adverse events were registered.

*2.4. Statistical Analysis*

All analyses were performed with the open-source statistical R environment (version 3.4.3, the R Foundation for Statistical Computing, Vienna, Austria). Because the study was not powered to allow for inferential statistical comparisons within groups, the focus of the analysis was to identify possible trends across them by summary descriptive statistics.

## 3. Results

A total of 6 eyes of 6 patients (1 man and 5 women) with mean age of 80 (75.0; 83.5) years were included in the study. The demographics and clinical characteristics of patients are reported in Table 1.

**Table 1.** Baseline demographics and clinical characteristics of cases.

| Variables | |
|---|---|
| Patients, n | 6 |
| Age, median years (q1; q3) | 80.0 (75.0; 83.5) |
| Male/Female, n | 1/5 |
| Right eye/Left eye, n | 2/4 |
| Duration of AMD, median yrs (q1; q3) | 4.75 (2.62; 8.00) |

The preoperative mean duration of AMD in the patients was 4.75 (2.62; 8.00) years, and 3 subjects were injected with intravitreal Anti-VEGF at least once.

### 3.1. Functional Parameter: Best-Corrected Visual Acuity for Distance and Near

At baseline, the study eye mean BCDVA was 20.00 letters (20.00; 20.00), which corresponds to 1.00 logMAR (1.00; 1.00), while the fellow eyes had a mean BCDVA of 1.30 logMAR (1.09; 1.30). At six months postoperative follow-up mean BCDVA increased, in median, to 30.00 letters (30.00; 33.80) with an improvement of 10.00 letters (6.25; 13.80). In detail, we observed that 5 patients gained at least 1 line on ETDRS chart, 4 patients gained 2 lines or more, 2 patients gained 3 lines or more and 1 patient gained 6 lines, while only one patient had a BCDVA reduction (5 letters) at 6 months follow-up. However, this patient had a worsening of senile dementia in the post-operative period (Figure 1).

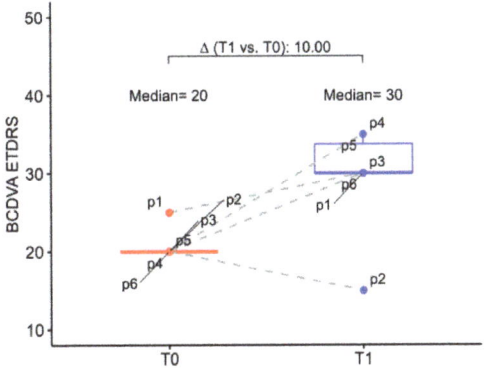

**Figure 1.** Box–whisker graphs of best corrected distance visual acuity in the patients at evaluation time points (T0) baseline and at 6 months (T1). Box–whisker plots show 25th and 75th percentile range (box) with 95% confidence interval (whiskers) and median values (transverse lines in box). Δ = absolute differences.

The baseline mean BCNVA in the study eye was 0.90 logMAR (0.83; 1.20), while the mean BCNVA in the fellow eye was 1.05 logMAR (1.00; 1.25). At six months postoperative follow-up BCNVA had a mean improvement of −0.30 logMAR (−0.55; −0.20) in the study eye. Overall, all patients have experienced an improvement of the BCNVA (Figure 2).

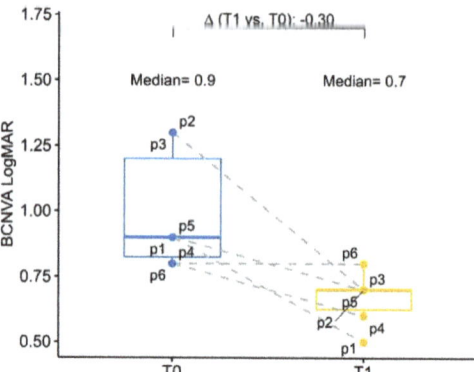

**Figure 2.** Box–whisker graphs of best corrected near visual acuity in the patients at evaluation time points (T0) baseline and at 6 months (T1). Box–whisker plots show 25th and 75th percentile range (box) with 95% confidence interval (whiskers) and median values (transverse lines in box). Δ = absolute differences.

*3.2. Anatomical Parameter and Endothelial Cell Density*

The baseline mean AC depth was 2.69 mm (2.66; 3.19) and 3.19 (3.08; 3.28) in the study eye and in the fellow eye, respectively. Anatomical changes after surgery were investigated both in terms of corneal endothelium-telescope distance (EC-IMTd) and in terms of corneal endothelium-interpupillary iris plane distance (EC-IPd). At 6 months follow-up mean EC-IMTd was 2.52 mm (2.23; 3.01), corresponding to a reduction of 0.64 mm (−1.25; −0.41) of AC depth. Six months after surgery mean EC-IPd was 3.40 (3.20; 3.56), representing an increase in depth of 0.68 mm (−0.31; 0.86). In five operated eyes EC-IPd > EC-IMTd, for only one eye EC-IMTd was slightly greater than EC-IPd, meaning that in this case, the telescopic optic was behind the iris plane (Figures 3 and 4).

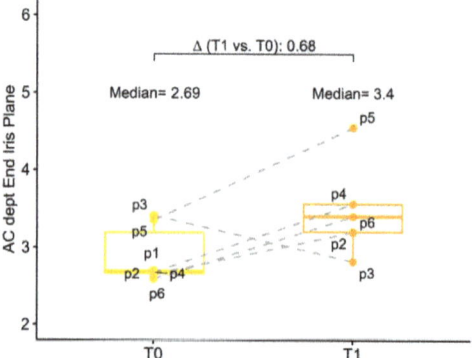

**Figure 3.** Box–whisker graphs of AC depth at evaluation time points (T0) baseline which correspond to the corneal endothelium-anterior capsule of the crystalline lens distance and at 6 months (T1) in terms of corneal endothelium-interpupillary iris plane distance in the patients. Box–whisker plots show 25th and 75th percentile range (box) with 95% confidence interval (whiskers) and median values (transverse lines in box). Δ = absolute differences.

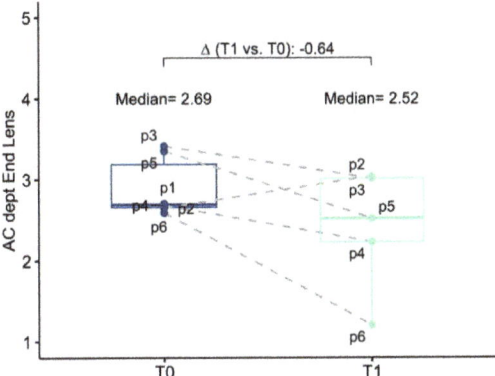

**Figure 4.** Box–whisker graphs of AC depth at evaluation time points (T0) baseline which correspond to the corneal endothelium-anterior capsule of the crystalline lens distance and at 6 months (T1) in terms of corneal endothelium–telescope distance in the patients. Box–whisker plots show 25th and 75th percentile range (box) with 95% confidence interval (whiskers) and median values (transverse lines in box). Δ = absolute differences.

No differences in post-operative functional or safety outcomes were observed in the patient with the telescopic optic behind the iris plane in comparison to the other study eyes. At the follow-up, fellow eye AC depth was unchanged from baseline.

At baseline, the mean ECD was 2488 (2248; 2874) and 2542 (2266; 2912) in the study eye and in the fellow eye, respectively. At 6 months follow-up mean study eye ECD was 2174 (1946; 2536). Compared to the baseline, ECD loss at 6 months follow-up was 12.6% (Figure 5).

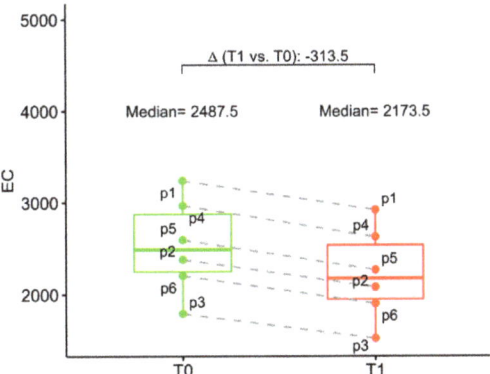

**Figure 5.** Box–whisker graphs of endothelial cell density in the patients at evaluation time points (T0) baseline and at 6 months (T1). Box–whisker plots show 25th and 75th percentile range (box) with 95% confidence interval (whiskers) and median values (transverse lines in box). Δ = absolute differences.

### 3.3. Intraocular Pressure

The baseline mean IOP was in the study eye 17.5 mmHg (16.2; 18.0). At 6 months follow-up mean IOP was 12.5 mmHg (12.0; 14.5), which represents a decrease of 4.50 mmHg (−5.75; −0.25).

As shown in Figure 6, we found an increased IOP in 5 patients at 7-day follow-up, which tends to decrease in four of them during subsequent follow-ups. One patient (P5) underwent YAG laser iridotomy treatment 8 days after surgery due to a sudden increase in blood pressure. One patient (P6) showed a trend of increasing IOP at the 15 day follow up and underwent YAG laser iridotomy treatment the same day. Thirty and 45 days postoperatively all patients reported a IOP lower than or equal to the preoperative one. At 3- and 6-month follow-ups, only one patient (P6) has higher IOP than in preoperative time (>21 mmHg) (Figure 6).

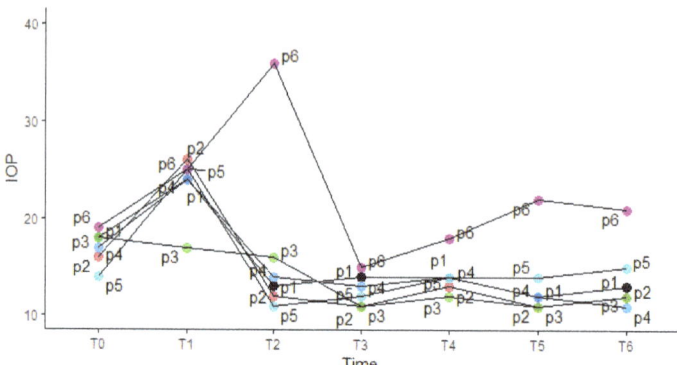

**Figure 6.** IOP trends at different times for each study eye. T0 = baseline; T1 = 7 days postoperative; T2 = 15 days postoperative; T3 = 30 days postoperative; T4 = 45 days postoperative; T5 = 3 months postoperative; T6 = 6 months postoperative.

Another patient (P4) underwent YAG laser iridotomy treatment 59 days after surgery due to an abrupt spike in IOP. Finally, all 3 patients (P4, P5, P6) who did not undergo intraoperative mechanical iridectomy required postoperative YAG laser iridotomy treatment for IOP management. Furthermore, 2 patients (P3 and P4) required post-operative prolonged topical glaucoma therapy, one of which (P4) for 3 months, while the other (P6) at the 6-month follow-up was still on therapy.

*3.4. Safety Outcomes*

No intraoperative complications have been reported. In post-operative time, common reported adverse events were corneal edema, which occurred in 2 patients, but persisted beyond 1 month after surgery in only one (P6), despite topical steroid therapy. One patient (P3) reported postoperative diplopia. As already mentioned, 3 patients required YAG laser iridotomy treatment for postoperative IOP management and 2 of them underwent prolonged topical glaucoma therapy. Finally, one patient (P6) was scheduled for surgical removal of the IMT™, due to poor IOP control consequent to the formation of irido-device synechiae for 360°.

## 4. Discussion

In this prospective multicentric case series, we evaluated functional and anatomical outcomes after SING IMT™ implantation in 6 patients. To the best of our knowledge, it is the first mid-term case series showing data after 6-month follow-up of SING IMT™ device implantation using FLACS surgery.

The largest analysis on the results of Galilean implantable miniature telescope for the treatment of dry AMD was conducted by the pilot study IMT-002, with an end-point at 24 months, and its subsequent extension to 60 months, study IMT-002-LT [12,14]. The authors reported a mean BCDVA improvement of 3.2 lines at 24 months and 2.4 lines at 60 months with first-generation IMT. Similarly, in our experience we found an average increase of 10.0 ETDRS letters (6.25; 13.8) at 6 months after surgery, corresponding to an improvement of 2 lines, but using new-generation IMT (SING-IMT™). On the other hand, if we do not consider the patient who showed post-operative dementia, who is the only one with vision worsening after surgery, the average BCDVA increase in our study population was 14 letters, which corresponded approximately to 3 lines. The age-stratified 12-month results of IMT-002 study highlighted as 79.8% of 75 years-old or elderly patients gained ≥2 lines. Considering the mean age of our study population, which was 80.0 (75.0; 83.5) years old, our findings revealed a BCDVA gain of at least 2 ETDRS lines in 66.7% of patients, which is 80% of patients, if we exclude from the analysis the one affected by dementia. A short-term retrospective case series on SING-IMT™ implants in 24 eyes was recently performed [17]. At three-months end-point follow-up, it reported a BCDVA improvements of ≥ 2 lines in the 70.83% of patients, which is comparable with our results. Despite this, it reported ≥ 3 lines gain in 58.33% of the implanted eye, while in our experience, only 2 patients out of 6 improved ≥ 3 lines on BCDVA. A possible explanation could be the elderly age range of our population (74–86), in fact, the 2 patients who gained 3 lines were respectively 74 and 78 years old, while only 1 of the 3 subjects aged over 80 increased the BCDVA by at least 10 letters.

Of note, duration of AMD seems to be a determining factor for the BCDVA improvement because none of the patients affected by the maculopathy for more than 5 years gained 3 letters.

All the patients of our study reported an improvement in BCNVA in the study eye at 6 months follow-up. Mean BCNVA improvements is −0.30 logMAR, corresponding to 3 lines ETDRS improvement for near vision. This visual improvement was comparable to that described in IMT-002 study showing 3.18 lines gained at 12 months and to that showed in Savastano's work reporting 3 month-results [12,13].

We aimed at investigating safety outcomes, as well. In literature the most common reported AE were inflammatory deposits on the device [12–15,18]. Differently, we did not find any inflammatory or pigmented deposits on the lens in our study population. Another frequent complication described in previous studies was corneal edema. IMT-002 study revealed a cumulative incidence of corneal edema of 7% within 30 days after implantation [14]. The incidence of corneal edema in our study was 33.3% (2/6), comparable with 29.2% rate of postoperative corneal edema reported by Toro et al. in their work on SING-IMT™ [18]. Elderly age range of our sample is a possible explanation for the higher rate of edema, also considering that in previous studies on first-generation IMT the rate of corneal edema increased with age of patients (7.1% in >75YO versus 4.3% in <75YO) within 30 days. The most common ocular complication highlighted from our findings was the post-operative IOP raise. First generation IMT™ safety evaluation revealed a cumulative incidence of treatment-needed IOP increasing of 28% within 7 days, while studies on SING-IMT™ reported a rate of 4.2% [14,18]. In our study cohort, 3 patients required post-operative IOP treatments, and two of them for at least 3 months consecutively. All the 3 eyes who experienced treatment needed IOP increasing had not undergone mechanical iridectomy during the surgery. Furthermore, we observed post-operative sudden rise of IOP, at different times, in all the 3 patients without intra-operative iridectomy, who required YAG laser iridotomy. In literature, post-operative iridotomy treatment was not reported to be needed to manage the abrupt rise of IOP, apart from one case in Savastano's work [13]. Comparing the IOP trends of patients underwent intraoperative iridectomy with others, we strongly suggest performing mechanical iridectomy during the surgery.

The mean loss of ECD rate with IMT™ was previously reported as 20% at 3 months, 13% to 25% at 1 year, and 29% at 2 years [14,15]. Previous study on SING-IMT™ reported a mean ECD decrease of 10.4% at 3 months [18]. We found a mean ECD loss of 12.6% at 6 months in the study eyes, similar to Toro et al. [18] findings. The main advantage of SING IMT™, if compared with the first generations IMT™, is the new device design and technique, allowing small corneal wound, the preloaded device, as well as the shorter surgery time. Further advantages expected from the use of FLACS could not be evaluated because we did not use assisted nuclear fragmentation and it is clearly known that the reduction of postoperative ECD loss is mainly due to a reduced cumulative dissipated energy during laser-assisted phacoemulsification [19]. However, the possibility of setting pre-operatively some anatomical parameters (e.g., the diameter of the capsulorhexis) increases surgical repeatability, predictability, shape accuration and strength of capsulorhexis, as well as reducing the risk of complications, compared to the manual procedure [20]. Moreover, FLACS was related to a lower overall variability of anterior chamber depth compared to conventional cataract surgery, with less postoperative IOL axial movements compared to the conventional tecnique [20,21].

The rate of IMT™ explantation is 5.8% (12/206) on 24-month follow-up [15]. In our study, only one patient was referred for SING-IMT™ explantation after 6-month follow-up. Age stratification identified elderly age as a possible predisposing factor to explantation, indeed 10 out of 12 patients who underwent this procedure were in the over 75 year old group [15]. Despite this, only 2 patients underwent explantation because of dissatisfaction.

## 5. Conclusions

The SING IMT™ device was effective in improving distance and near vision, without serious postoperative complications. These good results can be a hope to partially improve the quality of life of patients suffering from severe end stage macular atrophy. Despite this, a careful preoperative selection of patients is essential for maximizing the potential of the device, particularly considering the age and the duration of the disease. Further studies are needed to validate the long-term safety profile of the SING IMT™. We recommend intraoperative mechanical iridectomy in order to easily manage post-operative IOP and to avoid sudden IOP rise with its possible consequences. FLACS assistance during the surgery seems to be non-influential on the final outcomes. The limited size of the study cohort and the duration of the follow-up are the main limitations of this case series. However, it is a good starting point to better observe long-term functional results in such chronic and irreversible dry end-stage AMD conditions. Undoubtedly, a wider sample and a longer follow up could further strengthen our preliminary data.

**Supplementary Materials:** The following supporting information can be downloaded at: https://www.mdpi.com/article/10.3390/jcm13010076/s1.

**Author Contributions:** Validation, R.M., F.B.; formal analysis, M.D.N. and A.P.; investigation, V.P., G.B., L.V. and M.P.; data curation, F.P., K.C., I.P. and M.C.; writing—original draft preparation, M.G. and R.D.; writing—review and editing, R.M. and F.B. All authors have read and agreed to the published version of the manuscript.

**Funding:** This research received no external funding.

**Institutional Review Board Statement:** The work was approved by our Institutional Review Board.

**Informed Consent Statement:** Informed consent was obtained from all subjects involved in the study.

**Data Availability Statement:** All data will be available on request to the corresponding author.

**Conflicts of Interest:** The authors declare no conflict of interest.

## References

1. MitMitchell, P.; Liew, G.; Gopinath, B.; Wong, T.Y. Age-related macular degeneration. *Lancet* **2018**, *392*, 1147–1159. [CrossRef] [PubMed]
2. Guymer, R.H.; Campbell, T.G. Age-related macular degeneration. *Lancet* **2023**, *401*, 1459–1472. [CrossRef] [PubMed]
3. Khanani, A.M.; Thomas, M.J.; Aziz, A.A.; Weng, C.Y.; Danzig, C.J.; Yiu, G.; Kiss, S.; Waheed, N.K.; Kaiser, P.K. Review of gene therapies for age-related macular degeneration. *Eye* **2022**, *36*, 303–311. [CrossRef] [PubMed]
4. Schmidt-Erfurth, U.; Chong, V.; Loewenstein, A.; Larsen, M.; Souied, E.; Schlingemann, R.; Eldem, B.; Monés, J.; Richard, G.; Bandello, F. European Society of Retina Specialists. Guidelines for the management of neovascular age-related macular degeneration by the European Society of Retina Specialists (EURETINA). *Br. J. Ophthalmol.* **2014**, *98*, 1144–1167. [CrossRef] [PubMed]
5. Smith, W.; Assink, J.; Klein, R.; Mitchell, P.; Klaver, C.C.; Klein, B.E.; Hofman, A.; Jensen, S.; Wang, J.J.; de Jong, P.T. Risk factors for age- related macular degeneration: Pooled findings from three continents. *Ophthalmology* **2001**, *108*, 697–704. [CrossRef] [PubMed]

6. Wong, W.L.; Su, X.; Li, X.; Cheung, C.M.G.; Klein, R.; Cheng, C.Y.; Wong, T.Y. Global prevalence of age-related macular degeneration and disease burden projection for 2020 and 2040: A systematic review and meta-analysis. *Lancet Glob. Health* **2014**, *2*, e106–e116. [CrossRef] [PubMed]
7. United Nations Population Division. *World Population Prospects: The 2010 Revision Population Database*; United Nations Population Division: New York, NY, USA, 2010.
8. Macnamara, A.; Coussens, S.; Chen, C.; Schinazi, V.R.; Loetscher, T. The psychological impact of instrumental activities of daily living on people with simulated age-related macular degeneration. *BJPsych Open* **2022**, *8*, e152. [CrossRef] [PubMed]
9. Casten, R.J.; Rovner, B.W.; Tasman, W. Age-related macular degeneration and depression: A review of recent research. *Curr. Opin. Ophthalmol.* **2004**, *15*, 181–183. [CrossRef] [PubMed]
10. Singer, M.A.; Amir, N.; Herro, A.; Porbandarwalla, S.S.; Pollard, J. Improving quality of life in patients with end-stage age-related macular degeneration: Focus on miniature ocular implants. *Clin. Ophthalmol.* **2012**, *6*, 33–399. [CrossRef] [PubMed]
11. Lipshitz, I.; Sheah, A.; Loewenstein, A. The Implantable Miniaturized Telescope for patients with age-related macular degeneration: Design and surgical technique. *Oper. Tech. Cataract. Refract. Surg.* **2000**, *3*, 53–58.
12. Hudson, H.L.; Lane, S.S.; Heier, J.S.; Stulting, R.D.; Singerman, L.; Lichter, P.R.; Sternberg, P.; Chang, D.F.; IMT-002 Study Group. Implantable miniature telescope for the treatment of visual acuity loss resulting from end-stage age-related macular degeneration: 1-year results. *Ophthalmology* **2006**, *113*, 1987–2001. [CrossRef] [PubMed]
13. Savastano, A.; Ferrara, S.; Sasso, P.; Savastano, M.C.; Crincoli, E.; Caporossi, T.; De Vico, U.; Vidal Aroca, F.; Francione, G.; Sammarco, L.; et al. Smaller-Incision new-generation implantable miniature telescope: Three-months follow-up study. *Eur. J. Ophthalmol.* **2023**, 11206721231212545. [CrossRef] [PubMed]
14. Hudson, H.L.; Stulting, R.D.; Heier, J.S.; Lane, S.S.; Chang, D.F.; Singerman, L.J.; Bradford, C.A.; Leonard, R.E.; IMT002 Study Group. Implantable telescope for end-stage age-related macular degeneration: Long-term visual acuity and safety outcomes. *Am. J. Ophthalmol.* **2008**, *146*, 664–673.e1. [CrossRef] [PubMed]
15. Boyer, D.; Freund, K.B.; Regillo, C.; Levy, M.H.; Garg, S. Longterm (60-month) results for the implantable miniature telescope: Efficacy and safety outcomes stratified by age in patients with end-stage age-related macular degeneration. *Clin. Ophthalmol.* **2015**, *9*, 1099–1107. [CrossRef] [PubMed]
16. Grzybowski, A.; Wang, J.; Mao, F.; Wang, D.; Wang, N. Intraocular vision-improving devices in age-related macular degeneration. *Ann. Transl. Med.* **2020**, *8*, 1549. [CrossRef] [PubMed]
17. Dunbar, H.M.P.; Dhawahir-Scala, F.E. A Discussion of Commercially Available Intra-ocular Telescopic Implants for Patients with Age-Related Macular Degeneration. *Ophthalmol. Ther.* **2018**, *7*, 33–48. [CrossRef] [PubMed]
18. Toro, M.D.; Vidal-Aroca, F.; Montemagni, M.; Xompero, C.; Fioretto, G.; Costagliola, C. Three-Month Safety and Efficacy Outcomes for the Smaller-Incision New-Generation Implantable Miniature Telescope (SING IMT™). *J. Clin. Med.* **2023**, *12*, 518. [CrossRef] [PubMed]
19. Medhi, S.; Senthil Prasad, R.; Pai, A.; Muthukrishnan, G.R.; Mariammal, A.; Chitradevi, R.; Shekhar, M. Clinical outcomes of femtosecond laser-assisted cataract surgery versus conventional phacoemulsification: A retrospective study in a tertiary eye care center in South India. *Indian J. Ophthalmol.* **2022**, *70*, 4300–4305. [CrossRef] [PubMed]
20. Agarwal, K.; Hatch, K. Femtosecond Laser Assisted Cataract Surgery: A Review. *Semin. Ophthalmol.* **2021**, *36*, 618–627. [CrossRef] [PubMed]
21. Toto, L.; Mastropasqua, R.; Mattei, P.A.; Agnifili, L.; Mastropasqua, A.; Falconio, G.; Di Nicola, M.; Mastropasqua, L. Postoperative IOL Axial Movements and Refractive Changes After Femtosecond Laser-assisted Cataract Surgery Versus Conventional Phacoemulsification. *J. Refract. Surg.* **2015**, *31*, 524–530. [CrossRef] [PubMed]

**Disclaimer/Publisher's Note:** The statements, opinions and data contained in all publications are solely those of the individual author(s) and contributor(s) and not of MDPI and/or the editor(s). MDPI and/or the editor(s) disclaim responsibility for any injury to people or property resulting from any ideas, methods, instructions or products referred to in the content.

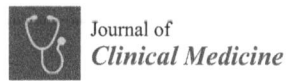

Article

# Immune Mediators Profiles in the Aqueous Humor of Patients with Simple Diabetic Retinopathy

Naoyuki Yamakawa [†], Hiroyuki Komatsu [†], Yoshihiko Usui *, Kinya Tsubota, Yoshihiro Wakabayashi and Hiroshi Goto

Department of Ophthalmology, Tokyo Medical University, 6-7-1 Nishi-shinjuku, Shinjuku-ku, Tokyo 160-0023, Japan; yamakawa@tokyo-med.ac.jp (N.Y.); v06058@gmail.com (H.K.); tsubnkin@hotmail.co.jp (K.T.); wbaki@tokyo-med.ac.jp (Y.W.); goto1115@tokyo-med.ac.jp (H.G.)
* Correspondence: usuyoshi@gmail.com; Tel.: +81-3-3342-6111
[†] These authors contributed equally to this work.

**Abstract:** Various immune mediators identified to date are associated with the development of advanced forms of diabetic retinopathy (DR), such as proliferative DR and diabetic macular edema, although the exact pathophysiological mechanisms of early stages of DR such as simple DR remain unclear. We determined the immune mediator profile in the aqueous humor of eyes with simple DR. Fifteen eyes of fifteen patients with simple DR were studied. Twenty-two eyes of twenty-two patients with cataracts and no DR served as controls. Undiluted aqueous humor samples were collected, and a cytometric bead array was used to determine the aqueous humor concentrations of 32 immune mediators comprising 13 interleukins (IL), interferon-γ, interferon-γ-inducible protein-10 (IP-10), monocyte chemoattractant protein-1, macrophage inflammatory protein (MIP)-1α, MIP-1β, regulated on activation, normal T cell expressed and secreted (RANTES), monokine induced by interferon-γ, basic fibroblast growth factor (bFGF), Fas ligand, granzyme A, granzyme B, interferon-inducible T-cell alpha chemoattractant (ITAC), fractalkine, granulocyte macrophage colony-stimulating factor, granulocyte colony-stimulating factor (G-CSF), vascular endothelial growth factor (VEGF), angiogenin, tumor necrosis factor-α, and CD40 ligand. Among the 32 immune mediators, 10 immune mediators, including bFGF, CD40 ligand, fractalkine, G-CSF, IL-6, IL-8, MIP-α, MIP-1β, and VEGF, showed significantly higher aqueous humor concentrations and the Fas ligand had significantly lower concentration ($p < 0.05$) in eyes with simple DR compared with control eyes. Of these 10 cytokines with significant concentration alteration, protein–protein interaction analysis revealed that 8 established an intricate interaction network. Various immune mediators may contribute to the pathogenesis of simple DR. Attention should be given to the concentrations of immune mediators in ocular fluids even in simple DR. Large-scale studies are warranted to assess whether altered aqueous humor concentrations of these 10 immune mediators are associated with an increased risk of progression to advanced stages of DR.

**Keywords:** diabetic retinopathy; simple diabetic retinopathy; immune mediator; cytokine; chemokine; growth factor

Citation: Yamakawa, N.; Komatsu, H.; Usui, Y.; Tsubota, K.; Wakabayashi, Y.; Goto, H. Immune Mediators Profiles in the Aqueous Humor of Patients with Simple Diabetic Retinopathy. *J. Clin. Med.* **2023**, *12*, 6931. https://doi.org/10.3390/jcm12216931

Academic Editor: Georgios D. Panos

Received: 30 September 2023
Revised: 2 November 2023
Accepted: 3 November 2023
Published: 5 November 2023

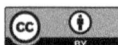

**Copyright:** © 2023 by the authors. Licensee MDPI, Basel, Switzerland. This article is an open access article distributed under the terms and conditions of the Creative Commons Attribution (CC BY) license (https://creativecommons.org/licenses/by/4.0/).

## 1. Introduction

Diabetic retinopathy (DR) is the major cause of blindness in the older population. Currently, 284.6 million people worldwide are estimated to have diabetes mellitus; approximately one third of those with diabetes are at risk of developing DR to some extent, and approximately one third of those with DR may advance to the vision-threatening stage [1]. Two major advanced forms of DR, diabetic macular edema and proliferative DR (PDR), develop from pre-retinal neovascularization (abnormal growth of new blood vessels) that causes the majority of diabetes-related severe visual impairment. Microaneurysms, retinal hemorrhages, and hard or soft exudates occur early in DR development, and characterize simple DR or non-proliferative DR. The progression of simple DR to subsequent stages like pre-PDR or macular edema varies among individuals. Several studies have estimated that the cumulative rate of progression from non-proliferative stages to vision-threatening stages ranges between 14 and 16% [2,3]. While the etiology remains poorly known, DR is clearly a complex multifactorial disease caused by a combination of genetic, environmental, and immunological factors [4–8]. Multiple immune mediators have been identified in eyes with PDR and diabetic macular edema, suggesting a pathogenetic role of the mediators.

However, there is no report to date which describes immune mediator concentrations in the ocular fluids of eyes with simple DR. Recently, two-color flow cytometry has been used for the simultaneous detection of many immune mediators using a very small volume of a sample such as aqueous humor [9]. The predominant advantage of cytometric bead array (CBA) technology lies in its ability to measure multiple parameters concurrently using a relatively small sample volume such as aqueous humor, making it faster and more cost-effective than ELISA technology. Previous studies on cytokines or chemokines associated with PDR or diabetic macular edema quantified a small number of cytokines or chemokines using the Enzyme-linked Immunosorbent Assay (ELISA) system [10,11]. Because single-assay measurements of immune mediators provide limited information, multiple immune mediators measured simultaneously must be analyzed to obtain a more comprehensive picture of DR.

The purpose of this study was to identify and quantify a wide spectrum of immune mediators including cytokines, chemokines, growth factors, and apoptosis-related molecules in aqueous humor samples collected from eyes with simple DR. Understanding how immune mediators are associated in the early stages of simple DR may shed light on the pathophysiology of DR progression and help to develop new biomarkers for early diagnosis.

## 2. Materials and Methods

### 2.1. Subjects

In this retrospective study, 15 patients (15 eyes) with simple DR were identified from the medical records between September 2011 and May 2022, and 22 patients (22 eyes) with cataract and no diabetic mellitus (DM) were included as disease controls. The 15 patients (11 males and 4 females) diagnosed with simple DR according to Davis classification were 65.8 ± 11.6 years of age; all had type 2 diabetes mellites (T2DM) with mean hemoglobin $A_{1C}$ (Hb$A_{1C}$) of 7.5 ± 1.4 and mean duration of diabetes of 12.1 ± 7.5 years (Table 1). The 22 cataract patients (9 males and 13 females) with no DR based on Davis classification were aged 72.1 ± 8.8 years. All patients were Japanese adults. The absence of diabetic macular edema was defined as no retinal thickening at the macula based on clinical and OCT examinations. This study was reviewed and approved by the institutional review board of Tokyo Medical University. Informed consent was obtained from each participant, who were provided with explanations regarding the purpose and methods of the study for effective disease control.

**Table 1.** Demographic and clinical data of patients with simple diabetic retinopathy (DR), and disease controls.

|  |  | Subject | Control |
|---|---|---|---|
| Number of eyes |  | 15 | 22 |
| Number of cases |  | 15 | 22 |
| Sex | Male | 11 | 9 |
|  | Female | 4 | 13 |
| Age (years) |  | 65.8 ± 11.6 | 72.1 ± 8.8 |
| HbA1c (%) |  | 7.5 ± 1.42 | — |

### 2.2. Measurements

Undiluted aqueous humor samples (approximately 100 μL) were collected via an anterior chamber tap with a 25 needle from patients with simple DR during outpatient consultation, and from cataract patients with no DM before cataract surgery. All samples were stored at −80 °C until use. The CBA Flex immunoassay kit (BD Biosciences, San Jose, CA, USA) was used to determine the aqueous humor concentrations of 32 immune mediators comprising interleukins (IL)-1α, IL-1β, IL-2, IL-3, IL-4, IL-5, IL-6, IL-8, IL-9, IL-10, IL-12p70, IL-17A, and IL-21, interferon (IFN)-γ, interferon-γ-inducible protein (IP)-10, monocyte chemoattractant protein (MCP)-1, macrophage inflammatory protein (MIP)-1α, MIP-1β, regulated on activation, normal T-cell expressed and secreted (RANTES), monokine induced by interferon-γ (Mig), basic fibroblast growth factor (bFGF), Fas ligand, granzyme A, granzyme B, interferon-inducible T-cell alpha chemoattractant (ITAC), fractalkine, granulocyte macrophage colony-stimulating factor (GM-CSF), granulocyte colony-stimulating factor (G-CSF), vascular endothelial growth factor (VEGF), angiogenin, tumor necrosis factor (TNF)-α, and CD40 ligand. This method allows the simultaneous detection of many analytes with a very small volume of sample (100 µL), as described previously [12].

### 2.3. Analysis for the Interaction of Altered Immune Mediators

To elucidate the interaction network of immune mediators with significantly altered expression levels in simple DR, we utilized Metascape [13] (https://metascape.org/, accessed on 5 November 2023). The STRING database ver.12 [14] (https://string-db.org/, accessed on 5 November 2023) was used to visualize the protein–protein interactions among the immune modulators with significantly altered aqueous humor concentrations in simple DR compared to disease controls.

### 2.4. Statistical Analysis

Statistical analyses were performed using JMP version 10 (SAS, Cary, NC, USA) and the graphs were generated using GraphPad Prism 9 (ver. 9.5.1). Two-group comparisons of categorical variables were performed using Fisher's exact test. Continuous variables were compared using Student's $t$-test or a Mann–Whitney U test depending on the normality of the data distribution. Specifically, we employed the non-parametric Mann–Whitney U test to analyze immune mediator concentrations since the data were not normally distributed. Data in the text and table are presented as mean ± standard deviation or median with interquartile range in parenthesis. Immune mediator concentrations below the lowest limit of detection were treated as 0 pg/mL in statistical analyses. The significance level for all tests was 5%.

## 3. Results

The demographic data of the simple DR group and control group are shown in Table 1. Table 2 presents the immune mediator concentrations in the simple DR group and control group. Aqueous humor concentrations [mean (interquartile range)] of nine immune mediators comprising bFGF, CD40 ligand, fractalkine, G-CSF, IL-6, IL-8, MIP-1α, MIP-1β, and VEGF were significantly higher in simple DR than in controls (Table 2). On the other hand, Fas ligand concentration in aqueous humor was significantly lower in simple DR than in controls. The aqueous humor concentrations of some immune mediators including Fas ligand and IL-9 in all patients with simple DR, and CD40 ligand, G-CSF, IL-1α, IL-5, IL-7, IL-9, TNF-α, and ITAC in all controls, were below the lowest limits of detection in all samples.

Table 2. Immune mediator levels in aqueous humor of patients with simple diabetic retinopathy.

| Name | Simple DR (n = 15) Median | Range | Controls (n = 22) Median | Range | p Values |
|---|---|---|---|---|---|
| Angiogenin (pg/mL) | 4468.9 | 1495–58426 | 5257 | 943–9489 | 0.614 |
| bFGF (pg/mL) | 9 | 0–301 | 0 | 0–38 | 0.026 |
| CD40 ligand (pg/mL) | 0 | 0–3.47 | 0 | 0–0 | 0.042 |
| Fas ligand (pg/mL) | 0 | 0–0 | 0 | 0–13.5 | 0.036 |
| Fractalkine (pg/mL) | 16.5 | 0–68 | 0 | 0–65 | 0.007 |
| G-CSF (pg/mL) | 0 | 0–38 | 0 | 0–0 | 0.042 |
| GM-CSF (pg/mL) | 0 | 0–4.86 | 0 | 0–4.8 | 0.819 |
| Granzyme A (pg/mL) | 0 | 0–6.51 | 0 | 0–13.5 | 0.262 |
| Granzyme B (pg/mL) | 0 | 0–133.44 | 0 | 0–13.5 | 0.725 |
| IFN-γ (pg/mL) | 0.5 | 0–3.93 | 0 | 0–6.64 | 0.939 |
| IL-1α (pg/mL) | 0 | 0–7.62 | 0 | 0–0 | 0.748 |
| IL-2 (pg/mL) | 0 | 0–76.6 | 0 | 0–17.8 | 0.593 |
| IL-3 (pg/mL) | 0 | 0–8.04 | 0 | 0–4.8 | 0.531 |
| IL-4 (pg/mL) | 0 | 0–9.23 | 0 | 0–2 | 0.915 |
| IL-5 (pg/mL) | 0 | 0–3.43 | 0 | 0–0 | 0.092 |
| IL-6 (pg/mL) | 15.9 | 0–11230 | 4.3 | 0–15.03 | <0.001 |
| IL-7 (pg/mL) | 0 | 0–112 | 0 | 0–0 | 0.181 |
| IL-8 (pg/mL) | 13.47 | 0–153 | 3 | 0–15.99 | 0.01 |
| IL-9 (pg/mL) | 0 | 0–0 | 0 | 0–0 | 1 |
| IL-10 (pg/mL) | 0 | 0–18.6 | 0 | 0–3.7 | 0.135 |
| IL-12p70 (pg/mL) | 0 | 0–96.8 | 0 | 0–13.5 | 0.075 |
| IL-17A (pg/mL) | 0 | 0–26.2 | 0 | 0–4.68 | 0.065 |
| IL-21 (pg/mL) | 0 | 0–181 | 0 | 0–17 | 0.829 |
| IP-10 (pg/mL) | 89.2 | 0–873 | 84.5 | 0–417 | 0.843 |
| MCP-1 (pg/mL) | 494.5 | 77–11859 | 327.8 | 72–780 | 0.152 |
| Mig (pg/mL) | 32 | 8–187 | 18.4 | 0–174 | 0.237 |
| MIP-1α (pg/mL) | 10.7 | 0–32.4 | 0 | 0–29 | 0.039 |
| MIP-1β (pg/mL) | 24.7 | 12.3–94.9 | 10.8 | 0–42 | 0.005 |
| RANTES (pg/mL) | 0.5 | 0–31.5 | 0 | 0–3.8 | 0.225 |
| TNF-α (pg/mL) | 0 | 0–0.84 | 0 | 0–0 | 0.748 |
| VEGF (pg/mL) | 34 | 0–159 | 11.9 | 0–69.3 | 0.033 |
| ITAC (pg/mL) | 0 | 0–17 | 0 | 0–0 | 0.511 |

Disease controls were patients with cataracts and no diabetic retinopathy. Immune mediator levels are expressed as median with interquartile range in parenthesis. bFGF, basic fibroblast growth factor; G-CSF, granulocyte-colony stimulating factor; GM-CSF, granulocyte macrophage-colony stimulating factor; IFN, interferon; IL, interleukin; IP-10, interferon gamma-induced protein 10 kDa; ITAC, interferon-inducible T-cell alpha chemoattractant; MCP, monocyte chemoattractant protein; Mig, monokine induced by interferon γ; MIP, macrophage inflammatory protein; RANTES, regulated upon activation, normal T expressed, and presumably secreted; TNF, tumor necrosis factor; VEGF, vascular endothelial growth factor.

Notably, the aqueous humor concentration of IL-8 in simple DR was significantly different compared to controls [13.47 (0–153) pg/mL versus 3 (0–15.99) pg/mL, $p = 0.01$] in this study. This aligns with previous reports, indicating a significant upregulation of aqueous humor IL-8 concentration in diabetic macular edema and PDR relative to controls [15,16]. Therefore, IL-8 upregulation may play a key role even in the very early stages of diabetic retinopathy.

In addition, we investigated the relationship among immune mediators with altered aqueous humor concentrations in simple DR. Among the 10 cytokines with significantly altered aqueous humor concentrations, a protein–protein interaction analysis using the STRING database revealed that eight were closely interconnected, forming a complex interaction network (Figure 1). These results suggest that diabetic retinopathy progresses via the interaction of multiple pathways, rather than through a single altered pathway.

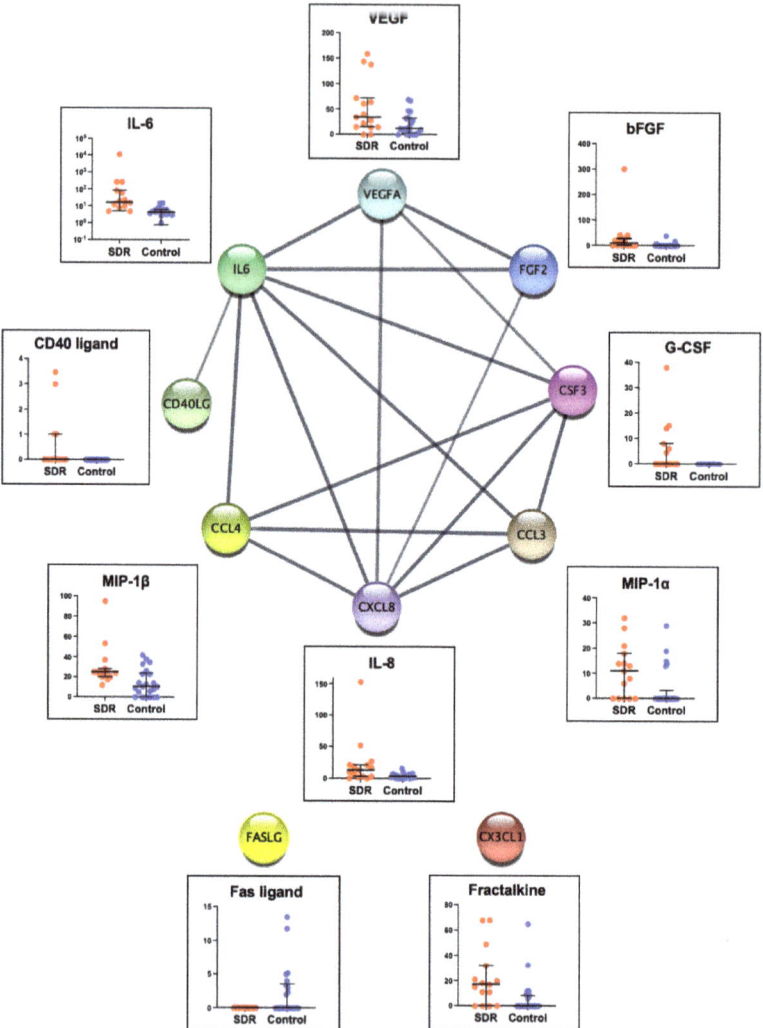

**Figure 1.** The graph generated from the STRING database represents protein–protein interactions among immune modulators that exhibited significant alterations in aqueous humor concentration in simple diabetic retinopathy. Each node, labeled by the cytokine name, is linked to an associated cytokine through a connection termed an "edge." Next to each node, a bar graph shows the aqueous humor concentration from this study. Among the 10 immune mediators, eight cytokines established edges with multiple cytokines. Conversely, Fas ligand and fractalkine showed no interactions with others.

## 4. Discussion

The etiology of DR remains largely unknown. Exposure to hyperglycemia over an extended period is considered to promote changes that cause vascular endothelial impairment. The early histologic features of DR are capillary basement membrane thickening, leukostasis, a loss of endothelial cells, and a loss of pericytes [17,18]. Sustained capillary occlusion causes hypoxia that is further accelerated by the release of VEGF and other immune mediators [19,20], leading to the development of intraretinal microvascular abnormalities, providing alternative collateral routes for blood to travel from the arteries to the veins. In up to 20% of patients with diabetes, ischemia of the inner retina secondary to the closure of parts of the retinal capillary bed leads to neovascularization on the surface of the retina and optic disc, signaling the presence of PDR [21].

Sustained hyperglycemia is considered to be the major initiating factor of DR. However, detailed mechanisms causing retinal abnormality remain unclear. The disease involves the progression of retinovascular damage with stepwise clinical progression from mild stages to advanced proliferative changes. The rate of progression varies among patients and depends mainly on systemic factors such as blood glucose level, blood pressure control, and blood lipid profile, which constitute independent risk factors of DR development [22]. Our results suggest that alterations to the aqueous humor concentrations of immune mediators in patients with simple DR may reflect the early stages of disease progression.

DR tends to cause ocular inflammation. Although the precise mechanisms underlying such chronic inflammation are not yet known, macrophages and many immune mediators including angiogenic growth factors, cytokines, and chemokines are involved in the onset and progression of DR. In advanced stages of DR, such as PDR and diabetic macular edema, immune cells and mediators play important roles in disease progression [19,20,23–25]. Indeed, macrophages have been shown to play a pivotal role in PDR and diabetic macular edema development, by invading the retina [24,26,27]. High levels of VEGF, a potent proangiogenic factor, are expressed in the retinas of diabetic patients, resulting in marked increases in intraocular VEGF concentration correlating with the presence of soft exudates, intraretinal microvascular abnormality, venous bleeding, venous loops, and neovascularization [19,28]. Genetic polymorphisms in VEGF-A have also been associated with an increased risk of developing proliferative DR, further corroborating the critical role of this factor in DR [29]. Vitreous and aqueous concentrations of VEGF and IL-6 may serve as biomarkers of disease progression, because they correlate with the severity of macular thickness alteration in diabetic macular edema [30]. The CD40 ligand is a member of the TNF receptor superfamily and is expressed on inflammatory cells, primarily activated CD4+ T cells, as a receptor for CD40. The CD40-CD40 ligand pathway plays a significant role in both autoimmunity and adaptive immunity [31,32], Studies have suggested that this pathway also contributes to the pathophysiology of diabetes mellitus [33,34]. Lamine et al. reported that circulating soluble CD40 ligand concentration in serum was associated with the severity of diabetic retinopathy in patients with T2DM [35]. In this study, the CD40 ligand concentration in aqueous humor was elevated in early-stage DR. Combined with previous research, this finding suggests the potential involvement of the CD40 ligand in diabetic retinopathy pathogenesis from the onset. Notably, the Fas ligand, an apoptosis-inducing ligand, was the sole cytokine showing a decrease in simple DR compared to controls. Previous in vitro studies demonstrated the suppression of Fas ligand expression by VEGF [36], which aligns with our observation of reduced Fas ligand concentrations in the aqueous humor of patients with simple DR.

Among the nine immune mediators that were upregulated in simple DR in this study, fractalkine, also known as chemokine CX3C Receptor 1, is particularly interesting for its dual roles as a chemotaxin and an activator of retinal microglia and infiltrating macrophages, as well as being a physiologically active compound that potently increases vascular permeability and promotes angiogenesis [37–39]. In addition, a previous study in mice suggested that microglia modulate neurovascular function in the retina, and dysfunction of the microglial–vascular function may potentially cause early vascular compromise, leading to the development of DR [40]. Therefore, the altered cytokines identified in this study may reflect the responses of various cells, including vascular endothelial cells, inflammatory cells, and retinal microglia, due to diabetic vascular abnormality.

Of the ten cytokines that showed significant alterations in simple DR in our study, nine immune mediators form a tightly interwoven and complex interaction network. This finding suggests that many immune mediators act synergistically, interacting to trigger the development of DR. Further research is warranted to uncover the functional roles of these 10 cytokines in the initiation and progression of early-stage DR.

This study has several limitations. First, because retrospectively collected samples were used, the time from HbA1c measurement or disease onset to aqueous humor collection varied among samples. This may suggest a variable degree of disease progression across the samples. Second, the single-center case–control study design may give rise to potential sampling or clinical biases, including collection bias, in specific periods related to geographic location, ethnicity, age, and sex distribution. Third, selection bias when using cataract patients instead of healthy controls is included as a limitation. Notably, the simple DR group in this study consisted of predominantly males, which is a potential bias. In addition, our sample size was small to detect the generalized alternation with simple DR. To address these concerns, future prospective multi-center studies on a global scale would be needed to validate the present findings.

## 5. Conclusions

The aqueous humor concentrations of 10 immune mediators comprising bFGF, CD40 ligand, Fas ligand, fractalkine, G-CSF, IL-6, IL-8, MIP-1$\alpha$, MIP-1$\beta$, and VEGF were altered in patients with simple DR. Although this is the first study of the aqueous humor immune mediator profile in simple DR, our results are mostly in agreement with previous studies showing that various immune mediators associated with inflammation and angiogenesis are related to the development of DR. Combinations of these immune mediators may also be useful biomarkers for the early detection of DR and the prediction of prognosis. Future large-scale studies are needed to evaluate whether altered aqueous humor concentrations of these cytokines or their interactions are associated with an increased risk of progression to advanced stages of DR.

**Author Contributions:** Conceptualization, Y.U. and H.G.; methodology, N.Y., H.K. and Y.W.; software, H.K. and K.T.; validation, N.Y.; formal analysis; N.Y. and H.K.; investigation, N.Y., H.K., Y.U., K.T. and Y.W.; resources, Y.U., K.T., Y.W. and H.G.; data curation, H.K. and K.T.; writing—original draft preparation, H.K.; writing—review and editing, N.Y., Y.U., K.T., Y.W. and H.G.; visualization, H.K.; supervision, Y.U. and H.G.; project administration, Y.U.; funding acquisition, Y.U. and H.G. All authors have read and agreed to the published version of the manuscript.

**Funding:** This research was supported in part by a Grant-in-Aid for Scientific Research (C) 16K11330, 19K09981, 19K09959, and 22K09840 from the Ministry of Education, Culture, Sports, Science, and Technology of Japan.

**Institutional Review Board Statement:** This study was conducted in accordance with the principles of the Declaration of Helsinki. This study was approved by the Ethics Committee of the Tokyo Medical University Hospital, Tokyo, Japan (SH3882).

**Informed Consent Statement:** Written informed consent was provided by all participants in the study.

**Data Availability Statement:** The data presented in this study are available on request from the corresponding author.

**Conflicts of Interest:** All of the authors declare they have no conflicts of interest.

## Abbreviations

DR: Diabetic retinopathy; PDR: proliferative diabetic retinopathy; SD: standard deviation.

## References

1. Zorena, K.; Raczynska, D.; Raczynska, K. Biomarkers in diabetic retinopathy and the therapeutic implications. *Mediat. Inflamm.* **2013**, *2013*, 193604. [CrossRef]
2. Sato, Y.; Lee, Z.; Hayashi, Y. Subclassification of preproliferative diabetic retinopathy and glycemic control: Relationship between mean hemoglobin A1C value and development of proliferative diabetic retinopathy. *Jpn. J. Ophthalmol.* **2001**, *45*, 523–527. [CrossRef]

3. Marques, I.P.; Madeira, M.H.; Messias, A.L.; Santos, T.; Martinho, A.C.-V.; Figueira, J.; Cunha-Vaz, J. Retinopathy Phenotypes in Type 2 Diabetes with Different Risks for Macular Edema and Proliferative Retinopathy. *J. Clin. Med.* **2020**, *9*, 1433. [CrossRef] [PubMed]
4. Omar, A.F.; Silva, P.S.; Sun, J.K. Genetics of diabetic retinopathy. *Semin. Ophthalmol.* **2013**, *28*, 337–346. [CrossRef]
5. Abcouwer, S.F.; Gardner, T.W. Diabetic retinopathy: Loss of neuroretinal adaptation to the diabetic metabolic environment. *Ann. N. Y. Acad. Sci.* **2014**, *1311*, 174–190. [CrossRef] [PubMed]
6. Boehm, M.R.; Oellers, P.; Thanos, S. Inflammation and immunology of the vitreoretinal compartment. *Inflamm. Allergy Drug Targets* **2011**, *10*, 283–309. [CrossRef] [PubMed]
7. Muramatsu, D.; Wakabayashi, Y.; Usui, Y.; Okunuki, Y.; Kezuka, T.; Goto, H. Correlation of complement fragment C5a with inflammatory cytokines in the vitreous of patients with proliferative diabetic retinopathy. *Graefe's Arch. Clin. Exp. Ophthalmol.* **2013**, *251*, 15–17. [CrossRef]
8. Wakabayashi, Y.; Usui, Y.; Shibauchi, Y.; Uchino, H.; Goto, H. Increased levels of 8-hydroxydeoxyguanosine in the vitreous of patients with diabetic retinopathy. *Diabetes Res. Clin. Pract.* **2010**, *89*, e59–e61. [CrossRef]
9. Maier, R.; Weger, M.; Haller-Schober, E.M.; El-Shabrawi, Y.; Theisl, A.; Barth, A.; Aigner, R.; Haas, A. Application of multiplex cytometric bead array technology for the measurement of angiogenic factors in the vitreous. *Mol. Vis.* **2006**, *12*, 1143–1147.
10. Song, Z.; Sun, M.; Zhou, F.; Huang, F.; Qu, J.; Chen, D. Increased intravitreous interleukin-18 correlated to vascular endothelial growth factor in patients with active proliferative diabetic retinopathy. *Graefe's Arch. Clin. Exp. Ophthalmol.* **2014**, *252*, 1229–1234. [CrossRef]
11. Funatsu, H.; Yamashita, H.; Noma, H.; Mimura, T.; Yamashita, T.; Hori, S. Increased levels of vascular endothelial growth factor and interleukin-6 in the aqueous humor of diabetics with macular edema. *Am. J. Ophthalmol.* **2002**, *133*, 70–77. [CrossRef] [PubMed]
12. Usui, Y.; Wakabayashi, Y.; Okunuki, Y.; Kimura, K.; Tajima, K.; Matsuda, R.; Ueda, S.; Ma, J.; Nagai, T.; Mori, H.; et al. Immune mediators in vitreous fluids from patients with vitreoretinal B-cell lymphoma. *Investig. Ophthalmol. Vis. Sci.* **2012**, *53*, 5395–5402. [CrossRef]
13. Zhou, Y.; Zhou, B.; Pache, L.; Chang, M.; Khodabakhshi, A.H.; Tanaseichuk, O.; Benner, C.; Chanda, S.K. Metascape provides a biologist-oriented resource for the analysis of systems-level datasets. *Nat. Commun.* **2019**, *10*, 1523. [CrossRef]
14. Szklarczyk, D.; Kirsch, R.; Koutrouli, M.; Nastou, K.; Mehryary, F.; Hachilif, R.; Gable, A.L.; Fang, T.; Doncheva, N.T.; Pyysalo, S.; et al. The STRING database in 2023: Protein–protein association networks and functional enrichment analyses for any sequenced genome of interest. *Nucleic Acids Res.* **2022**, *51*, D638–D646. [CrossRef]
15. Lee, W.J.; Kang, M.H.; Seong, M.; Cho, H.Y. Comparison of aqueous concentrations of angiogenic and inflammatory cytokines in diabetic macular oedema and macular oedema due to branch retinal vein occlusion. *Br. J. Ophthalmol.* **2012**, *96*, 1426–1430. [CrossRef]
16. Forooghian, F.; Kertes, P.J.; Eng, K.T.; Agron, E.; Chew, E.Y. Alterations in the intraocular cytokine milieu after intravitreal bevacizumab. *Investig. Ophthalmol. Vis. Sci.* **2010**, *51*, 2388–2392. [CrossRef] [PubMed]
17. Qazi, Y.; Maddula, S.; Ambati, B.K. Mediators of ocular angiogenesis. *J. Genet.* **2009**, *88*, 495–515. [CrossRef]
18. Mysona, B.A.; Shanab, A.Y.; Elshaer, S.L.; El-Remessy, A.B. Nerve growth factor in diabetic retinopathy: Beyond neurons. *Expert Rev. Ophthalmol.* **2014**, *9*, 99–107. [CrossRef] [PubMed]
19. Wakabayashi, Y.; Usui, Y.; Okunuki, Y.; Kezuka, T.; Takeuchi, M.; Goto, H.; Iwasaki, T. Correlation of vascular endothelial growth factor with chemokines in the vitreous in diabetic retinopathy. *Retina* **2010**, *30*, 339–344. [CrossRef]
20. Wakabayashi, Y.; Usui, Y.; Okunuki, Y.; Kezuka, T.; Takeuchi, M.; Iwasaki, T.; Ohno, A.; Goto, H. Increases of vitreous monocyte chemotactic protein 1 and interleukin 8 levels in patients with concurrent hypertension and diabetic retinopathy. *Retina* **2011**, *31*, 1951–1957. [CrossRef]
21. Arfken, C.L.; Reno, P.L.; Santiago, J.V.; Klein, R. Development of proliferative diabetic retinopathy in African-Americans and whites with type 1 diabetes. *Diabetes Care* **1998**, *21*, 792–795. [CrossRef]
22. Klein, R.; Klein, B.E.; Moss, S.E.; Cruickshanks, K.J. The Wisconsin Epidemiologic Study of Diabetic Retinopathy: XVII. The 14-year incidence and progression of diabetic retinopathy and associated risk factors in type 1 diabetes. *Ophthalmology* **1998**, *105*, 1801–1815. [CrossRef] [PubMed]
23. Kase, S.; Saito, W.; Ohno, S.; Ishida, S. Proliferative diabetic retinopathy with lymphocyte-rich epiretinal membrane associated with poor visual prognosis. *Investig. Ophthalmol. Vis. Sci.* **2009**, *50*, 5909–5912. [CrossRef] [PubMed]
24. Umazume, K.; Usui, Y.; Wakabayashi, Y.; Okunuki, Y.; Kezuka, T.; Goto, H. Effects of soluble CD14 and cytokine levels on diabetic macular edema and visual acuity. *Retina* **2013**, *33*, 1020–1025. [CrossRef]
25. Jonas, J.B.; Jonas, R.A.; Neumaier, M.; Findeisen, P. Cytokine concentration in aqueous humor of eyes with diabetic macular edema. *Retina* **2012**, *32*, 2150–2157. [CrossRef]
26. Kakehashi, A.; Inoda, S.; Mameuda, C.; Kuroki, M.; Jono, T.; Nagai, R.; Horiuchi, S.; Kawakami, M.; Kanazawa, Y. Relationship among VEGF, VEGF receptor, AGEs, and macrophages in proliferative diabetic retinopathy. *Diabetes Res. Clin. Pract.* **2008**, *79*, 438–445. [CrossRef] [PubMed]
27. Esser, P.; Heimann, K.; Wiedemann, P. Macrophages in proliferative vitreoretinopathy and proliferative diabetic retinopathy: Differentiation of subpopulations. *Br. J. Ophthalmol.* **1993**, *77*, 731–733. [CrossRef] [PubMed]

28. Crawford, T.N.; Alfaro, D.V., 3rd; Kerrison, J.B.; Jablon, E.P. Diabetic retinopathy and angiogenesis. *Curr. Diabetes Rev.* **2009**, *5*, 8–13. [CrossRef]
29. Al-Kateb, H.; Mirea, L.; Xie, X.; Sun, L.; Liu, M.; Chen, H.; Bull, S.B.; Boright, A.P.; Paterson, A.D. Multiple variants in vascular endothelial growth factor (VEGFA) are risk factors for time to severe retinopathy in type 1 diabetes: The DCCT/EDIC genetics study. *Diabetes* **2007**, *56*, 2161–2168. [CrossRef]
30. Owen, L.A.; Hartnett, M.E. Soluble mediators of diabetic macular edema: The diagnostic role of aqueous VEGF and cytokine levels in diabetic macular edema. *Curr. Diabetes Rep.* **2013**, *13*, 476–480. [CrossRef]
31. Zhang, B.; Wu, T.; Chen, M.; Zhou, Y.; Yi, D.; Guo, R. The CD40/CD40L system: A new therapeutic target for disease. *Immunol. Lett.* **2013**, *153*, 58–61. [CrossRef]
32. Elgueta, R.; Benson, M.J.; De Vries, V.C.; Wasiuk, A.; Guo, Y.; Noelle, R.J. Molecular mechanism and function of CD40/CD40L engagement in the immune system. *Immunol. Rev.* **2009**, *229*, 152–172. [CrossRef]
33. Cipollone, F.; Chiarelli, F.; Davì, G.; Ferri, C.; Desideri, G.; Fazia, M.; Iezzi, A.; Santilli, F.; Pini, B.; Cuccurullo, C.; et al. Enhanced soluble CD40 ligand contributes to endothelial cell dysfunction in vitro and monocyte activation in patients with diabetes mellitus: Effect of improved metabolic control. *Diabetologia* **2005**, *48*, 1216–1224. [CrossRef]
34. Linna, H.; Suija, K.; Rajala, U.; Herzig, K.H.; Karhu, T.; Jokelainen, J.; Keinänen-Kiukaanniemi, S.; Timonen, M. The association between impaired glucose tolerance and soluble CD40 ligand: A 15-year prospective cohort study. *Aging Clin. Exp. Res.* **2016**, *28*, 1243–1249. [CrossRef]
35. Lamine, L.B.; Turki, A.; Al-Khateeb, G.; Sellami, N.; Amor, H.B.; Sarray, S.; Jailani, M.; Ghorbel, M.; Mahjoub, T.; Almawi, W.Y. Elevation in Circulating Soluble CD40 Ligand Concentrations in Type 2 Diabetic Retinopathy and Association with its Severity. *Exp. Clin. Endocrinol. Diabetes* **2020**, *128*, 319–324. [CrossRef]
36. Berkkanoglu, M.; Guzeloglu-Kayisli, O.; Kayisli, U.A.; Selam, B.F.; Arici, A. Regulation of Fas ligand expression by vascular endothelial growth factor in endometrial stromal cells in vitro. *Mol. Hum. Reprod.* **2004**, *10*, 393–398. [CrossRef]
37. Liu, Y.; Zhao, T.; Yang, Z.; Li, Q. CX3CR1 RNAi inhibits hypoxia-induced microglia activation via p38MAPK/PKC pathway. *Int. J. Exp. Pathol.* **2014**, *95*, 153–157. [CrossRef] [PubMed]
38. Tang, Z.; Gan, Y.; Liu, Q.; Yin, J.-X.; Liu, Q.; Shi, J.; Shi, F.D. CX3CR1 deficiency suppresses activation and neurotoxicity of microglia/macrophage in experimental ischemic stroke. *J. Neuroinflammation* **2014**, *11*, 26. [CrossRef] [PubMed]
39. Zhang, M.; Xu, G.; Liu, W.; Ni, Y.; Zhou, W. Role of fractalkine/CX3CR1 interaction in light-induced photoreceptor degeneration through regulating retinal microglial activation and migration. *PLoS ONE* **2012**, *7*, e35446. [CrossRef] [PubMed]
40. Mills, S.A.; Jobling, A.I.; Dixon, M.A.; Bui, B.V.; Vessey, K.A.; Phipps, J.A.; Greferath, U.; Venables, G.; Wong, V.H.Y.; Wong, C.H.Y.; et al. Fractalkine-induced microglial vasoregulation occurs within the retina and is altered early in diabetic retinopathy. *Proc. Natl. Acad. Sci. USA* **2021**, *118*, e2112561118. [CrossRef] [PubMed]

**Disclaimer/Publisher's Note:** The statements, opinions and data contained in all publications are solely those of the individual author(s) and contributor(s) and not of MDPI and/or the editor(s). MDPI and/or the editor(s) disclaim responsibility for any injury to people or property resulting from any ideas, methods, instructions or products referred to in the content.

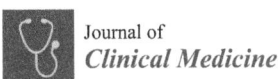 

*Systematic Review*

# Sympathetic Ophthalmia after Vitreoretinal Surgery without Antecedent History of Trauma: A Systematic Review and Meta-Analysis

Matteo Ripa [1,†], Georgios D. Panos [2,†], Robert Rejdak [3], Theodoros Empeslidis [4], Mario Damiano Toro [3,5,*], Ciro Costagliola [6], Andrea Ferrara [7], Stratos Gotzaridis [8], Rino Frisina [9] and Lorenzo Motta [1]

1. Department of Ophthalmology, William Harvey Hospital, East Kent Hospitals University NHS Foundation Trust, Ashford TN24 0LZ, UK; matteof12@gmail.com (M.R.)
2. Department of Ophthalmology, Queen's Medical Centre Campus, Nottingham University Hospitals, Nottingham NG7 2UH, UK
3. Department of General and Pediatric Ophthalmology, Medical University of Lublin, Ul. Chmielna 1, 20079 Lublin, Poland
4. Department of Ophthalmology, Stoneygate Eye Hospital, Leicester LE2 2PN, UK
5. Eye Clinic, Public Health Department, University of Naples Federico II, 80133 Naples, Italy
6. Eye Clinic, Department of Neurosciences, Reproductive and Dentistry Sciences, University of Naples Federico II, 80131 Naples, Italy
7. Department of Ophthalmology and Neuroscience, Medical School, University of Bari "Aldo Moro", 70121 Bari, Italy
8. My Retina Athens Eye Center, 11528 Athens, Greece
9. Ophthalmology Unit of Surgery, Department of Guglielmo da Saliceto Hospital, 29121 Piacenza, Italy
* Correspondence: toro.mario@email.it
† These authors contributed equally to this work.

**Abstract:** Background: To evaluate the morbidity frequency measures in terms of the cumulative incidence of sympathetic ophthalmia (SO) triggered by single or multiple vitreoretinal (VR) surgery procedures in eyes without an antecedent history of trauma and previous ocular surgery, except for previous or concomitant uneventful lens extraction, and to further investigate the relationship between VR surgery and SO. Methods: A literature search was conducted using PubMed, Embase, and Scopus from inception until 11 November 2022. The Joanna Briggs Institute (JBI) critical appraisal checklist for the case series and the Newcastle–Ottawa Scale were used to assess the risk of bias. The research was registered with the PROSPERO database (identifier, CRD42023397792). Meta-analyses were conducted using the measurement of risk and a 95% confidence interval (CI) for each study. Results: A random-effect meta-analysis demonstrated that the pooled cumulative incidence of SO triggered by single or multiple VR surgery procedures in eyes without an antecedent history of trauma and previous ocular surgery, except for previous or concomitant uneventful lens extraction among patients who developed SO regardless of the main trigger, was equal to 0.14 with a CI between 0.08 and 0.21 ($I^2$ = 78.25, z: 7.24, $p$ < 0.01). The pooled cumulative incidence of SO triggered by single or multiple VR surgery procedures in eyes without an antecedent history of trauma and previous ocular surgery, except for previous or concomitant uneventful lens extraction among patients who underwent VR surgery, was equal to 0.03 for every 100 people, with a confidence interval (CI) between 0.02% and 0.004% ($I^2$ = 27.77, z: 9.11, $p$ = 0.25). Conclusions: Despite postsurgical SO being a rare entity, it is a sight-threatening disease. VR surgery should be viewed as a possible inciting event for SO and considered when counseling patients undergoing VR surgery.

**Keywords:** pars plana vitrectomy; panuveitis; sympathetic ophthalmia; vitreoretinal surgery

## 1. Introduction

Sympathetic ophthalmia (SO) is a bilateral, diffuse, granulomatous panuveitis triggered by an ocular penetrating injury or ophthalmic surgery in one eye. The traumatized eye is defined as the "inciting" eye, whereas the fellow eye is referred to as the "sympathizing" eye [1]. After an initial eye injury, a sight-threatening inflammation may appear in both eyes after a variable period, with symptoms occurring from 1 week to 66 years after the initial event [2]. The exact pathogenesis of SO is still not entirely known despite some research showing an autoimmune T-cell-mediated reaction against the normally sequestered ocular antigens that become exposed to the systemic immune system by ocular trauma or surgery [3].

Despite being a potentially blinding disease, the morbidity frequency measures of SO need to be better delineated in the literature as SO is challenging to study due to its rarity and often delayed presentation. Nonetheless, in a recent meta-analysis of 24 studies, He et al. found that SO's estimated overall incidence proportion and incidence rate following open globe injury were 0.19% and 33 per 100,000 person-years, respectively [3]. Despite Marak et al. reporting the incidence of SO to be 0.1% after intraocular surgery, recent studies reported an increase in SO following surgical procedures [4].

Several surgical procedures have been reported as the primary triggers of SO, including cyclo-destructive procedures, cataract surgery, glaucoma filtration surgery, evisceration, and retinal laser photocoagulation [5]. Since the 1980s, the association between vitreoretinal (VR) surgery and SO has been investigated, and in recent years, ocular surgery, especially vitrectomy, has become an increasingly prevalent risk factor for SO [6–20]. However, most of these studies are heterogeneous, and they did not highlight well whether VR surgery alone or in combination with other surgical procedures in eyes with or without a history of previous ocular surgery or trauma represented the inciting event causing SO. To the best of our knowledge, no meta-analyses have investigated the morbidity frequency measures of SO triggered by single or multiple VR surgery procedures in eyes without an antecedent history of trauma and previous ocular surgery, except for previous or concomitant uneventful lens extraction. Therefore, we aimed to determine the pooled cumulative incidence of SO following single or multiple VR procedures in eyes that did not undergo either previous trauma or ocular surgery except for previous or concomitant uneventful lens extraction.

## 2. Materials and Methods

### 2.1. Search Strategy

We checked three databases from inception until 11 November 2022 (PubMed, Embase, and Scopus). The free text and controlled vocabulary were used to analyze the relationship between SO and VR surgery. Specifically, the Medical Subject Headings (MeSH) controlled vocabulary was used to search for articles in PubMed, and the Embase Subject Headings (Emtree) were used in the EMBASE. The search strategy combined the controlled vocabulary and the keywords according to the indications from each database. The keywords were selected based on readings related to the study's subject. The controlled vocabularies and keywords were used with Boolean operators to extend and direct the search. (For addition and restriction, the Boolean operators OR and AND were used.) The investigation was conducted using recognized and extended vocabulary without database filters to achieve a significant sample with a decreased potential loss. Our core search comprised the following terms: "retinal" OR "vitreoretinal surgery" AND "sympathetic ophthalmia". This continued until we reached a point when adding more terms provided no new results. In addition, we also hand-searched the bibliographies of included articles to identify further studies that were not found in the initial database search. The detailed search strategy and Preferred Reporting Items for Systematic Reviews and Meta-Analyses (PRISMA) Checklist are reported in Supplementary Materials S1 and S2.

### 2.2. Study Selection Data Extraction and Data Synthesis

Articles assessing the relationship between SO and VR surgery were included in this review. Specifically, we included all studies that explicitly addressed the presence of SO triggered by single or multiple VR surgery procedures in eyes without an antecedent history of trauma and previous ocular surgery, except for previous or concomitant uneventful lens extraction.

This review is reported following the Preferred Reporting Items for Systematic Reviews and Meta-Analyses (PRISMA) guidelines [21]. Two investigators (M.R. and L.M.) independently extracted baseline and outcome data. If consensus could not be reached, the two co-authors (M.R. and L.M.) discussed the inconsistencies for adjudication.

Articles were excluded if they were not available in the English language. In addition, all articles that did not investigate the morbidity frequency measures of SO after VR surgery procedures in eyes without an antecedent history of trauma and previous ocular surgery, except for previous or concomitant uneventful lens extraction, were excluded. Literature review studies, theses, case reports, dissertations; book chapters; technical reports; and letters from the publisher were not included in our analysis. Furthermore, studies were excluded if the study did not offer a clear description of SO assessment. Reasons for exclusion were documented. This study was registered in The International Prospective Register of Systematic Reviews (PROSPERO) (CRD42023397792).

SO was diagnosed if there were evidence of two of the following criteria in the sympathizing eye (SE) with a history of trauma or surgery preceding the onset of uveitis: (1) bilateral anterior granulomatous or non-granulomatous uveitis (i.e., anterior segment inflammation, (2) vitritis, (3) characteristic involvement of posterior segment showing choroiditis, yellowish-white choroidal lesions (Dalen–Fuchs nodules), papillitis, vasculitis, sunset glow fundus, or exudative retinal detachment, (4) diffuse choroidal thickening in the posterior pole on B-scan ultrasonography, and (5) able to pinpoint areas of hyper- or hypo-fluorescence on fluorescein angiography with late pooling of dye.

VR surgery procedures included: scleral buckle with or without subretinal fluid (SRF) drainage, pars plana vitrectomy with or without endolaser, cryopexy, gas or silicon oil injection, pneumatic retinopexy, or a combination of them.

We extracted the following data from each article: the first author, year published, country, study design, mean/median age of patients that developed SO after VR surgery, study period (years), total number of cases of SO in the report regardless of the main trigger, number of cases of SO after trauma in the report, number of cases of SO after VR surgery in the report (±lens extraction), VR and other surgical procedures performed, total number of VR procedures in the report, and other relevant parameters evaluated.

We used Covidence systematic review software© (Veritas Health Innovation, Melbourne, Australia), available at www.covidence.org [22], (accessed on 11 November 2022) to record and evaluate the study data between 11 October 2012 and 11 November 2022.

*2.3. Risk of Bias Assessment*

Two authors (M.R. and L.M.) independently appraised each cross-sectional and cohort study's methodological quality using the Newcastle–Ottawa scale (NOS) [23]. The Joanna Briggs Institute (JBI) critical appraisal checklist for the case series was used for the quality assessment of the case series [24]. Quality assessment data individually appraised by each of the reviewers were compared. M.R. and L.M. discussed the discrepancies for adjudication if consensus could not be achieved.

*2.4. Assessment of Quality of Evidence*

The Grading of Recommendations Assessment, Development, and Evaluation (GRADE) profiler version 3.6 was used to assess the quality of evidence for each outcome, along with the consensus of two authors (M.R. and L.M.) using the GRADE system. The quality of studies is initially rated as high in this system, but it can be downgraded due to (1) bias risk, (2) inconsistency, (3) indirectness, (4) imprecision, and (5) publication bias. This system categorizes evidence into four levels of quality: high, moderate, low, and very low [25,26].

*2.5. Statistical Analysis*

A random-effects meta-analysis of pooled cumulative incidence and their 95% confidence intervals of SO triggered by single or multiple VR surgery procedures in eyes without an antecedent history of trauma and previous ocular surgery, except for previous or concomitant uneventful lens extraction among patients who developed SO regardless of the main trigger, and a random-effects meta-analysis of the pooled incidence of proportion and their 95% confidence intervals of SO triggered by single or multiple VR surgery procedures in eyes without an antecedent history of trauma and previous ocular surgery, except for previous or concomitant uneventful lens extraction among patients who underwent VR surgery were obtained based on the exact binomial distributions (i.e., number of "events" versus a number of "non-events" in a sample) with Freeman–Tukey double-arcsine transformation using the "metaprop" command in STATA (STATA Corp, College Station, TX, USA), version 17.0. To characterize potential causes of variability, we performed subgroup analyses by stratifying the data by geographic region to investigate further the proportion of surgically induced SO.

According to Barker et al., a high $I^2$ in the context of proportional meta-analysis does not necessarily mean that data are inconsistent, and the results of this test should be interpreted conservatively. Therefore, we did not perform further analysis except for subgroup analyses. Tests to evaluate publication bias, such as Egger's test and funnel plots, were not performed as Egger's test and funnel plots were developed in the context of comparative data, and there is no evidence that proportional data adequately adjusts for these tests [27]. Statistical significance was determined by a two-sided *p*-value of 0.05.

## 3. Results

*3.1. Study Selection*

Figure 1 illustrates the flow chart of our analysis selection and identification process.

The search yielded 358 indexed articles (121, 153, and 82 records from PubMed, Embase, and Scopus, respectively). A search of the reference list yielded one other article. After duplication removal, we screened a total of 208 articles. After the title and abstract screening, we excluded 188 studies, and only 20 full-text studies were retrieved and assessed for final eligibility. Furthermore, an additional 5 articles were excluded because SO was neither triggered by VR surgery procedures in eyes without an antecedent history of trauma nor epidemiologic SO rates after VR surgery were investigated, resulting in 15 studies included in the systematic review [6–20].

Among the 15 studies included in the qualitative analysis, all [6–20] except two studies [11,16] reported the exact number of SO over a specific period. Indeed, these studies reported only SO's clinical presentation, course, and outcomes following vitreoretinal surgeries. Therefore, we excluded both studies from our quantitative synthesis. Finally, the two pooled incidence of proportion meta-analyses included 13 [6–10,12–15,17–20] and 3 studies [9,14,20], respectively, with a total of 99 SO after VR surgery alone or with a previous or concomitant uneventful lens extraction in eyes without an antecedent history of trauma and ocular surgery.

*3.2. Study Characteristics*

A summary of the main characteristics, including the first author, year published, country, study design, mean/median age of patients that developed SO after VR surgery, study period (years), total number of cases of SO in the report regardless of the main trigger, number of cases of SO after trauma in the report, number of cases of SO after VR surgery in the report (±lens extraction), VR and other surgical procedures performed, total number of VR procedures in the report, and other relevant parameters evaluated are summarized in Table 1.

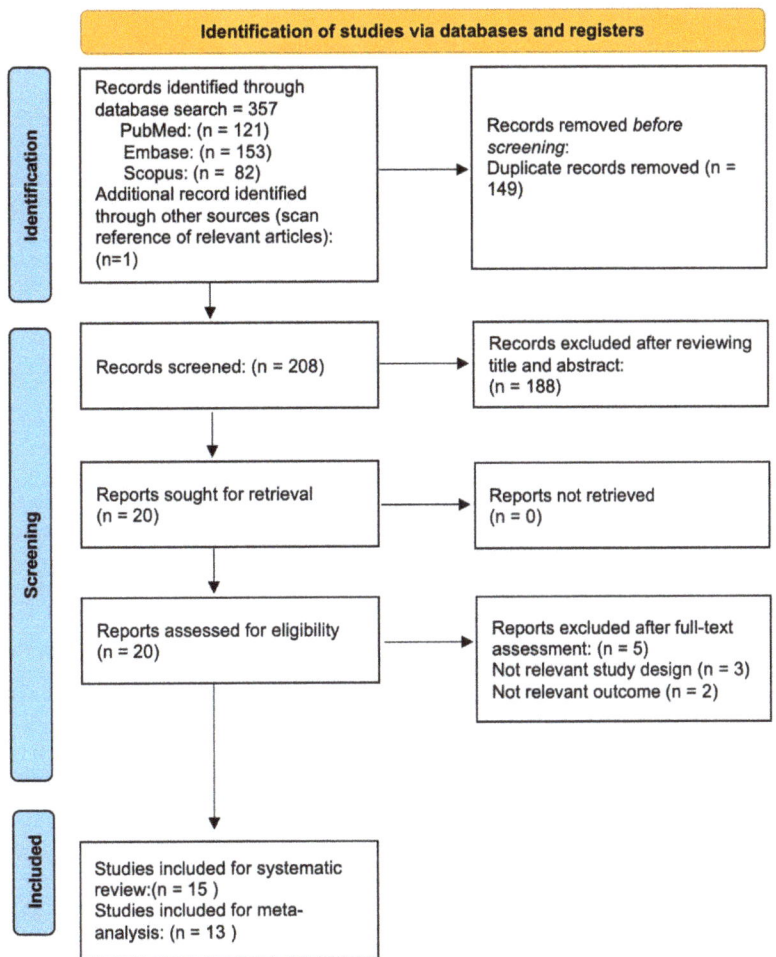

**Figure 1.** Flow diagram of the study selection process.

We assessed eight cross-sectional studies [6,7,9,10,12–15], one longitudinal study [11], and six case series [8,16–18,20]. Overall, three studies recruited data exclusively from the European population [6,11,14], four exclusively from the American (north and south) populations (north and south) countries [7,9,15,16], seven exclusively from the Asian population [8,10,12,13,17,18,20], and only one study analyzed the demographic profile of patients with SO in a multicenter collaborative retrospective study whose data were retrieved from the UK, Singapore, and India [19] (Figure 2).

The review of clinical records of all patients diagnosed and treated as SO ranged from sixty [9] to two hundred and fifty-two months [12], with a total of 99 cases of SO triggered by single or multiple VR surgery procedures in eyes without an antecedent history of trauma and previous ocular surgery, except for previous or concomitant uneventful lens extraction and an overall denominator of 826 patients who developed SO regardless of the main trigger in the study period analyzed with a median age of $55.26 \pm 14.74$. According to the articles that reported the exact number of VR procedures (denominator), only 37 patients developed the SO after 121.511 VR operations in the study period analyzed [9,14,20].

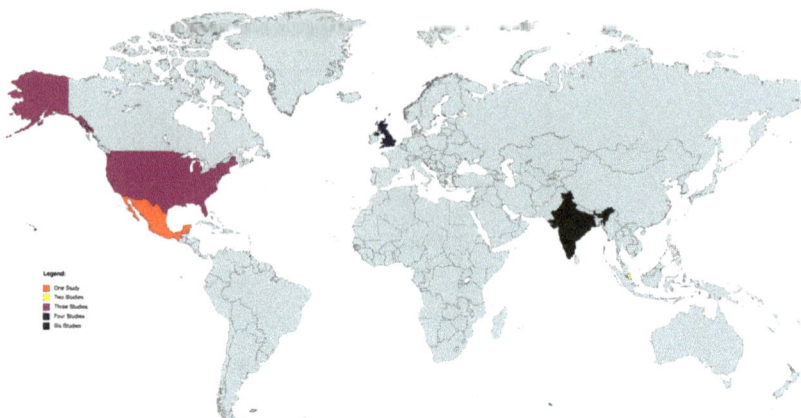

**Figure 2.** World map of studies included. Map generated through MapChart (MapChart, 2021).

All studies [6–20] except two retrieved data regardless of age. Indeed, Only Kumar et al. and Dutta Majumder et al. assessed the clinical features, management, visual outcome, and ocular complications in the sympathizing eye in pediatric patients with SO [8,13].

Only three studies reported total VR surgical operations performed over the study period, totaling 121.511 VR procedures [9,14,20].

Eleven studies reported the data of either SO after VR procedures alone or after VR surgery, plus previous or concomitant uneventful lens extraction [6,7,9,10,12,13,15–18,20]. The other four reported the total number of SO exclusively caused by VR procedures alone and uneventful lens extraction in eyes without any history of trauma and previous ocular surgery [8,11,14,19]. Five studies reported the data of SO either triggered by trauma alone or trauma followed by surgery [6,8,13,17,18].

According to data retrieved from all included studies, the total number of SO after VR procedures alone in eyes without an antecedent history of trauma and previous ocular surgery was 77, whereas the SO after VR surgery procedures in eyes that underwent VR procedures and either previous or concomitant uneventful lens extraction was 22.

Nine studies reported the data of SO triggered by different surgical operations [6,7,9,10,12,15,16,18,19]. To be specific, only 65 cases of SO had as the main trigger different surgical procedures such as cataract surgery, glaucoma filtration surgery, diode laser trans-scleral cyclophotoablation (TCP), neodymium: yttrium–argon–garnet- (YAG)-TCP and penetrating keratoplasty (PKP) alone or combined with PPV or SB.

Despite not being the primary purpose of the current research, trauma was the main trigger of SO in 255 cases, ranging from 0 to 94 in the included studies.

### 3.3. Meta-Analyses of Cumulative Incidence and Subgroups Meta-Analysis

A proportional random meta-analysis was performed to estimate the cumulative incidence of SO triggered by single or multiple VR surgery procedures in eyes without an antecedent history of trauma and previous ocular surgery, except for previous or concomitant uneventful lens extraction among patients who developed SO regardless of the main trigger. The total population (all patients that developed SO in the included studies) was equal to 817, and the sample size varied between 18 and 197 [6–10,12–15,17–20].

The pooled cumulative incidence of SO triggered by single or multiple VR surgery procedures in eyes without an antecedent history of trauma and previous ocular surgery, except for previous or concomitant uneventful lens extraction among patients who developed SO regardless of the main trigger, was equal to 0.14 with a confidence interval (CI) between 0.08 and 0.21 ($I^2 = 78.25$, z: 7.24, $p < 0.01$) (Figure 3).

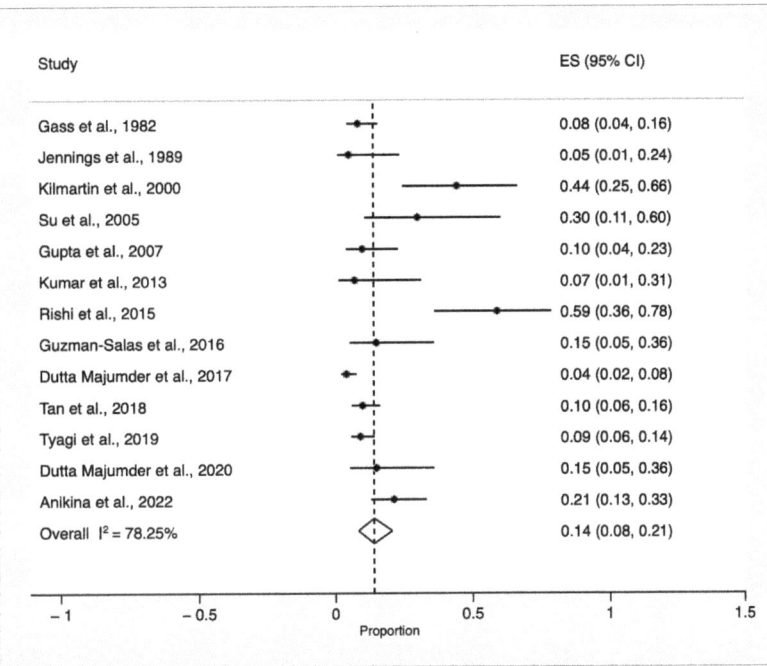

**Figure 3.** Proportional meta-analysis of cumulative sympathetic ophthalmia (SO) incidence triggered by single or multiple vitreoretinal (VR) surgery procedures in eyes without an antecedent history of trauma and previous ocular surgery, except for previous or concomitant uneventful lens extraction among patients who developed SO regardless of the main trigger [6–10,12–15,17–20]. ES: effect size, CI: confidence Interval.

Due to the expected heterogeneity among studies ($I^2$ = 78.25%), we planned a subgroup analysis. Subgroup analyses stratified by categorical study-level characteristics are reported in Figure 4. Therefore, we included geographic region (Europe vs. America vs. Asia) to investigate further the cumulative incidence of SO triggered by single or multiple VR surgery procedures in eyes without an antecedent history of trauma and previous ocular surgery, except for previous or concomitant uneventful lens extraction among patients who developed SO regardless of the main trigger. One study retrieved data from three countries (India, Singapore, and the UK). As most of the data were harvested and retrieved in India (89 out of 130), we considered this study in the Asian subgroup for the analysis [19]. The test for subgroup differences indicated a statistically significant subgroup effect ($p < 0.01$), meaning that this variable statistically significantly impacts the VR-induced SO. However, despite the analysis, substantial unexplained heterogeneity existed between the subgroups (High: $I^2$ = 74.68%) (Figure 4).

A proportional random meta-analysis was performed to estimate the pooled cumulative incidence of SO triggered by single or multiple VR surgery procedures in eyes without an antecedent history of trauma and previous ocular surgery, except for previous or concomitant uneventful lens extraction among patients who underwent VR procedures. The total population was equal to 121.511, and the sample size varied between 39,391 and 41,365. The pooled cumulative incidence of SO triggered by single or multiple VR surgery procedures in eyes without an antecedent history of trauma and previous ocular surgery, except for previous or concomitant uneventful lens extraction among patients who underwent VR surgery, was equal to 0.03 for every 100 people, with a confidence interval (CI) between 0.02% and 0.004% ($I^2$ = 27.77, z: 9.11, $p$ = 0.25) (Figure 5).

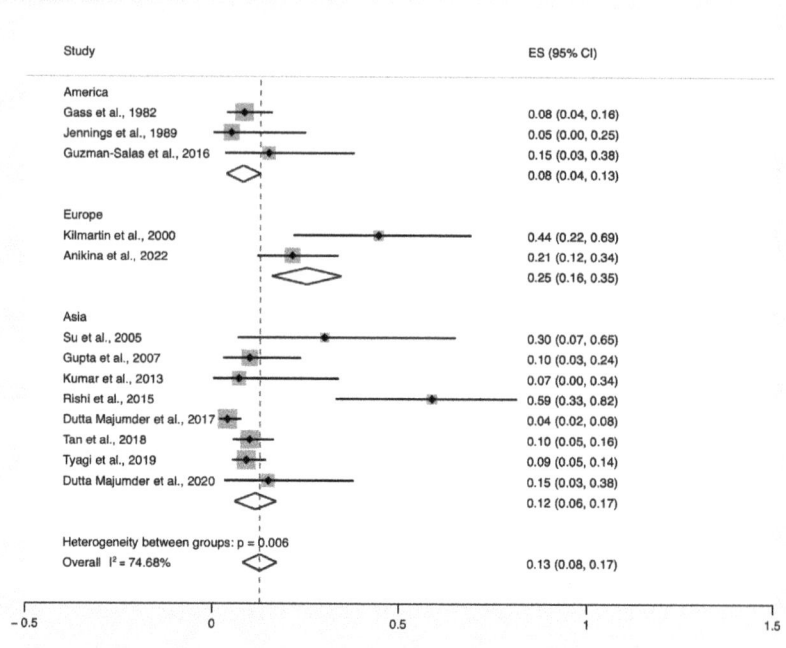

**Figure 4.** Proportional subgroup meta-analysis of cumulative sympathetic ophthalmia (SO) incidence triggered by single or multiple vitreoretinal (VR) surgery procedures in eyes without an antecedent history of trauma and previous ocular surgery, except for previous or concomitant uneventful lens extraction among patients who developed SO regardless of the main trigger according to the geographic area [6–10,12–15,17–20]. ES: effect size, CI: confidence interval.

### 3.4. Risk of Bias and GRADE Assessment

Tables S1 and S2, available in Supplementary Material S3, summarize all studies' risk of bias evaluation. Most studies scored 1 or 2 in the major domains of the quality scale used. The quality rating of the cross-sectional studies averaged 7.5 (95% CI 7.13 to 7.86) of the maximum score on the Newcastle–Ottawa Scale [6,7,9,10,12–15]. The quality rating of the longitudinal study [11] averaged 7 (95% CI 7 to 7) of the maximum score on the Newcastle–Ottawa Scale.

Overall, four cross-sectional studies reached a total score between 8 and 10 [6,9,10,14] and four reached a total score of 7 [7,12,13,15]. The longitudinal research achieved a score of 7 out of 9. According to the JBI critical appraisal checklist for case series, the quality of the included studies was moderate to good. All case series scored 7 out of 10 quality criteria or higher. Notably, two case series scored 8 out of 10 quality criteria as they extensively provided information regarding population demographics [19,20].

The quality of evidence for our primary outcome (pooled cumulative incidence of SO triggered by single or multiple VR surgery procedures in eyes without an antecedent history of trauma and previous ocular surgery, except for previous or concomitant uneventful lens extraction among patients who developed SO regardless of the main trigger) was low according to the GRADE methodology (Table S3 available in Supplementary Material S3.

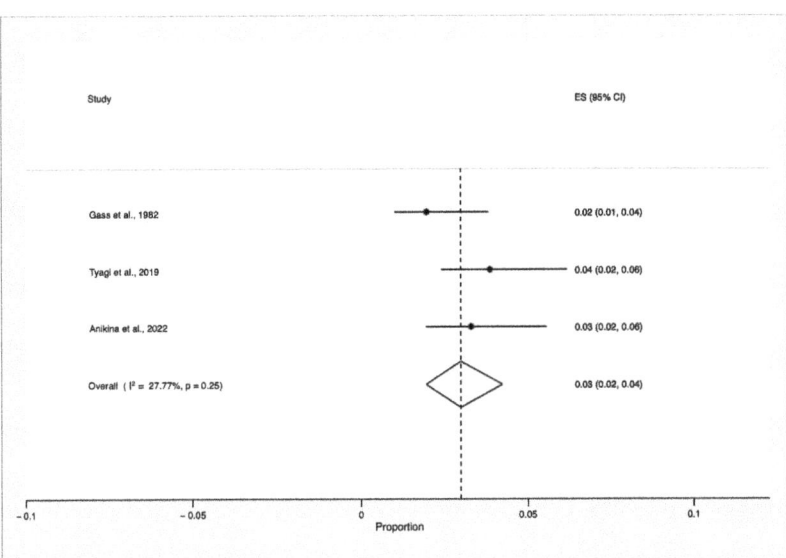

**Figure 5.** Proportional meta-analysis of cumulative sympathetic ophthalmia (SO) incidence triggered by single or multiple vitreoretinal (VR) surgery procedures in eyes without an antecedent history of trauma and previous ocular surgery, except for previous or concomitant uneventful lens extraction among patients who underwent VR surgery [9,14,20]. ES: effect size, CI: confidence interval.

Table 1. Characteristics of studies included in the systematic review.

| Study Name | Year of Publication | Country | Age of SO Patients after VR Surgery (Average ± SD) | Study Design | Duration (y.) | Number of SO Cases in the Study | Number of Cases of SO after Trauma (N and %) in the Study | Number of Cases of SO after Surgery (N and %) in the Study | Number of Cases of SO after VR Surgery (±Lens Extraction) (N and %) in the Study | Number of Cases of SO after Other Surgeries (N and %) in the Study | VR Procedures | Other Surgeries: | Total Number of VR Procedures in the Study | Other Relevant Parameters Evaluated: |
|---|---|---|---|---|---|---|---|---|---|---|---|---|---|---|
| Gass et al. [9] | 1982 | USA | 52 ± 13.98 | Cross-Sectional | Five years | 1. Survey of eye pathology laboratories: 53  2. Armed Forces Institute of Pathology: 33  3. Survey of retinal surgeons: 9 | 1. Survey of eye pathology laboratories: 29 (54.7%)  2. Armed Forces Institute of Pathology: not stated  3. Survey of retinal surgeons: 3 (33.3%) | 1. Survey of eye pathology laboratories: 24 (45.3%)  2. Armed Forces Institute of Pathology: 1 (3%)  3. Survey of retinal surgeons: 4 (44.4%) | 1. Survey of eye pathology laboratories: Exclusively Retinal Surgery: 3 (5.7%) Retinal Surgery + Lens extraction: 3 (5.7%)  2. Armed Forces Institute of Pathology: Retinal Surgery + Lens extraction: 1 (3%)  3. Survey of retinal surgeons: Exclusively Retinal Surgery: 1 (11.1%) | 1. Survey of eye pathology laboratories: 14 (26.4%)  2. Armed Forces Institute of Pathology: not stated  3. Survey of retinal surgeons: not stated | 1. Survey of eye pathology laboratories: SB: 3 (5.7%)  2. Armed Forces Institute of Pathology: 0  3. Survey of retinal surgeons: PPV: 1 (11.1%) | 1. Survey of eye pathology laboratories: Cataract extraction. 10 Filtering operation 3, Combined cataract extraction and filtering operation 1  2. Armed Forces Institute of Pathology: not stated  3. Survey of retinal surgeons: not stated | 1. Survey of eye pathology laboratories: 22,840 (surgical specimens)  2. Armed Forces Institute of Pathology: 3,000 eyes  3. Survey of retinal surgeons: 14,915 vitrectomies | / |
| Jennings et al. [7] | 1989 | USA | 62.3 ± 7.76 | Cross-Sectional | 11-year period: 1974 to 1985 | 20 | 16 (80%) | 3 (15%) | Exclusively Retinal Surgery: 1 (5%) | 2 (10%) | PPV: 1 (5%) | 2 (10%) Extracapsular Extraction with vitreous loss, 2 steroid injections, and 2 vitrectomies. Extracapsular Extraction with a dropped nucleus. | Not stated | SO from onset to last Observation in patients after VR surgery: 12.33 ± 14.46 months |

Table 1. *Cont.*

| Study Name | Year of Publication | Country | Age of SO Patients after VR Surgery (Average ± SD) | Study Design | Duration (y.) | Number of SO Cases in the Study | Number of Cases of SO after Trauma (N and %) in the Study | Number of Cases of SO after Surgery (N and %) in the Study | Number of Cases of SO after VR Surgery (±Lens Extraction) (N and %) in the Study | Number of Cases of SO after Other Surgeries (N and %) in the Study | VR Procedures | Other Surgeries: | Total Number of VR Procedures in the Study | Other Relevant Parameters Evaluated: |
|---|---|---|---|---|---|---|---|---|---|---|---|---|---|---|
| Kilmartin et al. [6] | 2000 | UK | 66 ± 10.2 | Cross-Sectional | July 1997 to September 1998, 14 months | 18 | Exclusively Trauma: 6 (33%) Trauma + Surgery: 2 (11.1%) | 10 (56%) | Exclusively Retinal Surgery: 6 (33%) 3 of these patients having undergone just one PPV Retinal Surgery + Lens extraction: 2 (11.1%) | 3 (16.7%) | PPV RD: 5 (27.8%) Ext RD: 1 (5.5%) | Trabeculectomy: 1 (5.5%) Ext beam DTX, PPV X2, Enucl: 1 (5.5%) Ext RD, PPV RD, Cyclodiodetx: 1 (5.5%) | Not stated | / |
| Pollack et al. [16] | 2001 | USA | 48.87 ± 21.79 | Case series | Not stated | 8 | 0 | 8 (100%) | Exclusively Retinal Surgery: 1 (12.5%) Retinal Surgery + Lens extraction: 6 | 1 (12.5%) | PPV: 1 PPV + SB + Lens Extraction:6 | Tectonic PKP, PPV: 1 (12.5%) | Not Stated | Time from PPV to onset of symptoms of SO: median of 7 months. Follow-up from onset of symptoms: 10.5 months Initial VA in sympathizing eye: 0.67 ± 0.56 LogMAR Final VA in the sympathizing eye: 0.47 ± 0.59 |

Table 1. Cont.

| Study Name | Year of Publication | Country | Age of SO Patients after VR Surgery (Average ± SD) | Study Design | Duration (y.) | Number of SO Cases in the Study | Number of Cases of SO after Trauma (N and %) in the Study | Number of Cases of SO after Surgery (N and %) in the Study | Number of Cases of SO after VR Surgery (±Lens Extraction) (N and %) in the Study | Number of Cases of SO after Other Surgeries (N and %) in the Study | VR Procedures | Other Surgeries | Total Number of VR Procedures in the Study | Other Relevant Parameters Evaluated |
|---|---|---|---|---|---|---|---|---|---|---|---|---|---|---|
| Grigoropoulos et al. [11] | 2006 | UK | Not stated | Cohort | Not stated | 1 | 0 | 0 | 1 | 0 | PPV + 210° retinectomy. | None | 1142 operations performed on the 304 eyes. | VA was limited to PL and the eye was hypotonus. Thirty-one months after the initial procedure and 9 months after the last procedure, the fellow eye developed SO. VA in the fellow eye decreased from 6/9 to 6/18 and remained stable |
| Su et al. [18] | 2005 | Singapore | 63 ± 19.98 | Case series | 1993–2003, ten years | 10 (1.08%) | Exclusively Trauma: 1 (10%) Trauma + Surgery: 3 (30%) | 6 (60%) | Exclusively Retinal Surgery: 1 (10%) Retinal Surgery + Lens extraction: 2 (20%) | 3 (30%) | Not stated | TCP: 2 YAG-TCP: 1 | 924 | Retinal surgery patients: Patient 1: initial VA in SE: 0.4 LogMAR Final VA in SE: 0.7 LogMAR Patient 2: initial VA in SE: 0.4 LogMAR Final VA in SE: 0.5 LogMAR Patient 3: initial VA in SE: HM Final VA in SE: NPL Interval between IE and onset of symptoms: (mean ± SD): 29 ± 32.3 months |

Table 1. Cont.

| Study Name | Year of Publication | Country | Age of SO Patients after VR Surgery (Average ± SD) | Study Design | Duration (y.) | Number of SO Cases in the Study | Number of Cases of SO after Trauma (N and %) in the Study | Number of Cases of SO after Surgery (N and %) in the Study | Number of Cases of SO after VR Surgery (±Lens Extraction) (N and %) in the Study | Number of Cases of SO after Other Surgeries (N and %) in the Study | VR Procedures | Other Surgeries | Total Number of VR Procedures in the Study | Other Relevant Parameters Evaluated: |
|---|---|---|---|---|---|---|---|---|---|---|---|---|---|---|
| Gupta et al. [10] | 2007 | India | Not stated | Cross-Sectional | June 1989–August 2004, 15 years and 2 months | 40 | 30 (75%) | 10 (25%) | Exclusively Retinal Surgery: 4 (10%) | 6 (15%) | PPV: 2 (5%) SB: 2 (5%) | Lens extraction: 5 (12.5%) Glaucoma Filtration Surgery: 1 (2.5%) | Not stated | / |
| Kumar et al. [13] | 2013 | India | Not stated (pediatric age) | Cross-Sectional | 2001–2011, ten years | 14 | Exclusively Trauma: 13 (92.9%) | 1 (7.1%) | Exclusively Retinal Surgery: 1 (7.1%) | 0 | PPV: 1 (7.1%) | / | 2511 pediatric patients with open globe injuries | / |
| Rishi et al. [17] | 2015 | India | 39.4 ± 14.72 | Comparative case series | 1995–2011, 16 years | 17 | Trauma + VR surgery: 7 (41.2%) | 10 (58.8%) | Exclusively Retinal Surgery: 5 (29.4%) Retinal Surgery + Lens extraction: 5 (29.4%) | 0 | SB: 3 SB + PPV: 2 | None | Not stated | Initial VA in SE (mean ± SD): 0.78 ± 0.72 Final VA in SE (mean ± SD): 0.26 ± 0.55 Follow-up (mean ± SD): 45 ± 52.74 months Duration of symptoms 22.5 days Interval between surgery and SO (mean ± SD): 38.1 ± 52.79 months Average Follow-up period 34 months |
| Guzman-Salas et al. [15] | 2016 | Mexico | Not Stated | Cross-Sectional | 2007–2013, 6 years | 20 | 10 (50%) | 10 (50%) | Exclusively Retinal Surgery: 3 (15%) | 7 (45%) | Retinopexy | Lens Extraction: 6 (30%) Ahmed valve implantation 1 (5%) | Not Stated | / |

Table 1. Cont.

| Study Name | Year of Publication | Country | Age of SO Patients after VR Surgery (Average ± SD) | Study Design | Duration (y.) | Number of SO Cases in the Study | Number of Cases of SO after Trauma (N and %) in the Study | Number of Cases of SO after Surgery (N and %) in the Study | Number of Cases of SO after VR Surgery (±Lens Extraction) (N and %) in the Study | Number of Cases of SO Surgeries after Other Surgeries (N and %) in the Study | VR Procedures | Other Surgeries: | Total Number of VR Procedures in the Study | Other Relevant Parameters Evaluated: |
|---|---|---|---|---|---|---|---|---|---|---|---|---|---|---|
| Dutta Majumder et al. [12] | 2017 | India | Not Stated | Cross-Sectional | June 1994–November 2015: 21 years and 5 months | 197 | Not Stated | 14 (7.1%) | Exclusively Retinal Surgery: 8 (4.1%) | 6 (3%) | SB: 4 (2%) PPV: 4 (2%) | Lens Extraction: 1 (0.5%) Lens Extraction + Anterior Vitrectomy: 3 (1.5%) Trabeculectomy: 1 (0.5%) PKP: 1 (0.5%) | Not Stated | / |
| Tyagi et al. [20] | 2019 | India | 41.14 ± 16.53 | Retrospective case series | 2005–2015, ten years | 175 | 0 | 16 (9.1%) | Exclusively Retinal Surgery: 13 (7.4%) Retinal Surgery + Lens extraction: 3 (1.7%) | Not Stated | PPV: 8 (4.6%) SB + PPV: 5 (2.9%) | Not Stated | 41.365 PPV | Time interval from surgery to diagnosis (mean): 154 days 2. VA: Initial VA in SE (mean ± SD): 1.03 ± 0.56 LogMar Final VA in SE (mean ± SD): 0.43 ± 0.57 LogMar Duration of follow-up of (mean) 25.8 months Duration from surgery (days): 1943 ± 349.28 |
| Tan et al. [19] | 2018 | India UK Singapore | Not Stated | Retrospective Multicenter Case Series | 1995–2014, 9 years | 130 | 94 (72.3%) | 36 (27.9%) | 13 (36.1%) | 23 | Not Stated | Lens Extraction 11 (30.5%) Glaucoma surgery 6 (16.7%) Others: 6 (16.7%) | Not Stated | / |

**Table 1.** *Cont.*

| Study Name | Year of Publication | Country | Age of SO Patients after VR Surgery (Average ± SD) | Study Design | Duration (y.) | Number of SO Cases in the Study | Number of Cases of SO after Trauma (N and %) in the Study | Number of Cases of SO after Surgery (N and %) in the Study | Number of Cases of SO after VR Surgery (±Lens Extraction) (N and %) in the Study | Number of Cases of SO after Other Surgeries (N and %) in the Study | VR Procedures | Other Surgeries: | Total Number of VR Procedures in the Study | Other Relevant Parameters Evaluated: |
|---|---|---|---|---|---|---|---|---|---|---|---|---|---|---|
| Dutta Majumder et al. [8] | 2020 | India | Not Stated (Pediatric Age) | Retrospective Case Series | December 1997–January 2017, 19 years, 1 month | 20 | Exclusively Trauma: 13 (65%) Trauma + Surgery: 4 (20%) | 3 (15%) | 3 (15%) | 0 | Not Stated | None | Not Stated | / |
| Anikina et al. [14] | 2022 | UK | | Cross-Sectional | January 2000 and December 2015, 15 year period | 61 | 40 (65.6%) | 21 (34.4%) as main trigger | 13 (21.3%) as main trigger | Not Stated | 10 multiple procedures: SB: 6 PPV: 21 (1 of the cases involved a combination). | Not Stated | 39.391 VR procedures SO after a single VR procedure was estimated to be 0.008%, rising to 6.67% with 7 procedures | / |

Abbreviations: DTX: radiotherapy, PPV: pars plana vitrectomy, Enucl = enucleation, Cyclodiodetx = cyclodiodetherapy, RD: retinal detachment, Ext = external, PKP: penetrating keratoplasty, SB: scleral buckle, LogMAR: Logarithm of the Minimum Angle of Resolution, PL: perception light, TCP: diode laser trans-scleral cyclophotoablation, Yag: neodymium:yttrium-argen-garnet, HM: hand movement, NPL: non-perception light, VR: vitreoretinal, SO: sympathetic ophthalmitis, SD: standard deviation, SE: sympathizing eye, IE: inciting event, y: years, N: number; VA: visual acuity.

## 4. Discussion

Our systematic review and meta-analysis aimed to evaluate the morbidity frequency measures in terms of the cumulative incidence of SO triggered by single or multiple VR surgery procedures in eyes without an antecedent history of trauma and previous ocular surgery, except for previous or concomitant uneventful lens extraction, and to further investigate the relationship between VR surgery and SO.

Analyzing data from thirteen studies, we found that the cumulative incidence of SO after single or multiple VR surgery in eyes with no history of trauma or previous ocular surgery, except for previous or concomitant uneventful lens extraction, was equal to 14% (CIs: 0.08–0.21%, $p < 0.01$) among patients who developed SO regardless of the main trigger [6–10,12–15,17–20].

The proportion of surgically induced SO has been increasing over the years, as previously stated by Su et al. [18], who found that SO occurred in 70% of their patients following ocular surgery, especially VR. Indeed, uveal protein release might occur during different VR surgical steps, such as the creation of sclerotomies, cryo-retinopexy, or subretinal and fluid drainage. This trend has increased, according to data reported by Hakin et al. [28], Jennings et al. [7], and Kilmartin et al. [6], from 17% to 56% from 1974 to 1998. Tan et al. also observed this increasing trend [19]. Among several reasons, the increase in surgically induced SO could be attributed to the advancements in vitreoretinal surgery. Indeed, more cases that would have previously been dismissed are now being operated on by ophthalmologists, including complicated cases that require multiple surgeries or procedures. The high level of advancement in VR surgery has also raised patient expectations, and more patients are likely to undergo numerous procedures on the same eye. In contrast, in their retrospective analysis, Dutta et al. [8], evaluating the clinical pattern of postsurgical SO in a tertiary eye care center in India, found a relatively lower proportion of surgically induced SO (7.10% had surgically induced SO). These data were consistent with those of Kumar et al. [13], who found a proportion of surgically induced SO of 7.1% in the pediatric population in an Indian center. This may be partially explained, considering that most Indian people reside in rural areas, where they often have poor access to personal protective equipment at work and have disproportionately low levels of awareness of eye safety. According to these data, our subgroup meta-analysis showed a higher rate of VR-induced SO in European countries compared to Asian countries, 25% (CIs: 0.16–0.35) vs. 12% (CIs: 0.06–0.17), $p < 0.01$. No reliable data could be obtained from American countries, as most of the studies were conducted before 1990 [7,9], and only in that year, de Juan and Hickingbotham developed the first 25-gauge (0.5 mm diameter) vitrectomy system based on conventional sclerotomy methods [29].

Unfortunately, repeated surgical procedures result in higher levels of uveal protein release. In 2022, Anikina et al. supported the increased proportion of surgically induced SO, analyzing the role of multiple VR surgery procedures and the type of VR intervention. They found that only eight (13%) patients had undergone a single event before their SO diagnosis. Specifically, VR surgery was performed before the diagnosis of SO in 25 of 61 cases, representing 41% of their entire cohort [14]. In addition, they suggested that the greater-than-average surgical complexity in VR surgery was responsible for many cases of VR-induced SO. Indeed, out of 25 VR procedures performed, there was a 29% retinectomy rate of PPV and a 57% rate of the use of silicone oil tamponade, and the higher number of procedural steps as well as the increased length of surgical time allowed a higher ocular antigen exposure to the immune system, potentially leading to SO.

With regard to different numbers of VR procedures, the authors were the first to analyze the effect of multiple VR procedures on the incidence of SO, demonstrating that performing two VR procedures on a patient raised the incidence of SO by a ten-fold increase in comparison to only performing one VR procedure on a patient. There was an exponential increase in risk according to the number of procedures, with 6.67% of patients who underwent seven VR procedures developing SO. Furthermore, despite pars plana vitrectomy being associated with twice the risk as compared to external retinal detachment repair surgeries [30], Dutta et al. [12] found that the incidence of SO following pars plana vitrectomy and scleral buckle surgery was the same, as previously published by Gupta et al. [10]. Indeed, patients undergoing scleral buckle surgery also face the risk of developing SO, as these procedures are usually associated with subretinal drainage, which may expose uveal antigens [12].

The pooled cumulative incidence of SO triggered by single or multiple VR surgery procedures in eyes without an antecedent history of trauma and previous ocular surgery, except for previous or concomitant uneventful lens extraction among patients who underwent VR surgery procedures, was equal to 0.03% (CIs: 0.004–0.02%, $p = 0.25$). Our results are consistent with the most recent data retrieved and published by Anikina et al., who analyzed 39,391 VR procedures performed over 15 years. They found 13 cases of SO triggered by VR surgery alone, corresponding to 1 in 3030 (0.03%) cases [14]. Accordingly, in 2019 Tyagi et al. found 16 cases of SO after VR surgery alone, corresponding to 1 in 2585 (0.04%) cases [20].

One of our systematic review and meta-analyses' strengths is that we included many studies retrieving data from patients of different countries covering a considerable period, making our findings generalizable. Moreover, we systematically evaluated all reports without timespan restriction, analyzing data from 40-year time studies. Our subgroup analyses did not significantly alter our results. Nevertheless, this systematic review and meta-analysis has several limitations. First, we limited our literature search to the English language, and no articles in Chinese and Japanese, including data from those populations, were retrieved. Therefore, the Asian subgroup mostly included articles whose data were retrieved in South Asia. Second, we only included thirteen studies in our meta-analysis. Third, we included in our meta-analysis, data of patients regardless of age combining data from the pediatric and adult populations; fourth, the meta-analysis included data collected after hand-searching the numerical data that could increase the risk of biases. Fifth, we found high heterogeneity, which our subgroup meta-analysis model only partially explained. This implies that other unknown sources of heterogeneity were present and may have heavily biased our results. Sixth, we recruited studies from different periods where the surgical instruments and techniques differed according to the technological advances of that era. Seventh, most of the included studies were retrospective and had intrinsic limitations, producing biased or inaccurate estimates. Eighth, due to the nature of the included studies, heterogeneous incidence rates, selection bias from different types of VR surgeries and VR diseases, and the inclusion of survey studies that are not methodologically comparable to retrospective studies could be an additional source of biases. In addition, in the oldest studies, the definition of SO was elusive or ill-defined, particularly in cases that manifested long after the surgery. The follow-up times in each study were variable, although SO can develop up to 66 years after the inciting injury. Finally, we synthesized data from patients that underwent single or multiple VR surgeries.

## 5. Conclusions

To the best of our knowledge, this is the first meta-analysis synthesizing the morbidity frequency measures of SO triggered by single or multiple VR surgery procedures in eyes without an antecedent history of trauma and previous ocular surgery, except for previous or concomitant uneventful lens extraction.

Although postsurgical sympathetic ophthalmitis is rare, it is a bilateral blinding disease. Despite its success and low incidence rate, VR surgery should be viewed as a possible inciting event for SO. Hence, ophthalmologists may consider counseling patients who require surgical single or multiple procedures about this risk. This could lead to better decision making and a more accurate process of consent for surgery.

**Supplementary Materials:** The following supporting information can be downloaded at: https://www.mdpi.com/article/10.3390/jcm12062316/s1, Supplementary Material S1: Detailed Research Strategy Material; Supplementary Material S2: PRISMA Checklist [31]; Supplementary Material S3: Risk of bias evaluation and GRADE assessment.

**Author Contributions:** Conceptualization: M.R.; methodology, M.R. and L.M.; software, M.R.; validation, L.M., G.D.P., M.D.T., R.R., C.C., R.F., A.F., T.E., S.G. and M.R.; formal analysis, M.R.; investigation, M.R.; resources, M.R.; data curation, M.R.; writing—original draft preparation, M.R.; writing—review and editing, M.R.; visualization, M.R.; supervision, L.M.; project administration, M.R. All authors have read and agreed to the published version of the manuscript.

**Funding:** This research received no external funding.

**Institutional Review Board Statement:** Not applicable.

**Informed Consent Statement:** Not applicable.

**Data Availability Statement:** Not applicable.

**Conflicts of Interest:** The authors declare no conflict of interest.

## References

1. Lucchini, S.; Govetto, A.; Carini, E.; Casalino, G.; Donati, S.; Radice, P. Presumed sympathetic ophthalmia following scleral buckling surgery: A case report and review of the literature. *Eur. J. Ophthalmol.* **2022**, *14*, 11206721221145212. [CrossRef]
2. Vote, B.J.; Hall, A.; Cairns, J.; Buttery, R. Changing trends in sympathetic ophthalmia. *Clin. Exp. Ophthalmol.* **2004**, *32*, 542–545. [CrossRef]
3. Galor, A.; Davis, J.L.; Flynn, H.W.; Feuer, W.J.; Dubovy, S.R.; Setlur, V.; Kesen, M.R.; Goldstein, D.A.; Tessler, H.H.; Ganelis, I.B.; et al. Sympathetic ophthalmia: Incidence of ocular complications and vision loss in the sympathizing eye. *Am. J. Ophthalmol.* **2009**, *148*, 704–710. [CrossRef] [PubMed]
4. Marak, G.E. Recent advances in sympathetic ophthalmia. *Surv. Ophthalmol.* **1979**, *24*, 141–156. [CrossRef]
5. Lam, S.; Tessler, H.H.; Lam, B.L.; Wilensky, J.T. High incidence of sympathetic ophthalmia after contact and noncontact neodymium: YAG cyclotherapy. *Ophthalmology* **1992**, *99*, 1818–1822. [CrossRef]
6. Kilmartin, D.J.; Dick, A.D.; Forrester, J.V. Prospective surveillance of sympathetic ophthalmia in the UK and Republic of Ireland. *Br. J. Ophthalmol.* **2000**, *84*, 259–263. [CrossRef] [PubMed]
7. Jennings, T.; Tessler, H.H. Twenty cases of sympathetic ophthalmia. *Br. J. Ophthalmol.* **1989**, *73*, 140–145. [CrossRef]
8. Majumder, P.D.; Mistry, S.; Sridharan, S.; George, A.E.; Rao, V.; Ganesh, S.K.; Biswas, J. Pediatric sympathetic ophthalmia: 20 years of data from a tertiary eye center in India. *J. Pediatr. Ophthalmol. Strabismus* **2020**, *57*, 154–158. [CrossRef] [PubMed]
9. Gass, J.D.M. Sympathetic ophthalmia following vitrectomy. *Am. J. Ophthalmol.* **1982**, *93*, 552–558. [CrossRef]
10. Gupta, V.; Gupta, A.; Dogra, M.R. Posterior sympathetic ophthalmia: A single centre long-term study of 40 patients from North India. *Eye* **2008**, *22*, 1459–1464. [CrossRef] [PubMed]
11. Grigoropoulos, V.G.; Benson, S.; Bunce, C.; Charteris, D.G. Functional outcome and prognostic factors in 304 eyes managed by retinectomy. *Graefes Arch. Clin. Exp. Ophthalmol.* **2007**, *245*, 641–649. [CrossRef]
12. Dutta Majumder, P.; Anthony, E.; George, A.E.; Ganesh, S.K.; Biswas, J. Postsurgical sympathetic ophthalmia: Retrospective analysis of a rare entity. *Int. Ophthalmol.* **2018**, *38*, 2487–2493. [CrossRef]
13. Kumar, K.; Mathai, A.; Murthy, S.I.; Jalali, S.; Sangwan, V.; Reddy Pappuru, R.; Pathangay, A. Sympathetic ophthalmia in pediatric age group: Clinical features and challenges in management in a tertiary center in Southern India. *Ocul. Immunol. Inflamm.* **2014**, *22*, 367–372. [CrossRef] [PubMed]
14. Anikina, E.; Wagner, S.K.; Liyanage, S.; Sullivan, P.; Pavesio, C.; Okhravi, N. The risk of sympathetic ophthalmia after vitreoretinal surgery. *Ophthalmol. Retina* **2022**, *6*, 347–360. [CrossRef]
15. Guzman-Salas, P.J.; Serna-Ojeda, J.C.; Guinto-Arcos, E.B.; Pedroza-Seres, M. Characteristics of sympathetic ophthalmia in a single international center. *Open Ophthalmol. J.* **2016**, *10*, 154. [CrossRef] [PubMed]
16. Pollack, A.L.; McDonald, H.R.; Ai, E.; Green, W.R.; Halpern, L.S.; Jampol, L.M.; Leahy, J.M.; Johnson, R.N.; Spencer, W.H.; Stern, W.H.; et al. Sympathetic ophthalmia associated with Pars Plana Vitrectomy without antecedent penetrating trauma. *Retina* **2001**, *21*, 146–154. [CrossRef] [PubMed]
17. Rishi, E.; Rishi, P.; Appukuttan, B.; Walinjkar, J.; Biswas, J.; Sharma, T. Sympathetic ophthalmitis following vitreoretinal surgery: Does antecedent trauma make a difference? *Indian J. Ophthalmol.* **2015**, *63*, 692–698. [CrossRef]
18. Su, D.H.W.; Chee, S.P. Sympathetic ophthalmia in Singapore: New trends in an old disease. *Graefes Arch. Clin. Exp. Ophthalmol.* **2006**, *244*, 243–247. [CrossRef]
19. Tan, X.L.; Seen, S.; Dutta Majumder, P.; Ganesh, S.K.; Agarwal, M.; Soni, A.; Biswas, J.; Aggarwal, K.; Mahendradas, P.; Gupta, V.; et al. Analysis of 130 cases of sympathetic ophthalmia—A retrospective multicenter case series. *Ocul. Immunol. Inflamm.* **2018**, *27*, 1259–1266. [CrossRef]
20. Tyagi, M.; Agarwal, K.; Reddy Pappuru, R.R.; Dedhia, C.; Agarwal, H.; Nayak, S.; Panchal, B.; Kaza, H.; Basu, S.; Pathengay, A.; et al. Sympathetic ophthalmia after vitreoretinal surgeries: Incidence, clinical presentations and outcomes of a rare disease. *Semin. Ophthalmol.* **2019**, *34*, 157–162. [CrossRef]

21. Page, M.J.; McKenzie, J.E.; Bossuyt, P.M.; Boutron, I.; Hoffmann, T.C.; Mulrow, C.D.; Shamseer, L.; Tetzlaff, J.M.; Akl, E.A.; Brennan, S.E.; et al. The PRISMA 2020 statement: An updated guideline for reporting systematic reviews. *BMJ* **2021**, *372*, 105906. [CrossRef]
22. Cleo, G.; Scott, A.M.; Islam, F.; Julien, B.; Beller, E. Usability and acceptability of four systematic review automation software packages: A mixed method design. *Syst. Rev.* **2019**, *8*, 145. [CrossRef] [PubMed]
23. Lo, C.K.L.; Mertz, D.; Loeb, M. Newcastle-Ottawa Scale: Comparing reviewers' to authors' assessments. *BMC Med. Res. Methodol.* **2014**, *14*, 45. [CrossRef] [PubMed]
24. Munn, Z.; Barker, T.H.; Moola, S.; Tufanaru, C.; Stern, C.; McArthur, A.; Stephenson, M.; Aromataris, E. Methodological quality of case series studies: An introduction to the JBI critical appraisal Tool. *JBI Evid. Synth.* **2020**, *18*, 2127–2133. [CrossRef] [PubMed]
25. Balshem, H.; Helfand, M.; Schünemann, H.J.; Oxman, A.D.; Kunz, R.; Brozek, J.; Vist, G.E.; Falck-Ytter, Y.; Meerpohl, J.; Norris, S.; et al. GRADE guidelines: 3. rating the quality of evidence. *J. Clin. Epidemiol.* **2011**, *64*, 401–406. [CrossRef]
26. Guyatt, G.H.; Oxman, A.D.; Vist, G.E.; Kunz, R.; Falck-Ytter, Y.; Alonso-Coello, P.; Schünemann, H.J. GRADE: An emerging consensus on rating quality of evidence and strength of recommendations. *BMJ* **2008**, *336*, 924–926. [CrossRef]
27. Barker, T.H.; Borges Migliavaca, C.; Stein, C.; Colpani, V.; Falavigna, M.; Aromataris, E.; Munn, Z. Conducting proportional meta-analysis in different types of systematic reviews: A guide for synthesisers of evidence. *BMC Med. Res. Methodol.* **2021**, *21*, 189. [CrossRef]
28. Hakin, K.N.; Pearson, R.V.; Lightman, S.L. Sympathetic ophthalmia: Visual results with modern immunosuppressive therapy. *Eye* **1992**, *6 Pt 5*, 453–455. [CrossRef] [PubMed]
29. De Juan, E.; Hickingbotham, D. Refinements in microinstrumentation for vitreous surgery. *Am. J. Ophthalmol.* **1990**, *109*, 218–220. [CrossRef] [PubMed]
30. Haruta, M.; Mukuno, H.; Nishijima, K.; Takagi, H.; Kita, M. Sympathetic ophthalmia after 23-gauge transconjunctival sutureless vitrectomy. *Clin. Ophthalmol.* **2010**, *4*, 1347–1349. [CrossRef]
31. Moher, D.; Liberati, A.; Tetzlaff, J.; Altman, D.G.; The PRISMA Group. Preferred Reporting Items for Systematic Reviews and Meta-Analyses: The PRISMA Statement. *PLoS Med.* **2009**, *6*, e1000097. [CrossRef] [PubMed]

**Disclaimer/Publisher's Note:** The statements, opinions and data contained in all publications are solely those of the individual author(s) and contributor(s) and not of MDPI and/or the editor(s). MDPI and/or the editor(s) disclaim responsibility for any injury to people or property resulting from any ideas, methods, instructions or products referred to in the content.

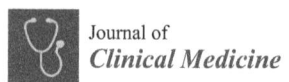 

*Article*

# Effect of Changes in Surgical Strategies for the Treatment of Primary Rhegmatogenous Retinal Detachment on Functional and Anatomical Outcomes: A Retrospective Analysis of 812 Cases from the Years 2004 to 2012

Aleksandra Sedova [1], Christoph Scholda [1], Thomas Huebl [1], Irene Steiner [2], Stefan Sacu [1], Michael Georgopoulos [1], Ursula Schmidt-Erfurth [1] and Andreas Pollreisz [1,*]

[1] Department of Ophthalmology and Optometry, Medical University of Vienna, 1090 Vienna, Austria
[2] Center for Medical Data Science (CeDAS), Institute of Medical Statistics, Medical University of Vienna, 1090 Vienna, Austria
* Correspondence: andreas.pollreisz@meduniwien.ac.at

**Abstract:** Background: At the Department of Ophthalmology and Optometry at the MUV surgical method (scleral buckling, vitrectomy, combined vitrectomy/scleral buckling) and timing (daytime, nighttime) for the treatment of primary rhegmatogenous retinal detachment (RRD) changed continuously in the years 2004 to 2012. This study aims to evaluate changes in surgical strategies over time including their impact on functional and anatomical outcomes. Methods: Retrospective evaluation of patients operated on primary RRD between the years 2004 and 2012. Baseline demographic data, month 3 best-corrected visual acuity (BCVA), surgical method, single success surgery, surgical timing, and intraoperative complications were analyzed. Results: Overall, 812 eyes of 812 patients with a mean (±SD) age of 58.1 ± 13.3 years were included. A total of 413 (51%) patients presented with macula-on and 359 (44%) with macula-off RRD. Month 3 BCVA increased over time, both in macula-on or macula-off groups ($p < 0.001$). The rate of complete retinal reattachment 3 months postoperatively increased significantly from 65% in 2004 to 83% in 2012 in both groups. Scleral buckling surgeries decreased continuously from 95% to 16% with an appropriate increase in vitrectomies as well as a decrease in surgeries during nighttime (68% in 2004, 6% in 2012) with equal or better visual and functional outcomes. Conclusion: Our data showed that improving functional and single-success surgery outcomes in patients operated on for primary RRD. In the years 2004 to 2012, surgical techniques shifted from scleral buckling to primary vitrectomy and were increasingly scheduled during the daytime.

**Keywords:** primary rhegmatogenous retinal detachment; retinal detachment surgery outcomes; scleral buckling; vitrectomy; combined vitrectomy/scleral buckling

**Citation:** Sedova, A.; Scholda, C.; Huebl, T.; Steiner, I.; Sacu, S.; Georgopoulos, M.; Schmidt-Erfurth, U.; Pollreisz, A. Effect of Changes in Surgical Strategies for the Treatment of Primary Rhegmatogenous Retinal Detachment on Functional and Anatomical Outcomes: A Retrospective Analysis of 812 Cases from the Years 2004 to 2012. *J. Clin. Med.* **2023**, *12*, 2278. https://doi.org/10.3390/jcm12062278

**Academic Editor:** Georgios D. Panos

Received: 13 February 2023
Revised: 9 March 2023
Accepted: 13 March 2023
Published: 15 March 2023

**Copyright:** © 2023 by the authors. Licensee MDPI, Basel, Switzerland. This article is an open access article distributed under the terms and conditions of the Creative Commons Attribution (CC BY) license (https://creativecommons.org/licenses/by/4.0/).

## 1. Introduction

Rhegmatogenous retinal detachment (RRD) is the most commonly occurring form of retinal detachment with the incidence ranging between 6.3 and 17.9 cases per 100,000 subjects per year [1]. It is defined as a pathological accumulation of fluid between the neurosensory retina and the retinal pigment epithelium caused by retinal tears and tractional forces allowing fluid influx [2]. RRD is a vision-threatening condition mainly affecting individuals over 50 years old and requiring retinal reattachment surgery [3]. Men are 1.3 to 2.3 times more likely to be diagnosed with RRD [1]. Timing of a surgical intervention is of uppermost importance for the visual outcome and is also dependent on the presence of macular detachment [4,5]. In cases with macula-off RRD, detachment of the macula causes photoreceptor cell death through apoptosis, which is responsible for poor visual outcomes [6]. Cells undergoing apoptosis are already found within 24 h following RRD, reaching a peak at 2 days and then dropping gradually over the following 5 days [6].

There are different methods for surgical repair available, including pars plana vitrectomy, scleral buckling, and pneumatic retinopexy [7,8]. Scleral buckling was first introduced by Custodis in 1949, widely popularized by Charles Schepens in the 1950s, and improved by Lincoff in the 1960s [9,10]. In the 1970s, pars plana vitrectomy was developed by Robert Machemer and proved to be equally effective as scleral buckling for the management of RRD [11–13]. In 1986, pneumatic retinopexy was firstly proposed by Hilton and Grizzard as a procedure for selected RRD cases, for which hospitalization is not needed [14]. All these techniques have undergone significant improvements since their introduction, with vitrectomy being the most commonly used surgical approach to date [15].

The aim of this retrospective study was to evaluate the effects of surgical method (scleral buckling vs. vitrectomy) and scheduling of surgery (routine daytime program vs. emergency surgery outside routine program including nighttime) on functional and anatomical outcomes in eyes with primary rhegmatogenous retinal detachment in a single tertiary referral center.

## 2. Materials and Methods

### 2.1. Subjects

This retrospective study was conducted at the Department of Ophthalmology and Optometry at the Medical University of Vienna (MUV) according to the Declaration of Helsinki, including current revisions and Good Clinical Practice (GCP) guidelines. The study protocol was approved by the Ethics Committee of MUV (Ethics number: EK1766/2016). Clinical records of all eyes treated for primary rhegmatogenous retinal detachment with either encircling scleral buckling, segmental scleral buckling or vitrectomy between the years 2004 and 2012 were reviewed by a vitreoretinal surgeon (A.P.). Exclusion criteria included cases with symptoms of retinal detachment for more than 4 weeks (due to expected inferior visual, functional, and morphological outcomes in macula-off patients) history of any prior vitreoretinal surgery, proliferative vitreoretinopathy stage C or higher, giant retinal tear, traumatic or post-traumatic retinal detachment, endophthalmitis or uveitis in the case history, retinoschisis-related detachment, and presence of retinal diseases (diabetic retinopathy, age-related macular degeneration, epiretinal membrane, macular hole), contralateral eye already presented with retinal detachment, incomplete data in the patient charts, follow-up visits less than 2 months after surgery (some patients prefer having their follow-up visits at their local eye center for travel distance reasons). Data collected included age, sex, surgical method, duration of surgery, presence of macula detachment (macula-off), preoperative and postoperative (3 months postoperatively) Snellen best corrected visual acuity (BCVA), intraoperative complications, lens status, single surgery anatomical outcome success, and timepoint of surgical intervention (daytime, nighttime). Single surgery anatomical success was defined as a complete attachment of the retina 2–3 months postoperatively after a single procedure. For analysis, the patients were divided into two groups depending on the presence of macula detachment (macula-on and macula-off groups). Further, surgeons were divided into two groups depending on their specialization: vitreoretinal surgery specialist and general ophthalmic surgeon. A total of 198 patients did not show up for their scheduled follow-up visit 3 months post-surgery. Re-surgeries were excluded from the analyses.

### 2.2. Surgical Procedure

The surgeries were performed by a total of 13 vitreoretinal surgery specialists and 17 general ophthalmic surgeons with all procedures done under general anesthesia. After disinfection of eyelids and periorbital skin with 5% polyvidone-iodine solution, polyvidone-iodine eye drops were applied at the beginning and at the end of surgery.

A 23-gauge ($n$ = 306, 78%) or 20-gauge ($n$ = 88, 22%) pars plana vitrectomy was performed with the OS3 surgery system (Oertli Instruments, Berneck, Switzerland) using peristaltic pump settings and a single-use pneumatic stripper (SPS) by all surgeons. For the 23-gauge system valved Oertli trocars were used, while for the 20-gauge system a trocar-free approach was applied. Every patient received a complete vitrectomy with cryo- or endolaser coagulation and gas (SF6, C2F6, or C3F8) or silicone oil filling.

The standard procedure for the scleral buckling procedure is as follows. After the opening of the conjunctiva at the limbus, the retinal tear was coagulated with cryocoagulation under indirect ophthalmoscopy. A scleral explant (radial or circumferential sponge, encircling silicone band) was fixated with 4-0 mersilene sutures. Subretinal drainage was performed based on the surgeon's discretion. The conjunctiva was closed with 7-0 vicryl sutures. In some cases, the vitrectomy procedure was combined with scleral buckling.

For analysis, the time of surgery was divided into a routine daytime program, which included surgeries performed between 7 am and 4 pm and an outside routine program encompassing surgeries between 4 pm and 7 am.

*2.3. Statistical Analysis*

Quantitative variables are reported as mean ± standard deviation. For qualitative variables, absolute frequencies and percentages are reported.

To analyze if BCVA at baseline changed over time, a univariate linear model was calculated with the year (2004–2012) as the independent variable for the entire sample and the two subgroups (macula-on and macula-off).

The effect of surgeon specialization (general ophthalmic surgeon/VR surgery specialist), scheduling of surgery (routine surgical program/outside routine surgical program), surgical method (vitrectomy/buckle/vitrectomy + buckle surgery), and year of surgery (2004–2012) on BCVA at month 3, was analyzed by linear models adjusted for BCVA at baseline. Additionally, a linear model with stepwise variable selection using the AIC criterion was calculated (R-function step), including all the independent variables mentioned above, whereby the interaction between year (2004–2012) and surgery before 2009 (yes/no) was additionally included as an independent variable. The null hypothesis of the interaction term is that the slope of the regression line does not differ between the years 2004–2008 and 2009–2012. The final model with the selected variables was then calculated using all valid observations. If the F-test of the surgical method revealed a $p$-value < 0.05, pairwise comparisons were conducted. The dichotomous endpoints "single success surgery" and "intraoperative complications" were analyzed analogously by calculating logistic regression models. Due to the small number of patients with intraoperative complications, no multivariable logistic regression model was calculated for this endpoint.

Statistical analyses were carried out with R 4.0.5. For all analyses, the significance level has been set to 0.05. Estimates are reported with 95% confidence limits. No adjustment for multiple testing was done. Hence, the interpretation of the $p$-values is descriptive.

## 3. Results

Eight-hundred and twelve eyes from 812 patients receiving surgical treatment for rhegmatogenous retinal detachment between the years 2004 and 2012 were eligible for inclusion in this retrospective study. The mean participant age at diagnosis was 58.1 ± 13.3. Out of these patients, 294 were female (36%). A total of 502 eyes (62%) were phakic, 294 eyes (36%) pseudophakic, and 16 eyes (2%) aphakic. Out of all operated eyes, 433 (53%) were right eyes. In addition, 413 (51%) patients presented with macula-on retinal detachment, and 359 (44%) patients with macula-off. In the surgical records of 40 (5%) patients, there was no indication regarding macula status. The number of macula-on patients was 45, 48, 45, 50, 40, 45, 51, 40, and 49, respectively in the 9 years ranging from 2004 to 2012. The number of macula-off patients was 27, 30, 37, 36, 48, 57, 43, 32, and 49, respectively analyzed in the same time period.

*3.1. Choice of Surgical Method over Time*

The number of performed vitrectomies increased continuously from 2004 to 2012 with an appropriate decrease in scleral buckling surgeries (Figure 1). While in the year 2004, 5% of surgeries were performed with vitrectomy, this number increased to 84% 8 years later. The number of performed 20-gauge vitrectomies was 5, 9, 11, 8, 14, 10, 21, 4, and 6, respectively between the years 2004 and 2012. The number of 23-gauge vitrectomies was 0, 0, 7, 21, 22, 45, 60, 67, and 84, respectively during the same time period. Scleral buckling procedures decreased from 92% of all surgeries in 2004 to 8% in the year 2012 (number of performed buckles between 2004 and 2012: 71, 68, 62, 60, 51, 47, 19, 9, and 8, respectively). Combined procedures of vitrectomy and scleral buckling were performed in 2, 10, 12, 11, 10, 13, 10, 2, and 8 cases, respectively, between 2004 and 2012 with no trend regarding frequency observable over these years. See Table 1 for detailed information about surgery type and intraocular tamponade.

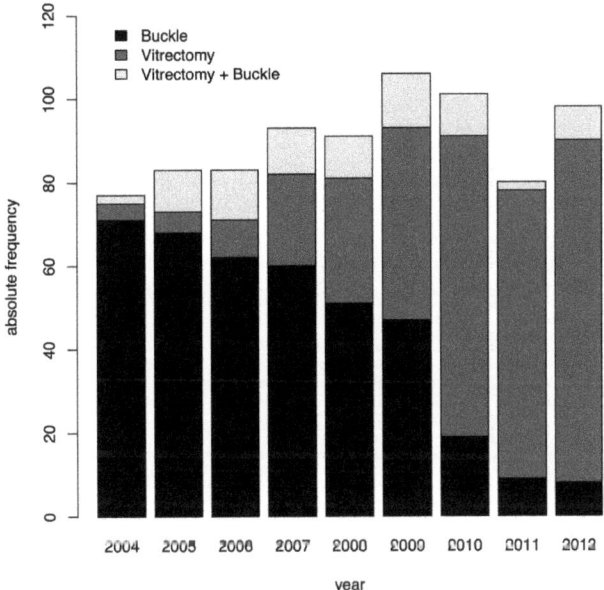

**Figure 1.** A bar chart showing the increasing number of performed vitrectomies (dark grey) in the years 2004 to 2012 with a simultaneous decrease of scleral buckle surgeries (black). The number of combined procedures (vitrectomy + scleral buckle) is shown in light grey.

**Table 1.** The number of performed procedures between the years 2004 and 2012 grouped according to the surgical method and gas/silicone oil filling ($n$ = number of surgeries per year; % = percentage per year).

| Year | Vitrectomy | | Scleral Buckling | Combined Vitrectomy/Scleral Buckling | |
|---|---|---|---|---|---|
| | Gas | Silicone Oil | | Gas | Silicone Oil |
| 2004 | $n = 0$ (0%) | $n = 4$ (5%) | $n = 71$ (92%) | $n = 1$ (1%) | $n = 1$ (1%) |
| 2005 | $n = 5$ (6%) | $n = 0$ (0%) | $n = 68$ (82%) | $n = 3$ (4%) | $n = 7$ (8%) |
| 2006 | $n = 9$ (11%) | $n = 0$ (0%) | $n = 62$ (75%) | $n = 8$ (10%) | $n = 4$ (5%) |
| 2007 | $n = 20$ (22%) | $n = 2$ (2%) | $n = 60$ (65%) | $n = 7$ (8%) | $n = 4$ (4%) |
| 2008 | $n = 25$ (27%) | $n = 5$ (5%) | $n = 51$ (56%) | $n = 8$ (9%) | $n = 2$ (2%) |
| 2009 | $n = 45$ (42%) | $n = 1$ (1%) | $n = 47$ (44%) | $n = 12$ (11%) | $n = 1$ (1%) |
| 2010 | $n = 70$ (69%) | $n = 2$ (2%) | $n = 19$ (19%) | $n = 8$ (8%) | $n = 2$ (2%) |
| 2011 | $n = 68$ (85%) | $n = 1$ (1%) | $n = 9$ (11%) | $n = 2$ (2%) | $n = 0$ (0%) |
| 2012 | $n = 79$ (81%) | $n = 3$ (3%) | $n = 8$ (8%) | $n = 6$ (6%) | $n = 2$ (2%) |

The number of performed vitrectomies was 5, 9, 18, 29, 36, 55, 81, 71, and 91 in the 9 years ranging from 2004 to 2012. The number of scleral buckle surgeries was 71, 74, 65, 63, 55, 51, 20, 9, and 7 in the same time period. Combined vitrectomy and scleral buckle procedures were performed in 2, 10, 12, 11, 10, 13, 10, 2, and 8 eyes during that time frame.

A total of 170 eyes (21%) required additional surgery due to not having an attached retina after the first surgery.

### 3.2. Scheduling of Surgery

In the years from 2008 to 2012, the majority of RD surgeries were performed during the routine surgical program ($n$ = 81%), while between 2004 and 2007 only 43% of cases were scheduled during the daytime. In the year 2004, 68% of eyes were operated outside the routine program including nighttime, four years later this number dropped to 25%, decreasing further within the next 4 years and reaching 6% in 2012. In the years 2004 to 2008 about 58% of procedures during the routine surgical program were performed by surgeons specialized in vitreoretinal surgery. From 2009 onwards this number increased to over 96%.

See Table 2 for a detailed overview of performed surgeries according to group and surgeon specialisation.

**Table 2.** The number of surgeries performed between the years 2004 and 2012 grouped according to time of surgery and surgeon specialization. $n$ = number of surgeries per year; % = percentage per year.

| | Routine Program (7 a.m.–4 p.m.) | | | | | | Outside Routine Program (4 p.m.–7 a.m.) | | | | | |
|---|---|---|---|---|---|---|---|---|---|---|---|---|
| | All Surgeons | | Vitreoretinal Surgery Specialists | | General Ophthalmic Surgeons | | All Surgeons | | Vitreoretinal Surgery Specialists | | General Ophthalmic Surgeons | |
| Year | $n$ | % of All Surgeries | $n$ | % of Surgeries in Routine Program | $n$ | % of Surgeries in Routine Program | $n$ | % of All Surgeries | $n$ | % of Surgeries Outside Routine Program | $n$ | % of Surgeries Outside Routine Program |
| 2004 | 24 | 32 | 10 | 42 | 14 | 58 | 52 | 68 | 16 | 31 | 36 | 69 |
| 2005 | 34 | 41 | 10 | 29 | 24 | 71 | 49 | 59 | 14 | 29 | 35 | 71 |
| 2006 | 39 | 47 | 19 | 49 | 20 | 51 | 44 | 53 | 16 | 36 | 28 | 64 |
| 2007 | 49 | 53 | 34 | 69 | 15 | 31 | 44 | 47 | 18 | 41 | 26 | 59 |
| 2008 | 68 | 75 | 51 | 75 | 17 | 25 | 23 | 25 | 12 | 52 | 11 | 48 |
| 2009 | 80 | 79 | 75 | 94 | 5 | 6 | 21 | 21 | 10 | 48 | 11 | 52 |
| 2010 | 83 | 82 | 80 | 96 | 3 | 4 | 18 | 18 | 14 | 78 | 4 | 22 |
| 2011 | 67 | 86 | 67 | 100 | 0 | 0 | 11 | 14 | 11 | 100 | 0 | 0 |
| 2012 | 89 | 94 | 86 | 97 | 3 | 3 | 6 | 6 | 6 | 100 | 0 | 0 |

The average time from the first presentation at the clinic to surgery increased from 0.5 to 1.48 days from 2004 to 2012.

### 3.3. Visual Acuity Outcomes

#### 3.3.1. Visual Acuity at Baseline

Among all macula-on and macula-off patients, BCVA at baseline did not change significantly over time (mean change per year [95% CI]: 0.00097 [−0.009; 0.011], $p$ = 0.9). Within macula-off patients, the change of BCVA at baseline over time was statistically not significant either (mean change per year [95% CI]: 0.0044 [−0.00054; 0.0093], $p$ = 0.08). Within macula-on patients, there was a borderline significant increase over time (0.011 [0.00005; 0.022], $p$ = 0.050). Patients with unknown macula status at the time of surgery due to incomplete medical records were excluded from this analysis.

#### 3.3.2. Visual Acuity 3 Months Postoperatively in Macula-On Patients

In the macula-on patients, BCVA 3 months postoperatively significantly increased over time (mean change per year adjusted for visual acuity at baseline [95% CI]: 0.021 [0.009; 0.032], $p$ = 0.0005; Figure 2A). BCVA 3 months postoperatively was on average significantly higher in patients after vitrectomy compared to scleral buckling (mean difference adjusted for visual acuity at baseline [95% CI]: 0.064 [0.002; 0.126], $p = 0.04$) and significantly lower in patients after combined vitrectomy/scleral buckling compared to vitrectomy (−0.142 [−0.264; −0.019], $p = 0.02$), whereas the difference between combined vitrectomy/scleral buckling vs. scleral buckling was not statistically significant (−0.078 [−0.197; 0.042], $p = 0.2$). Surgeons' specialization in retinal surgery (0.02 [−0.04; 0.08], $p = 0.5$), scheduling of surgery (−0.02 [−0.08; 0.04], $p = 0.5$) had no significant effect on BCVA at month 3. In the stepwise linear regression model, only BCVA at baseline and year of surgery remained in the model.

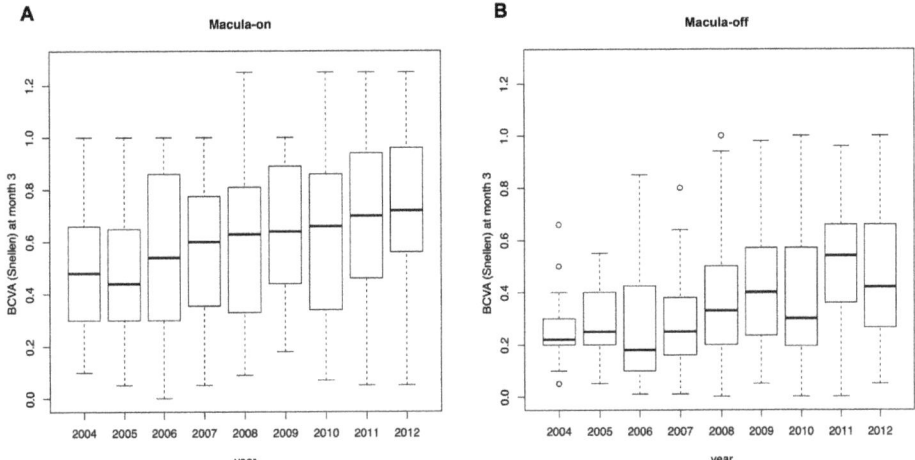

**Figure 2.** Box plots of BCVA (Snellen) at baseline and at month 3 in macula-on (**A**) and macula-off (**B**) patients grouped by year of surgery. In the box plots, the inferior boundary of the box indicates the 25th percentile, a black line within the box marks the median, and the superior boundary of the box indicates the 75th percentile. Outliers are defined as values that are smaller/greater than 1.5 times the interquartile range (IQR) from the box. Whiskers above and below the box indicate the minimum and the maximum, respectively, if no outliers are present. In the case of outliers, the whiskers extend to the smallest/largest value within the interval [25th percentile − 1.5 IQR; 75th percentile + 1.5 IQR].

### 3.3.3. Visual Acuity 3 Months Postoperatively in Macula-Off Patients

In the macula-off patients, univariate analyses adjusted for BCVA at baseline revealed a significant effect on BCVA 3 months postoperatively of surgery year (0.027 [0.017; 0.038], $p < 0.0001$; Figure 2B), surgeons' specialization in retinal surgery (0.13 [0.07; 0.19], $p < 0.0001$) and surgical method (F-test: $p < 0.0001$), but not of the scheduling of surgery (−0.009 [−0.075; 0.058], $p = 0.8$). In the stepwise linear regression model, the variables BCVA at baseline (0.55 [0.33; 0.77], $p < 0.0001$), surgeons' specialization in retinal surgery, surgery time, and surgical method were selected. BCVA 3 months postoperatively was higher for surgeries performed by surgeons specialized in retinal surgery compared to general ophthalmic surgeons (0.098 [0.032; 0.16], $p = 0.004$). Scheduling of surgery did not have any statistically significant effect on BCVA 3 months postoperatively (0.062 [−0.005; 0.13], $p = 0.07$). BCVA 3 months postoperatively was significantly higher in patients after vitrectomy compared to scleral buckling (0.115 [0.054; 0.177], $p = 0.0003$) and significantly lower after combined vitrectomy/scleral buckling compared to vitrectomy (−0.135 [−0.213; −0.058], $p = 0.0007$), whereas the comparison of combined vitrectomy/scleral buckling with scleral buckling was not statistically significant (−0.02 [−0.099; 0.059], $p = 0.6$).

### 3.4. Single Surgery Anatomical Success

The rate of complete retinal reattachment after a single procedure increased from 64% (46/72 eyes) in 2004 to 83% (81/98 eyes) in 2012 regardless of the surgical method. See

Table 3 for detailed information. Patients with missing macula status in medical records at the time of surgery were excluded from this analysis.

**Table 3.** The number of single surgery anatomical success surgeries from 2004 to 2012 grouped according to macula status and surgical method ($n$ = number of surgeries with single surgery anatomical success per year; % = percentage per year). Patients with missing macula status are not included.

| Year | Macula-On | Macula-Off | Vitrectomy | Scleral Buckling | Combined Vitrectomy/Scleral Buckling |
|---|---|---|---|---|---|
| 2004 | $n$ = 27 (60%) | $n$ = 19 (70%) | $n$ = 3 (100%) | $n$ = 41 (61%) | $n$ = 2 (100%) |
| 2005 | $n$ = 26 (54%) | $n$ = 20 (67%) | $n$ = 1 (20%) | $n$ = 38 (59%) | $n$ = 7 (78%) |
| 2006 | $n$ = 29 (64%) | $n$ = 25 (68%) | $n$ = 8 (89%) | $n$ = 38 (62%) | $n$ = 8 (67%) |
| 2007 | $n$ = 32 (64%) | $n$ = 23 (64%) | $n$ = 13 (72%) | $n$ = 37 (64%) | $n$ = 5 (50%) |
| 2008 | $n$ = 28 (70%) | $n$ = 36 (75%) | $n$ = 19 (66%) | $n$ = 36 (72%) | $n$ = 9 (100%) |
| 2009 | $n$ = 31 (69%) | $n$ = 45 (79%) | $n$ = 34 (77%) | $n$ = 31 (67%) | $n$ = 11 (92%) |
| 2010 | $n$ = 39 (76%) | $n$ = 37 (86%) | $n$ = 54 (82%) | $n$ = 13 (72%) | $n$ = 9 (90%) |
| 2011 | $n$ = 32 (80%) | $n$ = 25 (78%) | $n$ = 51 (82%) | $n$ = 5 (62%) | $n$ = 1 (50%) |
| 2012 | $n$ = 38 (78%) | $n$ = 43 (88%) | $n$ = 70 (85%) | $n$ = 5 (62%) | $n$ = 6 (75%) |

3.4.1. Single Surgery Anatomical Success in Macula-On Patients

In the univariate logistic regression models, surgeons' specialization in retinal surgery (OR [95% CI]: 2.2 [1.42; 3.33], $p$ = 0.0003), surgical method (F-test: $p$ = 0.005), and year of surgery (OR [95% CI]: 1.15 [1.06; 1.25], $p$ = 0.001) had a significant effect on single surgery success, but not scheduling of surgery (0.81 [0.53; 1.24], $p$ = 0.3). The odds for single success surgery were higher in vitrectomy compared to scleral buckling (OR [95% CI]: 2.12 [1.34; 3.34], $p$ = 0.001), whereas the comparisons with combined vitrectomy/scleral buckling were not statistically significant (vitrectomy + buckle vs. buckle: $p$ = 0.25, vitrectomy + buckle vs. vitrectomy: $p$ = 0.64). In the stepwise logistic regression model, surgeons' specialization in retinal surgery and year of surgery remained in the model. According to this final model, the odds for single success surgery were 1.13 times higher (95% CI: [1.01; 1.26], $p$ = 0.03) for surgeons specializing in retinal surgery compared to general ophthalmic surgeons and increased with increasing surgery year, but the effect of surgery years did not reach statistical significance (OR [95% CI]: 1.017 [0.997; 1.038], $p$ = 0.1).

3.4.2. Single Surgery Anatomical Success in Macula-Off Patients

Surgeons' specialization in retinal surgery (2.4 [1.40; 3.98], $p$ = 0.001), surgical method (F-test: $p$ = 0.01), and year of surgery (1.17 [1.06; 1.29], $p$ = 0.003), but not the scheduling of surgery (0.81 [0.45; 1.43], $p$ = 0.5) had a significant effect on single surgery success. The odds for single surgery success were higher in patients after vitrectomy compared to scleral buckling (OR [95% CI]: 2.11 [1.24; 3.57], $p$ = 0.006), but the comparisons with combined vitrectomy/scleral buckling were not statistically significant (vitrectomy + scleral buckling compared to scleral buckling: 2.02 [0.91; 4.5], $p$ = 0.09, vitrectomy + scleral buckling compared to vitrectomy: 0.96 [0.42; 2.2], $p$ = 0.9). In the stepwise logistic regression model, surgeons' specialization in retinal surgery (OR [95% CI]: 1.13 [0.999; 1.27], $p$ = 0.053) and surgery year (OR [95% CI]: 1.02 [0.996; 1.04], $p$ = 0.1) remained in the model, but these variables failed to reach statistical significance.

*3.5. Intraoperative Complications*

Among macula-on and macula-off patients operated on in the years 2004–2008, intraoperative complications, such as vitreous hemorrhage, iatrogenic retinal defects, choroidal hemorrhage, displacement of infusion cannula, and scleral perforation when placing scleral sutures occurred in 24 out of 406 eyes (5.9%). Among macula-on and macula-off patients operated on in the years 2009–2012, intraoperative complications occurred in 16 out of 366 eyes (4.4%). In the macula-on patients as well as in macula-off patients, intraoperative complications did not change significantly over time ($p = 0.5/p = 0.4$). In the macula-on/macula-off groups, surgeons' specialization in retinal surgery ($p = 0.7/p = 0.2$), surgical method ($p = 0.5/p = 0.6$), scheduling of surgery ($p = 0.3/p = 0.9$) had no significant effect on intraoperative complications. Patients with missing information in the medical records regarding macula status at the time of surgery were not included in this analysis.

## 4. Discussion

In our study, we evaluated changes in surgical strategies for the treatment of RRD and their impact on functional and anatomical outcomes. Between 2004 and 2012 we observed a shift in surgical methods from scleral buckling towards vitrectomy as well as in surgical scheduling towards a routine daytime program. These changes in treatment strategies led to an improvement in functional and single-surgery success outcome.

In 2008, a new strategy for the treatment of RRD was implemented in our department. The modified approach called for surgery with a delay of no longer than 24 h for macula-on and 48 h for patients presenting with macula-off RRD. This strategy provided better planning and an opportunity to perform surgery during a routine daytime program preferably by vitreoretinal surgery specialists.

The macula status at the time of surgery is the main prognostic factor for visual outcome. Several studies have shown visual prognosis to be directly correlated with the duration of macula-off RRD, while others demonstrated that a surgery delay of up to 7–8 days does not affect visual results [4,16–20]. In cases with an attached macula, a timely surgical intervention is recommended in order to prevent detachment of the macula with worse visual outcomes [5,21]. Ehrlich et al. showed in a retrospective study of patients with macula-on RRD treated with small-gauge vitrectomy, that no statistically significant correlation was found between time to surgery and anatomical and visual outcomes. However, 83% of patients were operated on within 24 h of their presentation at the clinic. Similar results among patients with macula-on RRD yet managed with scleral buckling (56% of subjects treated within 24 h) were reported by Wykoff et al. [22]. In a prospective study by Ho et al. analyzing eyes with macula-on RRD, a shift of subretinal fluid towards the macula in 13% of eyes at the time of surgery was observed, leading to macular detachment only in 4% of eyes (2 cases within 24 h, 1 case at day 4) [23]. In this study, slightly over 60% of cases were treated within 24 h and 26% of surgeries were performed outside normal working hours [23]. These studies support our results that a minimal delay of the surgery (maximum 24 h for macula-on cases) does not worsen functional and visual outcomes.

Surgery for RRD performed as an emergency after regularly planned cases or during nighttime has an impact on the performance of staff due to fatigue, which may lead to higher complication rates [24]. Furthermore, having a surgical team available and keeping the facilities running during night hours usually results in higher costs [25].

In general, macula-on RRD has a better visual prognosis compared to macula-off RDD [26]. In our study, mean BCVA 3 months postoperatively improved significantly from 2004 to 2012, both in subjects with macula-on or macula-off detachments. Among macula-off patients treated after 2008, the mean BCVA 3 months postoperatively was significantly higher in the vitrectomy group compared to the scleral buckling group. Also, macula-on patients operated on after the year 2008 showed better visual outcomes in the vitrectomy group, but these changes were not statistically significant. In a prospective study with 199 macula-on patients treated with scleral buckling, Wykoff et al. showed that the median BCVA two months postoperatively was similar (0.67) to the one observed among our patients. In a retrospective study by Bourla et al., analyzing 25 patients with vitrectomy operations, the mean final BCVA was 0.7 in the macula-on group and 0.3 in the macula-off group, which corresponds to our results [27]. In our study, there was a minimal decrease in the mean BCVA in macula-on patients from baseline, which is clinically not significant and potentially caused by cataract formation. In the medical charts reviewed, cataract grades were not recorded and cataract surgeries were often performed in other centers with no access to these data.

In a large prospective study on 291 subjects with macula-off RRD, two thirds of patients demonstrated final BCVA to be over 0.33 Snellen [16]. Among these subjects, 77% were treated with vitrectomy. Another prospective study conducted by Heimann et al. showed a statistically significantly better final BCVA in the scleral buckling group (0.5 Snellen) compared to the vitrectomy group (0.33 Snellen) among phakic patients. Upon taking into account pseudophakic/aphakic patients, there was no difference in BCVA improvement between both treatment groups [28]. A systematic Cochrane Review comparing vitrectomy and scleral buckling in the treatment of RRD published in 2019 revealed similar outcomes regarding visual acuity [29].

In our study, the rate of complete retinal attachment 2–3 months postoperatively after a single procedure increased significantly over time from 65% in 2004 to 83% in 2012 in all subjects regardless of the treatment method. Single surgery success rates also improved regardless of macula-on or off status after 2008. Heimann et al. could show significantly better primary anatomical success rates in pseudophakic/aphakic patients treated with vitrectomy compared to the ones managed with buckling (72 vs. 53%) [28]. Another prospective study showed 69% single surgery anatomical success rates at month 6 in pseudophakic eyes treated with vitrectomy [30], while Bourla et al. demonstrated 98% single surgery success rates with vitrectomy [27]. Wykoff et al. reported primary anatomic success rates of 88% among macula-on patients operated with scleral buckling [22]. This rate is higher compared to our results (60% before 2008 and 78% after 2008). A potential explanation for the lower rates in our scleral buckling cohort could be that the majority of the procedures were performed during nighttime by general ophthalmic surgeons not specialized in retinal detachment cases. A recent systematic Cochrane Review conducted by Znaor et al. concluded that there is no difference between vitrectomy and scleral buckling in terms of final anatomical success rates [29]. Overall, the shift of surgeries for RRD in our clinic towards optimized surgical settings during the daytime is associated with reduced re-detachment rates.

There are several limitations to this study. First, the study was retrospective in design and therefore factors such as amblyopia, location and number of retinal holes, and the differentiation between PVR grades A and B were not reliably evaluable in the medical records. Secondly, from 2009 onwards there were fewer general ophthalmic surgeons performing retinal detachment surgeries. Thirdly, due to the grouping together of surgeons in our analyses, study outcomes may have been affected by different surgical skills and experience. Fourthly, due to the short follow-up period, there is a possibility of a missed retinal reattachment more than 3 months postoperatively if the patient did not visit our clinic. The strengths of this retrospective study are the number of patients included and the single center setting with uniform surgical systems used by the surgeons.

## 5. Conclusions

In conclusion, our retrospective analysis showed continuous improving anatomical and functional outcomes in patients treated for primary macula-on or off RRD when shifting surgical methods from scleral buckling to vitrectomy and scheduling of surgeries preferentially in the routine daytime program.

**Author Contributions:** A.S.: data processing, drafting, and revision of the paper. C.S.: project design, project oversight, and revision of the paper. T.H.: data collection and data processing. I.S.: statistical analysis, data processing, and revision of the paper. S.S., M.G. and U.S.-E.: project oversight and revision of the paper. A.P.: project design, project oversight, and final revision of the paper. A.P. is the guarantor of the project. All authors have read and agreed to the published version of the manuscript.

**Funding:** This research received no external funding.

**Institutional Review Board Statement:** This retrospective study was conducted at the Department of Ophthalmology and Optometry at the Medical University of Vienna (MUV) according to the Declaration of Helsinki, including current revisions and Good Clinical Practice (GCP) guidelines. The study protocol was approved by the Ethics Committee of MUV (Ethics number: EK1766/2016).

**Informed Consent Statement:** Due to retrospective study design, informed written consent was not required by the Ethics Committee.

**Data Availability Statement:** The datasets generated during and/or analyzed during the current study are available from the corresponding author on reasonable request.

**Conflicts of Interest:** Andreas Pollreisz: consultant at Oertli Instruments. The other authors declare no potential conflict of interest.

# References

1. Mitry, D.; Charteris, D.G.; Fleck, B.W.; Campbell, H.; Singh, J. The Epidemiology of Rhegmatogenous Retinal Detachment: Geographical Variation and Clinical Associations. *Br. J. Ophthalmol.* **2010**, *94*, 678–684. [CrossRef] [PubMed]
2. Kuhn, F.; Aylward, B. Rhegmatogenous Retinal Detachment: A Reappraisal of Its Pathophysiology and Treatment. *Ophthalmic Res.* **2013**, *51*, 15–31. [CrossRef] [PubMed]
3. Nielsen, B.R.; Alberti, M.; Bjerrum, S.S.; la Cour, M. The Incidence of Rhegmatogenous Retinal Detachment Is Increasing. *Acta Ophthalmol.* **2020**, *98*, 603–606. [CrossRef] [PubMed]
4. Van Bussel, E.; Van Der Valk, R.; Bijlsma, W.R.; La Heij, E.C. Impact of Duration of Macula-off Retinal Detachment on Visual Outcome: A Systematic Review and Meta-Analysis of Literature. *Retina* **2014**, *34*, 1917–1925. [CrossRef]
5. Ehrlich, R.; Niederer, R.; Ahmad, N.; Polkinghorne, P. Timing of Acute Macula-on Rhegmatogenous Retinal Detachment Repair. *Retina* **2013**, *33*, 105–110. [CrossRef]
6. Arroyo, J.G.; Yang, L.; Bula, D.; Chen, D.F. Photoreceptor Apoptosis in Human Retinal Detachment. *Am. J. Ophthalmol.* **2005**, *139*, 605–610. [CrossRef]
7. Adelman, R.A.; Parnes, A.J.; Ducournau, D. Strategy for the Management of Uncomplicated Retinal Detachments: The European Vitreo-Retinal Society Retinal Detachment Study Report 1. *Ophthalmology* **2013**, *120*, 1804–1808. [CrossRef]
8. Adelman, R.A.; Parnes, A.J.; Sipperley, J.O.; Ducournau, D. Strategy for the Management of Complex Retinal Detachments: The European Vitreo-Retinal Society Retinal Detachment Study Report 2. *Ophthalmology* **2013**, *120*, 1809–1813. [CrossRef]
9. Schepens, C.L.; Okamura, I.D.; Brockhurst, R.J. The Scleral Buckling Procedures: 1. Surgical Techniques and Management. *AMA Arch. Ophthalmol.* **1957**, *58*, 797–811. [CrossRef]
10. Custodis, E. Die Behandlung Der Netzhautablösung Durch Umschriebene Diathermiekoagulation Und Einer Mittels Plombenaufnähung Erzeugten Eindellung Der Sklera Im Bereich Des Risses. *Klin. Monbl. Augenheilkd. Augenarztl. Fortbild.* **1956**, *129*, 476–495.
11. Machemer, R.; Buettner, H.; Norton, E.; Parel, J. Vitrectomy: A Pars Plana Approach. *Trans. Am. Acad. Ophthalmol. Otolaryngol.* **1971**, *75*, 813–820.
12. Machemer, R.; Parel, J.M.; Norton, E.W.; Buettner, H. Vitrectomy: A Pars Plana Approach. Technical Improvements and Further Results. *Trans. Am. Acad Ophthalmol Otolaryngol.* **1972**, *76*, 462–466. [PubMed]
13. Machemer, R.; Parel, J.M.; Buettner, H. A New Concept for Vitreous Surgery. 1. Instrumentation. *Am. J. Ophthalmol.* **1972**, *73*, 1–7. [CrossRef] [PubMed]
14. Hilton, G.F.; Grizzard, W.S. Pneumatic Retinopexy: A Two-Step Outpatient Operation without Conjunctival Incision. *Ophthalmology* **1986**, *93*, 626–641. [CrossRef] [PubMed]
15. Nemet, A.; Moshiri, A.; Yiu, G.; Loewenstein, A.; Moisseiev, E. A Review of Innovations in Rhegmatogenous Retinal Detachment Surgical Techniques. *J. Ophthalmol.* **2017**, *2017*, 4310643. [CrossRef]
16. Mitry, D.; Awan, M.A.; Borooah, S.; Syrogiannis, A.; Lim-Fat, C.; Campbell, H.; Wright, A.F.; Fleck, B.W.; Charteris, D.G.; Yorston, D.; et al. Long-Term Visual Acuity and the Duration of Macular Detachment: Findings from a Prospective Population-Based Study. *Br. J. Ophthalmol.* **2013**, *97*, 149–152. [CrossRef]
17. Burton, T.C. Recovery of Visual Acuity after Retinal Detachment Involving the Macula. *Trans. Am. Ophthalmol. Soc.* **1982**, *80*, 475–497.
18. Park, D.H.; Choi, K.S.; Sun, H.J.; Lee, S.J. Factors Associated with Visual Outcome After Macula-Off Rhegmatogenous Retinal Detachment Surgery. *Retina* **2018**, *38*, 137–147. [CrossRef]
19. Liu, F.; Meyer, C.H.; Mennel, S.; Hoerle, S.; Kroll, P. Visual Recovery After Scleral Buckling Surgery in Macula-Off Rhegmatogenous Retinal Detachment. *Ophthalmologica* **2006**, *220*, 174–180. [CrossRef]
20. Ross, W.H. Visual Recovery After Macula-Off Retinal Detachment. *Eye* **2002**, *16*, 440–446. [CrossRef]
21. Salicone, A.; Smiddy, W.E.; Venkatraman, A.; Feuer, W. Visual Recovery After Scleral Buckling Procedure for Retinal Detachment. *Ophthalmology* **2006**, *113*, 1734–1742. [CrossRef] [PubMed]
22. Wykoff, C.C.; Smiddy, W.E.; Mathen, T.; Schwartz, S.G.; Flynn, H.W.; Shi, W. Fovea-Sparing Retinal Detachments: Time to Surgery and Visual Outcomes. *Am. J. Ophthalmol.* **2010**, *150*, 205–210.e2. [CrossRef] [PubMed]

23. Ho, S.F.; Fitt, A.; Frimpong-Ansah, K.; Benson, M.T. The Management of Primary Rhegmatogenous Retinal Detachment Not Involving the Fovea. *Eye* **2006**, *20*, 1049–1053. [CrossRef] [PubMed]
24. Slack, P.S.; Coulson, C.J.; Ma, X.; Webster, K.; Proops, D.W. The Effect of Operating Time on Surgeons' Muscular Fatigue. *Ann. R. Coll. Surg. Engl.* **2008**, *90*, 651–657. [CrossRef]
25. Hartz, A.J.; Burton, T.C.; Gottlieb, M.S.; McCarty, D.J.; Williams, D.F.; Prescott, A.; Klein, P. Outcome and Cost Analysis of Scheduled versus Emergency Scleral Buckling Surgery. *Ophthalmology* **1992**, *99*, 1358–1363. [CrossRef]
26. Williamson, T.H.; Shunmugam, M.; Rodrigues, I.; Dogramaci, M.; Lee, E. Characteristics of Rhegmatogenous Retinal Detachment and Their Relationship to Visual Outcome. *Eye* **2013**, *27*, 1063–1069. [CrossRef]
27. Bourla, D.H.; Bor, E.; Axer-Siegel, R.; Mimouni, K.; Weinberger, D. Outcomes and Complications of Rhegmatogenous Retinal Detachment Repair with Selective Sutureless 25-Gauge Pars Plana Vitrectomy. *Am. J. Ophthalmol.* **2010**, *149*, 630–634.e1. [CrossRef]
28. Heimann, H.; Bartz-Schmidt, K.U.; Bornfeld, N.; Weiss, C.; Hilgers, R.D.; Foerster, M.H. Scleral Buckling versus Primary Vitrectomy in Rhegmatogenous Retinal Detachment. A Prospective Randomized Multicenter Clinical Study. *Ophthalmology* **2007**, *114*, 2142–2154. [CrossRef]
29. Znaor, L.; Medic, A.; Binder, S.; Vucinovic, A.; Marin Lovric, J.; Puljak, L. Pars Plana Vitrectomy versus Scleral Buckling for Repairing Simple Rhegmatogenous Retinal Detachments. *Cochrane Database Syst. Rev.* **2019**, *3*, CD009562. [CrossRef]
30. Süsskind, D.; Neuhann, I.; Hilgers, R.D.; Hagemann, U.; Szurman, P.; Bartz-Schmidt, K.U.; Aisenbrey, S. Primary Vitrectomy for Rhegmatogenous Retinal Detachment in Pseudophakic Eyes: 20-Gauge versus 25-Gauge Vitrectomy. *Acta Ophthalmol.* **2016**, *94*, 824–828. [CrossRef]

**Disclaimer/Publisher's Note:** The statements, opinions and data contained in all publications are solely those of the individual author(s) and contributor(s) and not of MDPI and/or the editor(s). MDPI and/or the editor(s) disclaim responsibility for any injury to people or property resulting from any ideas, methods, instructions or products referred to in the content.

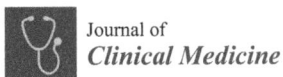

Review

# Trans-Scleral Plugs Fixated FIL SSF IOL: A Review of the Literature and Comparison with Other Secondary IOL Implants

Raffaele Raimondi [1,*], Tania Sorrentino [1], Raphael Kilian [2], Yash Verma [1], Francesco Paolo De Rosa [1], Giuseppe Cancian [1], Panos Tsoutsanis [1], Giovanni Fossati [1], Davide Allegrini [3] and Mario R. Romano [1,3]

[1] Department of Biomedical Sciences, Humanitas University, Via Rita Levi Montalcini 4, 20090 Pieve Emanuele, Italy
[2] Ophthalmic Unit, Department of Neurosciences, Biomedicine and Movement Sciences, University of Verona, 37129 Verona, Italy
[3] Eye Center, Humanitas Gavazzeni-Castelli, 24128 Bergamo, Italy
* Correspondence: raffor9@gmail.com; Tel.: +39-02-8224-7100

**Abstract: Purpose.** To revise the current literature on FIL SSF (Carlevale) intraocular lens, previously known as Carlevale lens, and to compare their outcomes with those from other secondary IOL implants. **Methods.** We performed a peer review of the literature regarding FIL SSF IOLs until April 2021 and analyzed the results only of articles with a minimum of 25 cases and a follow-up of at least 6 months. The searches yielded 36 citations, 11 of which were abstracts of meeting presentations that were not included in the analysis because of their limited data. The authors reviewed 25 abstracts and selected six articles of possible clinical relevance to review in full text. Of these, four were considered to be sufficiently clinically relevant. Particularly, we extrapolated data regarding the pre- and postoperative best corrected visual acuities (BCVA) and the complications related to the procedure. The complication rates were then compared with those from a recently published Ophthalmic Technology Assessment by the American Academy of Ophthalmology (AAO) on secondary IOL implants. **Results.** Four studies with a total of 333 cases were included for results analysis. The BCVA improved in all cases after surgery, as expected. Cystoid macular edema (CME) and increased intraocular pressure were the most common complications, with an incidence of up to 7.4% and 16.5%, respectively. Other IOL types from the AAO report included anterior chamber IOLs, iris fixation IOLs, sutured iris fixation IOLs, sutured scleral fixation IOLs, and sutureless scleral fixation IOLs. There was no statistically significant difference in the rates of postoperative CME ($p = 0.20$), and vitreous hemorrhage ($p = 0.89$) between other secondary implants and the FIL SSF IOL, whereas the rate of retinal detachment was significantly less with FIL SSF IOLs ($p = 0.04$). **Conclusion.** The results of our study suggest the implantation of FIL SSF IOLs is an effective and safe surgical strategy in cases where there is a lack of capsular support. In fact, their outcomes seem to be comparable to those obtained with the other available secondary IOL implants. According to published literature, the FIL SSF (Carlevale) IOL provides favorable functional results with a low rate of postoperative complications.

**Keywords:** Carlevale lens; secondary implant; scleral fixated intraocular lens; suture less fixation

Citation: Raimondi, R.; Sorrentino, T.; Kilian, R.; Verma, Y.; De Rosa, F.P.; Cancian, G.; Tsoutsanis, P.; Fossati, G.; Allegrini, D.; Romano, M.R. Trans-Scleral Plugs Fixated FIL SSF IOL: A Review of the Literature and Comparison with Other Secondary IOL Implants. *J. Clin. Med.* **2023**, *12*, 1994. https://doi.org/10.3390/jcm12051994

Academic Editor: Georgios D. Panos

Received: 18 December 2022
Revised: 26 February 2023
Accepted: 1 March 2023
Published: 2 March 2023

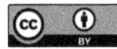

**Copyright:** © 2023 by the authors. Licensee MDPI, Basel, Switzerland. This article is an open access article distributed under the terms and conditions of the Creative Commons Attribution (CC BY) license (https://creativecommons.org/licenses/by/4.0/).

## 1. Introduction

Posterior capsular rupture is one of the most common complications of cataract surgery [1]. Different secondary intraocular lens (IOL) implants have been proposed in the absence of a capsular support (Figure 1), and even though open-loop anterior chamber IOLs are the only FDA-approved ones, several other options are also available. However, the question of which of these options produces the best outcomes remains a topic of debate.

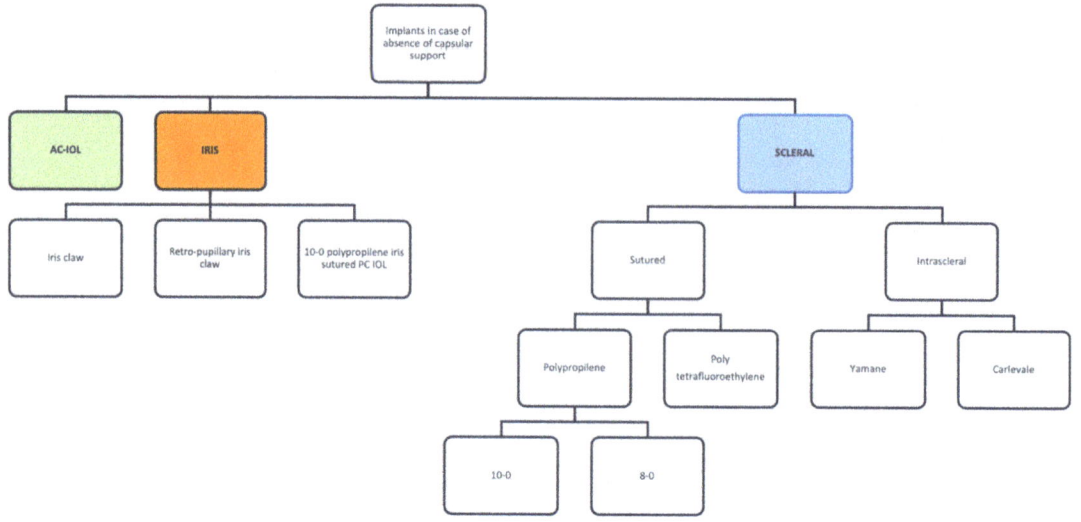

**Figure 1.** Schematic representation of implant options in the absence of capsular support.

Recently, a new trans-scleral plug IOL (FIL SSF) was introduced on the market and has shown to provide excellent clinical results [2].

### 1.1. Anterior Chamber IOLs

Flexible one-piece polymethyl methacrylate (PMMA) open-loop anterior chamber IOLs (ACIOLs) are foldable lenses whose haptics are placed against the scleral spur. Despite the short surgical time and the sutureless technique, the implantation site of such IOLs presents several drawbacks [3]. First, these lenses can lead to corneal endothelial damage, increasing the risk of endothelial decompensation [4]. Second, the trabecular meshwork might also be injured, and the IOL itself might rub against the iris, causing chronic inflammation, IOP increase, and an uveitis-glaucoma-hyphema syndrome. This is more frequent in case the ACIOL is not properly sized or flexible. Overall, these complications occur more commonly with close-looped AC IOLs rather than with open-looped ones [5,6]. Surgeons should refrain from using these implants on younger patients or patients who have a history of uveitis. Additionally, one-piece ACIOLs are not suitable for patients with shallow ACs, irideal abnormalities, or endothelial dysfunction [7].

### 1.2. Iris Fixation IOLs

There are two types of iris-fixated lenses: the iris-claw lens (EU Artisan; USA Verisyse Ophtec, Groningen, The Netherlands) and iris-sutured IOLs (the former being an evolution of the Worst iris-claw lens). The iris-claw lens is a PMMA lens whose haptics form clips grasping the irideal tissue at the midperipheral portion of the iris, in order not to interfere with the normal physiology of the iris (i.e., pupillary dilation and constriction) or that of the angular structures [6]. As for ACIOLs, the short surgical time and the independence from sutures are important advantages; however, they may still lead to possible complications such as endothelial cell loss, iris atrophy, lens dislocation, pupillary distortion, and macular edema [8]. Iris-claw lenses can be placed either at a pre-pupillary or at a retro-pupillary level. In addition to their location, these two do not show marked differences with regards to optical outcomes; however, retro-pupillary claw lenses have been noted to present a lower rate of endothelial cell loss [8].

Iris-sutured IOLs, on the other hand, can also be placed in the posterior chamber with the help of 10-0 polypropylene sutures securing their haptics on the iris. However, due to the fragility of the iris, some degree of lenticular mobility is always present, thus predisposing to pseudo-phacodonesis and tilting of the IOL. In addition, this procedure is much more cumbersome than the insertion of an open-loop AC IOL, especially when a limbal approach is used (i.e., when the procedure is not coupled with penetrating keratoplasty) [5,9].

*1.3. Scleral Fixation IOLs*

Scleral-fixated IOLs (SFIOLs) can be positioned either via transscleral sutures or with suture-independent techniques.

Sutured SFIOLs require either polypropylene (Prolene) or polytetrafluoroethylene (Gore-Tex) suture material to be passed through specific holes in the IOL haptics and eventually fixed at the sclera. Given the high risk of knot erosion that characterizes 10-0 Prolene sutures [10], which in turn increases the risk of endophthalmitis [10], 8-0 Prolene or Gore-Tex sutures are generally preferred.

Due to the risks associated with sutures, researchers have investigated sutureless methods for intrascleral fixation. The Yamane technique and the fibrin glue technique by Agarwal are among the most well-known, both of which use 3-piece IOLs off-label. The Yamane technique involves creating two angled sclerotomies at the end of two lamellar scleral dissections. The IOL's haptics are then brought outside onto the sclera, and their ends are cauterized using an ophthalmic cautery device to create a flange for each haptic. Finally, the haptics are secured in position within scleral tunnels created using a needle [11].

Agarwal's technique, on the other hand, is based on the generation of two partial-thickness scleral flaps, below which the haptics are externalized and eventually fixed with the help of fibrin glue [12].

Since the introduction of Yamane and Agarwal's techniques, a great deal of interest was raised in devising an approved sutureless SFIOL. This resulted in the conception of the FIL SSF IOL (Soleko, Rome, Italy), a foldable, one-piece, acrylic lens with 25% $H_2O$ and a UV filter. This IOL presents with two transcleral T-shaped plugs/haptics anchoring the lens to the sclera without the use of sutures and without requiring any adjustments in the positioning of the haptics [2,13]. FIL SSF IOLs minimize IOL tilting though a T-shaped harpoon and four scleral sulcus counterpressure points; however, in order to obtain a good IOL centration, a symmetrical positioning of the sclerotomies is mandatory [2,14,15].

The purpose of our study was to revise published results of this trans-scleral plug implant and to compare them with those highlighted in a recently published American Academy of Ophthalmology (AAO) ophthalmic technology assessment on various secondary IOL implants [7]. This review reports published outcomes of FIL SSF IOL and compares complication rates with the AAO ophthalmology technology assessment which does not include this IOL.

## 2. Methods

The peer-reviewed literature on FIL SSF IOLs was analyzed, and all articles regarding these were selected until April 2021. The research was conducted on Medline, on CENTRAL, and on the World Health Organization (WHO) International Clinical Trials Registry Platform (ICTRP) and was limited to studies published in English. The search strategy used the following MeSH terms and text words: sutureless scleral fixation, FIL SSF, sutureless scleral lens, and FIL SSF IOL.

The initial search yielded 36 citations, 11 of which were abstracts of meeting presentations that were not included in the analysis because of their limited data. The authors reviewed 25 abstracts and selected six articles of possible clinical relevance to review in full text. Of these, four were considered to be sufficiently clinically relevant. According to the AAO criteria [9] and to avoid the biases of smaller studies, only reports with at least 25 adult participants and a minimum 6-month mean follow-up were included in this analysis.

The panel methodologist (R.R.) assessed and assigned each study with a level of evidence rating according to the American Academy of Ophthalmology's guidelines and using the rating scale developed by the British Centre for Evidence-Based Medicine. Level I articles were well-designed and well-conducted randomized clinical trials, level II was assigned to well-designed and well-conducted cohort and case-control studies, and level III to case series. Since no articles satisfied the level I-level III evidence requirements, all articles were rated as having level II evidence.

Results from the analyzed studies were then compared to those extrapolated from a recently published ophthalmic technology assessment by the American Academy of Ophthalmology on intraocular lenses, in the absence of zonular support. Particularly, the complications that were compared, were only those for which every analyzed study had published results.

*Statistical Analysis*

To carry out the statistical analysis, we used the STATA/IC 16 software, and all data were expressed as mean—standard deviation. A one-way analysis of variance (ANOVA) was used to investigate any statistically significant differences between the means. The differences were considered statistically significant if $p$ value was <0.05.

## 3. Results

*3.1. Visual Outcomes*

A recent report by Barca et al. on 32 eyes implanted with a FIL SSF IOL found an increase in the mean BCVA from $0.46 \pm 0.29$ logMAR preoperatively to $0.13 \pm 0.12$ logMAR 8 months after the procedure ($p < 0.05$). In another study on 78 patients, Rossi et al. also found a significant increase in BCVA, i.e., from $0.86 \pm 0.56$ logMAR to $0.38 \pm 0.42$ logMAR at 6 months after scleral fixation of the IOL, ($p < 0.001$). Similar results on a much larger cohort of patients were reported by Georgalas et al. In their study, they followed up on 169 eyes for a mean 9-month period and reported an increase in mean BCVA from $0.58 \pm 0.49$ logMAR to $0.09 \pm 0.1$ logMAR, ($p = 0.0001$). In 2021, Vaiano et al. investigated the visual outcomes associated with FIL SSF IOL implantation in 54 eyes and found an improvement from $0.93 \pm 0.61$ logMAR to $0.42 \pm 0.34$ (logMAR), $0.42 \pm 0.37$ (logMAR), and $0.38 \pm 0.38$ (logMAR), respectively, at 3, 6, and 12 months from the surgery (Table 1).

**Table 1.** Weighted mean preoperative and postoperative best-corrected visual acuity by Carlevale lens technique.

| Authors | Total N. of Eyes | Mean Follow-Up | BCVA (logMAR) | |
|---|---|---|---|---|
| | | | Preoperative | Postoperative |
| Barca et al. [2] | 32 | 8 | $0.46 \pm 0.29$ | $0.13 \pm 0.12$ |
| Rossi et al. [14] | 78 | 6 | $0.86 \pm 0.56$ | $0.38 \pm 0.42$ |
| Georgalas et al. [13] | 169 | 9 | $0.58 \pm 0.49$ | $0.09 \pm 0.1$ |
| Vaiano et al. [16] | 54 | 12 | $0.42 \pm 0.34$ | $0.38 \pm 0.38$ |

*3.2. Complications*

The most frequent complication reported among the analyzed studies was increased intraocular pressure (IOP), followed by cystoid macular edema (CME). The mean endothelial cell loss was analyzed only by Barca et al. and was found to have decreased after the surgery (i.e., from $2307 \pm 406$ to $2208 \pm 372$, $p < 0.01$). The exact distribution of the complications among each group of study can be found in Table 2. Notably, no cases of lens tilt or lens decentration were reported. In addition, none of the studies reported the need for postoperative IOL explantation for any reason.

Table 2. Complications rates in the analyzed publications.

| Authors | Cystoid Macular Edema | IOP Increase | Reverse Pupillary Block | Vitreous Hemorrhage | Retinal Tears | Retinal Detachment | Corneal Decompensation | Haptic Exposure |
|---|---|---|---|---|---|---|---|---|
| Barca et al. [2] | 1 (3.1%) | 1 (3.1%) | 2 (6.2%) | 1 (3.1%) | | | | |
| Rossi et al. [14] | 4 (5.1%) | 2 (2.5%) | | | 2 (2.5%) | 2 (2.5%) | 1 (1.3%) | |
| Georgalas et al. [13] | | 28 (16.5%) | | 8 (4.7%) | | | | |
| Vaiano et al. [16] | 4 (7.4%) | | | | | 1 (1.8%) | | 2 (3.7%) |

### 3.3. Comparison with Other Secondary IOL Implants

The weighted data coming from our review and those coming from the AAO report on complications from secondary IOL implants are shown in Table 3, whereas the raw data from each single study can be found in Tables 4–6.

Table 3. Intraocular lens weighted complication means.

| Lens Type | Total N. of Eyes | CME | Vitreous Haemorrhage % | Retinal Detachment % |
|---|---|---|---|---|
| Carlevale | 333 | 5.4 | 4.4 | 2.2 |
| Anterior chamber IOL | 311 | 7.3 | 2.2 | 0.9 |
| Iris fixation, anterior | 254 | 4.2 | 1.2 | 0.4 |
| Iris fixation, posterior | 629 | 2.8 | 0.3 | 0.7 |
| Iris fixation suture | 639 | 16.2 | 0.7 | 2.0 |
| Scleral fixation suture | 1163 | 4.8 | 4.3 | 2.2 |
| Scleral fixation sutureless | 1331 | 4.5 | 3.4 | 0.5 |

Table 4. Cystoid macular edema incidence of complications of different implants.

| CME Carlevale | CME Angle | CME Iris Clip | CME Iris Suture | CME Scleral Suture | CME Sclera Sutureless |
|---|---|---|---|---|---|
| 3.1 [2] | 6.6 [17] | 7.7 [18] | 28 [19] | 7.3 [20] | 1.6 [21] |
| 5.1 [14] | 6.8 [22] | 3.1 [23] | 2.8 [24] | 6.3 [25] | 1.4 [26] |
| 7.4 [16] | 15 [27] | 0.9 [28] | 4.5 [31] | 5.7 [29] | 4.8 [26] |
| | 0 [30] | | 11.5 [35] | 10.4 [32] | 4 [33] |
| | 3.4 [34] | | 1.9 [38] | 8 [36] | 2.9 [37] |
| | | | | | 4.2 [39] |
| | | | | | 3 [40] |
| | | | | | 1 [11] |
| | | | | | 3.3 [38] |
| | | | | | 2. [38] |
| | | | | | 21.3 [41] |

Table 5. Vitreous hemorrhage incidence of complications of different implants.

| VH Carlevale | VH Angle | VH Iris Clip | VH Iris Suture | VH Scleral Suture | VH Sclera Sutureless |
|---|---|---|---|---|---|
| 3.1 [2] | 0 [17] | 2.6 [18] | 1.6 [42] | 4.8 [43] | 3.2 [21] |
| 4.7 [13] | 0 [22] | 1 [38] | 0.3 [19] | 3 [44] | 0 [33] |
| | 2.2 [30] | | | 2.9 [29] | 0 [37] |
| | 6.7 [45] | | | 8.3 [32] | 8.3 [39] |
| | | | | 7.8 [46] | 0 [40] |
| | | | | 5 [36] | 5 [11] |
| | | | | | 0 [38] |
| | | | | | 2.5 [38] |
| | | | | | 22.1 [41] |

Table 6. Retinal detachment incidence of complications of different implants.

| RD Carlevale | RD Angle | RD Iris Clip | RD Iris Suture | RD Scleral Suture | RD Sclera Sutureless |
|---|---|---|---|---|---|
| 2.5 [14] | 0 [17] | 0.8 [18] | 0.5 [42] | 8.2 [47] | 1 [26] |
| 1.8 [17] | 0 [22] | 0 [48] | 2.5 [19] | 6.3 [43] | 0 [26] |
| | 0 [27] | 3.2 [49] | 2.1 [24] | 4.9 [20] | 0 [33] |
| | 2.2 [30] | 0.3 [28] | 5.5 [31] | 4.2 [32] | 0 [37] |
| | 2.2 [45] | 1.5 [31] | | | 0 [39] |
| | | 0 [50] | | | 0 [40] |
| | | 1 [38] | | | 0 [11] |
| | | | | | 3.3 [38] |
| | | | | | 0 [38] |

Given that the cohorts of patients in the different studies might have had heterogeneous basal conditions determining the need for a secondary IOL implant, we felt that the comparison between the final BCVAs amongst the various studies might have been biased and decided to only compare the complication rates.

The results of the one-way ANOVA for the most extensively reported complications showed no statistically significant difference in the rates of CME ($p = 0.20$) and vitreous hemorrhage ($p = 0.89$) between other secondary implants and the FIL SSF IOL, whereas there was a statistically significant difference in the rate of retinal detachment ($p = 0.04$). However, the sample size was too small to perform a Wilcoxon rank-sum test and compare the means between the different techniques. (Figures 2–4).

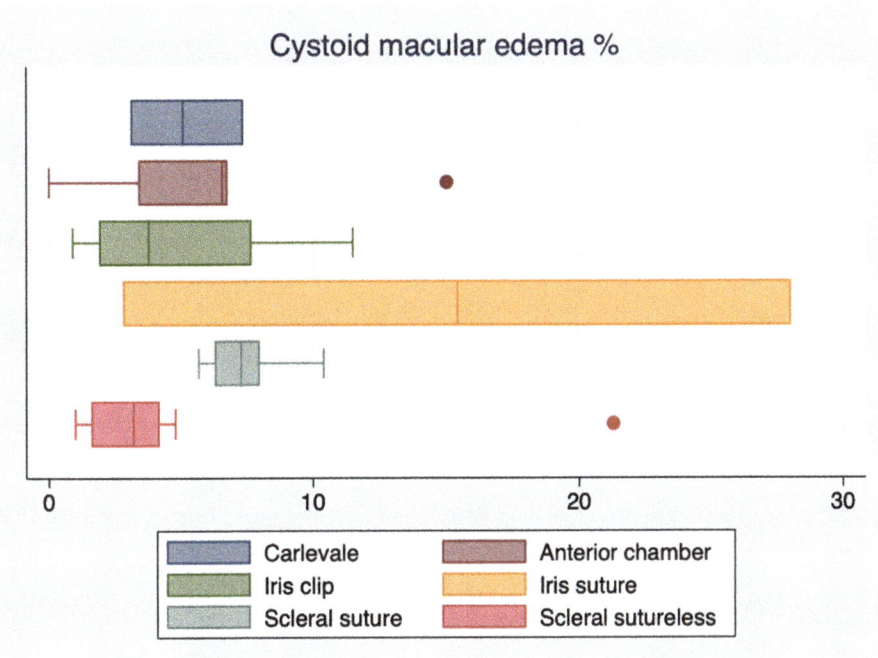

**Figure 2.** Boxplot of cystoid macular edema reported incidences.

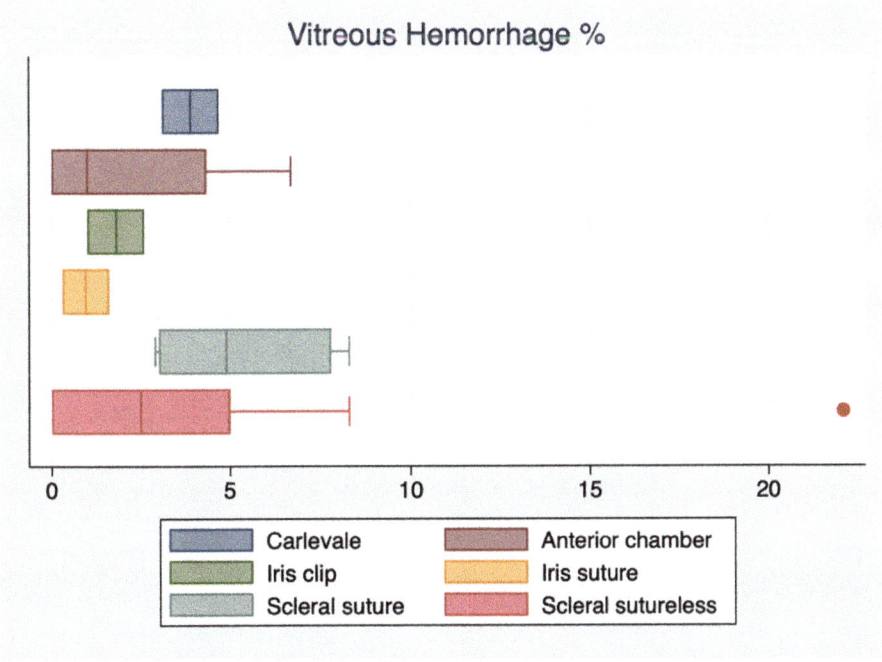

**Figure 3.** Boxplot of vitreous hemorrhage reported incidences.

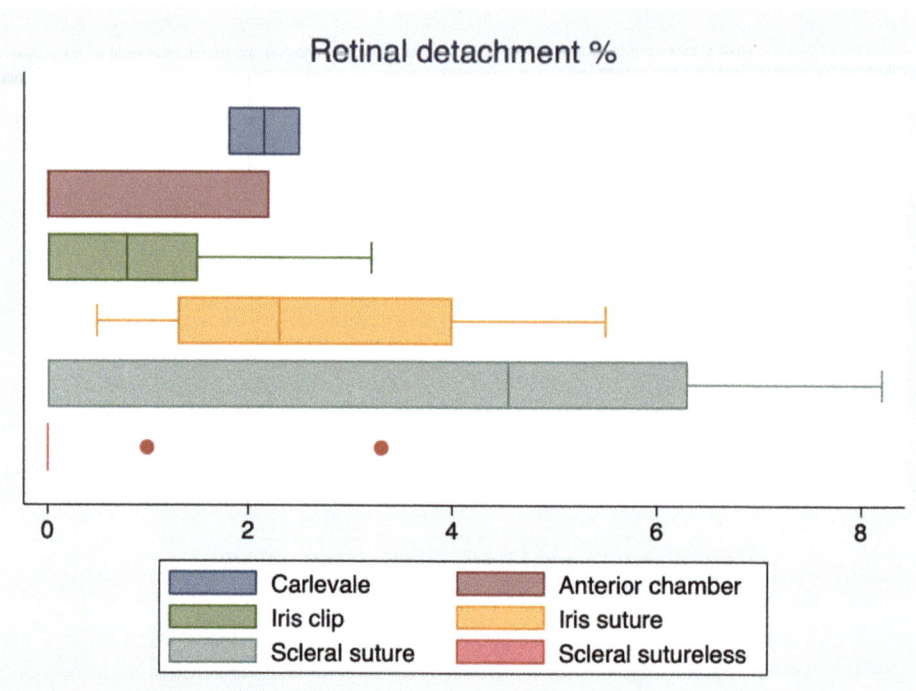

**Figure 4.** Boxplot of retinal detachment reported incidences.

## 4. Discussion

To our knowledge, the results of this review summarize for the first time the visual outcomes and complications of this new scleral-fixated IOL. Overall, the implantation of the FIL SSF IOL seems to be a safe and effective technique. In addition, similar outcomes are reported by different authors, which suggests a good reproducibility of the surgical technique.

When looking at the other secondary IOL implantation techniques included in the AAO technology assessment, several points need to be highlighted. Comparing FIL SSF IOLs with 10-0 propylene scleral-sutured posterior chamber IOLs, the former show a lower incidence of cystoid macular edema and of retinal detachment, although not statistically significant. In fact, for 10-0 propylene scleral-sutured posterior chamber IOLs, the AAO technology assessment reported a rate of macular edema and retinal detachment that varied between 5.7 and 10.4% and between 0 and 8.2%, respectively. Indeed, the surgical technique needed to implant a FIL SSF might be easier than that implying a scleral sutured IOL, so that the surgeon causes less damage to the posterior chamber structures, thus reducing the complication rate. Moreover, the FIL SSF IOL allows firm intrascleral fixation of haptics, granting the possibility of safe, extensive scleral indentation to detect any possible peripheral retinal tear. This may explain the low retinal detachment rates reported.

Intrascleral haptic fixation posterior chamber IOLs are another type of scleral-sutured lens that has been extensively studied in the literature. In most published studies, the rate of the main complications is comparable to that of FIL SSF IOLs, with the exception of the series published by Todorich et al. [41], which reported a 21.3% incidence of cystoid macular edema.

The 10-0 polypropylene iris-sutured posterior chamber IOLs, on the other hand, were reported to induce cystoid macular edema in up to 28% of cases [40], and to have a variable retinal detachment rate between 0.5 and 5.5%.

Unlike the above-described lenses, iris-claw IOLs are held in position by the fixation of their haptics to the iris. Even though some studies reported no incidence of cystoid macular edema, others have shown this complication occurring in up to 11.5% of patients. Moreover, postoperative uveitis has been described in a significant percentage of patients, i.e., 7.7% [18], whereas this complication has never been reported in studies regarding FIL SSF IOLs.

Along with a pretty high incidence of postoperative glaucoma (up to 16.7%) and cystoid macular edema (up to 15%), anterior chamber IOLs have also been described as being considerably affected by chronic uveitis (up to 20%). The results of our study show that these three major complications are less common when considering FIL SSF IOLs.

Nonetheless, the lack of comparative studies makes it difficult to compare the rate of complications of the FIL SSF IOLs with that of other IOL types implanted in the absence of zonular support. Despite lacking some precision (i.e., different studies might have had cohorts of patients with different basal conditions), in this study we proposed a simple and effective way of comparing the results of different secondary IOL implants. By analyzing the incidence of the major characteristic complications, it is evident that the FIL SSF IOL showed a good safety profile, which is comparable, and in certain instances superior, to other IOLs implanted in the absence of zonular support [51].

Indeed, the FIL SSF IOL is a foldable IOL, composed of 25% $H_2O$ acrylic and is designed to have flexible sclero-corneal plugs at the end of its two haptics, allowing it to be implanted posterior to the iris and to attach to the sclera in a sutureless fashion. It has an optic diameter of 6.5 mm, a total length of 13.2 mm, and is available in IOL powers ranging from −5.0 to +35.0 diopters [52].

The FIL SSF lens is a remarkable invention with a number of advantages that surpass the previously described implants. Specifically, it is designed to minimize lens tilting and associated multiple aberrations through its T-shaped harpoon and four scleral sulcus counterpressure points. This is in contrast to other types of lenses such as ACIOL, IFIOL, or SFIOL, which commonly require sutures for fixation, and subsequently expose patients to significant postoperative risks. These risks include corneal decompensation, erosion into angle structures, pupillary block, suprachoroidal or vitreous hemorrhage, retinal detachment, lens tilt or dislocation, and suture erosion, among others.

However, the FIL SSF lens has been shown to effectively reduce these risks by employing a sutureless scleral fixation (SSF) procedure during implantation, which not only ensures a simplified surgical process but also reduces intraoperative time. The innovative design and technology of the FIL SSF lens have revolutionized the field of secondary implants, offering a safer and more efficient alternative to traditional IOL implants. Furthermore, even though no previous study has ever evaluated the impact of this factor on the final BCVA, unlike other IOLs, where manipulation of the haptics is needed to achieve IOL centration, symmetrical positioning of the sclerotomies allows the FIL SSF IOLs to be placed in a secured, centrally aligned position, thus avoiding possible post-operative visual aberrations [2,14,15]. Moreover, it is important to highlight that the FIL SSF IOL is the only labeled IOL for scleral fixation, while other techniques use lenses labeled for capsular bag implants.

Future research adopting computational simulation can be useful to calculate and predict refractive outcomes in complicated cases; this technology is widely applied with success in other fields and can potentially boost results [53].

Among the drawbacks of the FIL SSF IOL is its hydrophilic nature. In fact, this may lead to IOL opacification if air or a gaseous tamponading agent is being used, or late opacification after implantation, which, on the contrary, is very rare with hydrophobic lenses [54]. Accordingly, for the labeling company, new research is currently in place to switch to a hydrophobic FIL SSF IOL. Lastly, in the analyzed literature, it was not possible to retrieve the distance from the limbus and the covering technique of the T-shape haptic that may impact the complication rate.

This review has several limitations. Firstly, in order to compare the outcomes with the AAO technology assessment, some studies were not included in this analysis, which limited the number of cases analyzed. Secondly, we were not able to compare functional results since improvement in BCVA is highly dependent on corneal and retinal status, which was not reported in the analyzed studies.

## 5. Conclusions

Numerous published studies have demonstrated that the FIL SSF IOL represents a secure and reliable device with a low incidence of complications. Moreover, its performance and efficacy appear to be on par with other available techniques currently in use. However, despite these promising findings, it is imperative to conduct further research in the form of prospective comparative studies in order to fortify the scientific evidence supporting the effectiveness of this technique.

**Author Contributions:** Conceptualization, D.A., P.T. and R.R.; methodology, T.S.; investigation, R.K.; resources, G.F. and Y.V.; data curation, F.P.D.R. and G.C.; writing—original draft preparation, R.R. and Y.V.; writing—review and editing, F.P.D.R. and M.R.R. All authors have read and agreed to the published version of the manuscript.

**Funding:** This research received no external funding.

**Institutional Review Board Statement:** Not applicable.

**Informed Consent Statement:** Ethics approval was deemed not necessary by the Humanitas ethics committee.

**Data Availability Statement:** Data generated or analyzed during this study are included in this article. Further enquiries can be directed to the corresponding author.

**Conflicts of Interest:** The authors declare no conflict of interest.

## References

1. Chen, M.; LaMattina, K.; Patrianakos, T.; Dwarakanathan, S. Complication rate of posterior capsule rupture with vitreous loss during phacoemulsification at a Hawaiian cataract surgical center: A clinical audit. *Clin. Ophthalmol.* **2014**, *8*, 375–378. [CrossRef] [PubMed]
2. Barca, F.; Caporossi, T.; de Angelis, L.; Giansanti, F.; Savastano, A.; Di Leo, L.; Rizzo, S. Trans-scleral plugs fixated IOL: A new paradigm for sutureless scleral fixation. *J. Cataract. Refract. Surg.* **2020**, *46*, 716–720. [CrossRef] [PubMed]
3. Lyle, W.A.; Jin, J.-C. Secondary Intraocular Lens Implantation: Anterior Chamber vs. Posterior Chamber Lenses. *Ophthalmic Surg. Lasers Imaging Retin.* **1993**, *24*, 375–381. [CrossRef]
4. Ravalico, G.; Botteri, E.; Baccara, F. Long-term endothelial changes after implantation of anterior chamber intraocular lenses in cataract surgery. *J. Cataract. Refract. Surg.* **2003**, *29*, 1918–1923. [CrossRef]
5. Dick, H.B.; Augustin, A.J. Lens implant selection with absence of capsular support. *Curr. Opin. Ophthalmol.* **2001**, *12*, 47–57. [CrossRef]
6. Smith, P.W.; Wong, S.K.; Stark, W.J.; Gottsch, J.D.; Terry, A.C.; Bonham, R.D. Complications of Semiflexible, Closed-Loop Anterior Chamber Intraocular Lenses. *Arch. Ophthalmol.* **1987**, *105*, 52–57. [CrossRef]
7. Shen, J.F.; Deng, S.; Hammersmith, K.M.; Kuo, A.N.; Li, J.Y.; Weikert, M.P.; Shtein, R.M. Intraocular Lens Implantation in the Absence of Zonular Support: An Outcomes and Safety Update: A Report by the American Academy of Ophthalmology. *Ophthalmology* **2020**, *127*, 1234–1258. [CrossRef]
8. Peralba, R.T.; Lamas-Francis, D.; Sarandeses-Diez, T.; Martínez-Pérez, L.; Rodríguez-Ares, T. Iris-claw intraocular lens for aphakia: Can location influence the final outcomes? *J. Cataract. Refract. Surg.* **2018**, *44*, 818–826. [CrossRef]
9. Wagoner, M.D.; Cox, T.A.; Ariyasu, R.G.; Jacobs, D.S.; Karp, C.L. Intraocular lens implantation in the absence of capsular support: A report by the American Academy of Ophthalmology. *Ophthalmology* **2003**, *110*, 840–859. [CrossRef]
10. Kim, J.; Kinyoun, J.L.; Saperstein, D.A.; Porter, S.L. Subluxation of transscleral sutured posterior chamber intraocular lens (TSIOL). *Am. J. Ophthalmol.* **2003**, *136*, 382–384. [CrossRef]
11. Yamane, S.; Sato, S.; Maruyama-Inoue, M.; Kadonosono, K. Flanged Intrascleral Intraocular Lens Fixation with Double-Needle Technique. *Ophthalmology* **2017**, *124*, 1136–1142. [CrossRef] [PubMed]

12. Agarwal, A.; Kumar, D.A.; Jacob, S.; Baid, C.; Agarwal, A.; Srinivasan, S. Fibrin glue–assisted sutureless posterior chamber intraocular lens implantation in eyes with deficient posterior capsules. *J. Cataract. Refract. Surg.* **2008**, *34*, 1433–1438. [CrossRef] [PubMed]
13. Georgalas, I.; Spyropoulos, D.; Gotzaridis, S.; Papakonstantinou, E.; Kandarakis, S.; Kanakis, M.; Karamaounas, A.; Petrou, P. Scleral fixation of Carlevale intraocular lens: A new tool in correcting aphakia with no capsular support. *Eur. J. Ophthalmol.* **2021**, *32*, 527–533. [CrossRef] [PubMed]
14. Rossi, T.; Iannetta, D.; Romano, V.; Carlevale, C.; Forlini, M.; Telani, S.; Imburgia, A.; Mularoni, A.; Fontana, L.; Ripandelli, G. A novel intraocular lens designed for sutureless scleral fixation: Surgical series. *Graefe's Arch. Clin. Exp. Ophthalmol.* **2020**, *259*, 257–262. [CrossRef] [PubMed]
15. Petrelli, M.; Schmutz, L.; Gkaragkani, E.; Droutsas, K.; Kymionis, G.D. Simultaneous penetrating keratoplasty and implantation of a new scleral-fixated, sutureless, posterior chamber intraocular lens (Soleko, Carlevale): A novel technique. *Cornea* **2020**, *39*, 1450–1452. [CrossRef] [PubMed]
16. Vaiano, A.S.; Hoffer, K.J.; Greco, A.; Greco, A.; D'Amico, G.; Pasqualitto, V.; Carlevale, C.; Savini, G. Long-term Outcomes and Complications of the New Carlevale Sutureless Scleral Fixation Posterior Chamber IOL. *J. Refract. Surg.* **2021**, *37*, 126–132. [CrossRef]
17. Dadeya, S.; Kamlesh, P.K.S. Secondary Intraocular Lens (IOL) Implantation: Anterior Chamber versus Scleral Fixation Long-Term Comparative Evaluation. *Eur. J. Ophthalmol.* **2003**, *13*, 627–633. [CrossRef]
18. De Silva, S.R.; Arun, K.; Anandan, M.; Glover, N.; Patel, C.K.; Rosen, P. Iris-claw intraocular lenses to correct aphakia in the absence of capsule support. *J. Cataract. Refract. Surg.* **2011**, *37*, 1667–1672. [CrossRef]
19. Farjo, A.A.; Rhee, D.J.; Soong, H.K.; Meyer, R.F.; Sugar, A. Iris-Sutured Posterior Chamber Intraocular Lens Implantation During Penetrating Keratoplasty. *Cornea* **2004**, *23*, 18–28. [CrossRef]
20. McAllister, A.S.; Hirst, L.W. Visual outcomes and complications of scleral-fixated posterior chamber intraocular lenses. *J. Cataract. Refract. Surg.* **2011**, *37*, 1263–1269. [CrossRef]
21. Scharioth, G.B.; Prasad, S.; Georgalas, I.; Tataru, C.; Pavlidis, M. Intermediate results of sutureless intrascleral posterior chamber intraocular lens fixation. *J. Cataract. Refract. Surg.* **2010**, *36*, 254–259. [CrossRef] [PubMed]
22. Evereklioglu, C.; Er, H.; Bekir, N.A.; Borazan, M.; Zorlu, F. Comparison of secondary implantation of flexible open-loop anterior chamber and scleral-fixated posterior chamber intraocular lenses. *J. Cataract. Refract. Surg.* **2003**, *29*, 301–308. [CrossRef] [PubMed]
23. Güell, J.L.; Verdaguer, P.; Elies, D.; Gris, O.; Manero, F.; Mateu-Figueras, G.; Morral, M. Secondary iris-claw anterior chamber lens implantation in patients with aphakia without capsular support. *Br. J. Ophthalmol.* **2014**, *98*, 658–663. [CrossRef] [PubMed]
24. Condon, G.P.; Masket, S.; Kranemann, C.; Crandall, A.S.; Ahmed, I.I.K. Small-Incision Iris Fixation of Foldable Intraocular Lenses in the Absence of Capsule Support. *Ophthalmology* **2007**, *114*, 1311–1318. [CrossRef] [PubMed]
25. Burcu, A.; Yalniz-Akkaya, Z.; Abay, I.; Acar, M.A.; Ornek, F. Scleral-Fixated Posterior Chamber Intraocular Lens Implantation in Pediatric and Adult Patients. *Semin. Ophthalmol.* **2013**, *29*, 39–44. [CrossRef]
26. Kumar, D.A.; Agarwal, A. Glued intraocular lens: A major review on surgical technique and results. *Curr. Opin. Ophthalmol.* **2013**, *24*, 21–29. [CrossRef] [PubMed]
27. Donaldson, K.E.; Gorscak, J.J.; Budenz, D.L.; Feuer, W.J.; Benz, M.S.; Forster, R.K. Anterior chamber and sutured posterior chamber intraocular lenses in eyes with poor capsular support. *J. Cataract. Refract. Surg.* **2005**, *31*, 903–909. [CrossRef] [PubMed]
28. Forlini, M.; Soliman, W.; Bratu, A.; Rossini, P.; Cavallini, G.M.; Forlini, C. Long-term follow-up of retropupillary iris-claw intraocular lens implantation: A retrospective analysis. *BMC Ophthalmol.* **2015**, *15*, 143. [CrossRef]
29. Mahmood, S.A.; Zafar, S.; Shakir, M.; Rizvi, S.F. Visual acuity after trans-scleral sutured posterior chamber intraocular lens. *J. Coll. Physicians Surg. Pak.* **2014**, *24*, 922–926.
30. Kwong, Y.Y.; Yuen, H.K.; Lam, R.F.; Lee, V.Y.; Rao, S.K.; Lam, D.S. Comparison of Outcomes of Primary Scleral-Fixated versus Primary Anterior Chamber Intraocular Lens Implantation in Complicated Cataract Surgeries. *Ophthalmology* **2007**, *114*, 80–85. [CrossRef]
31. Faria, M.Y.; Ferreira, N.P.; Pinto, J.M.; Cordeiro-Sousa, D.; Cardoso-Leal, I.; Neto, E.; Marques-Neves, C. Retropupillary iris claw intraocular lens implantation in aphakia for dislocated intraocular lens. *Int. Med. Case Rep. J.* **2016**, *9*, 261–265. [CrossRef] [PubMed]
32. Long, C.; Wei, Y.; Yuan, Z.; Zhang, Z.; Lin, X.; Liu, B. Modified technique for transscleral fixation of posterior chamber intraocular lenses. *BMC Ophthalmol.* **2015**, *15*, 127. [CrossRef] [PubMed]
33. Narang, P.; Narang, S. Glue-assisted intrascleral fixation of posterior chamber intraocular lens. *Indian J. Ophthalmol.* **2013**, *61*, 163–167. [CrossRef] [PubMed]
34. Jamwal, R. Bioavailable curcumin formulations: A review of pharmacokinetic studies in healthy volunteers. *J. Integr. Med.* **2018**, *16*, 367–374. [CrossRef] [PubMed]
35. Kumar, K.V.; Jayamadhury, G.; Potti, S.; Kumar, R.M.; Mishra, K.D.; Nambula, S.R. Retropupillary fixation of iris-claw lens in visual rehabilitation of aphakic eyes. *Indian J. Ophthalmol.* **2016**, *64*, 743–746. [CrossRef] [PubMed]
36. Yeung, L.; Wang, N.-K.; Wu, W.-C.; Chen, K.-J. Combined 23-gauge transconjunctival vitrectomy and scleral fixation of intraocular lens without conjunctival dissection in managing lens complications. *BMC Ophthalmol.* **2018**, *18*, 108. [CrossRef]
37. Yamane, S.; Inoue, M.; Arakawa, A.; Kadonosono, K. Sutureless 27-Gauge Needle–Guided Intrascleral Intraocular Lens Implantation with Lamellar Scleral Dissection. *Ophthalmology* **2014**, *121*, 61–66. [CrossRef]

38. Kelkar, A.; Shah, R.; Vasavda, V.; Kelkar, J.; Kelkar, S. Primary iris claw IOL retrofixation with intravitreal triamcinolone acetonide in cases of inadequate capsular support. *Int. Ophthalmol.* **2017**, *38*, 111–117. [CrossRef]
39. Kawaji, T.; Sato, T.; Tanihara, H. Sutureless intrascleral intraocular lens fixation with lamellar dissection of scleral tunnel. *Clin. Ophthalmol.* **2016**, *10*, 227–231. [CrossRef]
40. Zhang, Y.; He, F.; Jiang, J.; Li, Q.; Wang, Z. Modified technique for intrascleral fixation of posterior chamber intraocular lens without scleral flaps. *J. Cataract. Refract. Surg.* **2017**, *43*, 162–166. [CrossRef]
41. Todorich, B.; Stem, M.S.; Kooragayala, K.; Thanos, A.; Faia, L.J.; Williams, G.A.; Hassan, T.S.; Woodward, M.A.; Wolfe, J.D. Structural analysis and comprehensive surgical outcomes of the sutureless intrascleral fixation of secondary intraocular lenses in human eyes. *Retina* **2018**, *38*, S31–S40. [CrossRef] [PubMed]
42. Akpek, E.K.; Altan-Yaycioglu, R.; Karadayi, K.; Christen, W.; Stark, W.J. Long-term outcomes of combined penetrating keratoplasty with iris-sutured intraocular lens implantation. *Ophthalmology* **2003**, *110*, 1017–1022. [CrossRef] [PubMed]
43. Bading, G.; Hillenkamp, J.; Sachs, H.G.; Gabel, V.-P.; Framme, C. Long-term Safety and Functional Outcome of Combined Pars Plana Vitrectomy and Scleral-Fixated Sutured Posterior Chamber Lens Implantation. *Am. J. Ophthalmol.* **2007**, *144*, 371–377.e1. [CrossRef] [PubMed]
44. Kim, S.J.; Lee, S.J.; Park, C.H.; Jung, G.Y.; Park, S.H. Long-Term Stability and Visual Outcomes of a Single-Piece, Foldable, Acrylic Intraocular Lens for Scleral Fixation. *Retina* **2009**, *29*, 91–97. [CrossRef] [PubMed]
45. Chan, T.; Lam, J.K.; Jhanji, V.; Li, E.Y. Comparison of Outcomes of Primary Anterior Chamber Versus Secondary Scleral-Fixated Intraocular Lens Implantation in Complicated Cataract Surgeries. *Am. J. Ophthalmol.* **2015**, *159*, 221–226.e2. [CrossRef]
46. Kang, D.J.; Kim, H.K. Clinical analysis of the factors contributing to pupillary optic capture after transscleral fixation of posterior chamber intraocular lens for dislocated intraocular lens. *J. Cataract. Refract. Surg.* **2016**, *42*, 1146–1150. [CrossRef]
47. Vote, B.J.; Tranos, P.; Bunce, C.; Charteris, D.G.; Da Cruz, L. Long-Term Outcome of Combined Pars Plana Vitrectomy and Scleral Fixated Sutured Posterior Chamber Intraocular Lens Implantation. *Am. J. Ophthalmol.* **2006**, *141*, 308–312.e1. [CrossRef]
48. Mohammad-Rabie, H.; Malekifar, P.; Esfandiari, H. Visual Outcomes after Primary Iris Claw Artisan Intraocular Lens Implantation during Complicated Cataract Surgery. *Semin. Ophthalmol.* **2016**, *32*, 337–340. [CrossRef]
49. Schallenberg, M.; Dekowski, D.; Hahn, A.; Laube, T.; Steuhl, K.-P.; Meller, D. Aphakia correction with retropupillary fixated iris-claw lens (Artisan)—Long-term results. *Clin. Ophthalmol.* **2013**, *8*, 137–141. [CrossRef]
50. Choragiewicz, T.; Rejdak, R.; Grzybowski, A.; Nowomiejska, K.; Moneta-Wielgoś, J.; Ozimek, M.; Jünemann, A.G.M. Outcomes of Sutureless Iris-Claw Lens Implantation. *J. Ophthalmol.* **2016**, *2016*, 7013709. [CrossRef]
51. Schnurrbusch, U.E.K.; Welt, K.; Horn, L.-C.; Wiedemann, P.; Wolf, S. Histological findings of surgically excised choroidal neovascular membranes after photodynamic therapy. *Br. J. Ophthalmol.* **2001**, *85*, 1086–1091. [CrossRef] [PubMed]
52. Veronese, C.; Maiolo, C.; Armstrong, G.W.; Primavera, L.; Torrazza, C.; Della Mora, L.; Ciardella, A.P. New surgical approach for sutureless scleral fixation. *Eur. J. Ophthalmol.* **2020**, *30*, 612–615. [CrossRef] [PubMed]
53. Jamari, J.; Ammarullah, M.; Saad, A.; Syahrom, A.; Uddin, M.; van der Heide, E.; Basri, H. The Effect of Bottom Profile Dimples on the Femoral Head on Wear in Metal-on-Metal Total Hip Arthroplasty. *J. Funct. Biomater.* **2021**, *12*, 38. [CrossRef] [PubMed]
54. Marcovich, A.L.; Tandogan, T.; Bareket, M.; Eting, E.; Kaplan-Ashiri, I.; Bukelman, A.; Auffarth, G.U.; Khoramnia, R. Opacification of hydrophilic intraocular lenses associated with vitrectomy and injection of intraocular gas. *BMJ Open Ophthalmol.* **2018**, *3*, e000157. [CrossRef] [PubMed]

**Disclaimer/Publisher's Note:** The statements, opinions and data contained in all publications are solely those of the individual author(s) and contributor(s) and not of MDPI and/or the editor(s). MDPI and/or the editor(s) disclaim responsibility for any injury to people or property resulting from any ideas, methods, instructions or products referred to in the content.

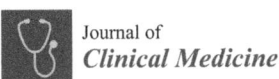 

Article

# Cystoid Macular Edema after Rhegmatogenous Retinal Detachment Repair with Pars Plana Vitrectomy: Rate, Risk Factors, and Outcomes

Malik Merad [1], Fabien Vérité [2], Florian Baudin [1], Inès Ben Ghezala [1], Cyril Meillon [1], Alain Marie Bron [1,3], Louis Arnould [1], Pétra Eid [1], Catherine Creuzot-Garcher [1,3] and Pierre-Henry Gabrielle [1,3,*]

1. Department of Ophthalmology, Dijon University Hospital, 21000 Dijon, France
2. Agathe Group INSERM U 1150, UMR 7222 CNRS, ISIR (Institute of Intelligent Systems and Robotics), Sorbonne Université, 75005 Paris, France
3. Eye and Nutrition Research Group, Centre des Sciences du Goût et de l'Alimentation, AgroSup Dijon, CNRS, INRAE, Université de Bourgogne Franche-Comté, 21000 Dijon, France
* Correspondence: phgabrielle@gmail.com; Tel.: +33-380-293-031

**Abstract:** (1) Background: The aim was to describe the rate and outcomes of cystoid macular edema (CME) after pars plana vitrectomy (PPV) for primary rhegmatogenous retinal detachment (RRD) and to identify risk factors and imaging characteristics. (2) Methods: A retrospective consecutive case study was conducted over a 5-year period among adult patients who underwent PPV for primary RRD repair. The main outcome measure was the rate of CME at 12 months following PPV. (3) Results: Overall, 493 eyes were included. The CME rate was 28% (93 patients) at 12 months. In multivariate analysis, eyes with worse presenting visual acuity (VA) (odds ratio [OR], 1.55; 95% CI, 1.07–2.25; $p = 0.02$) and grade C proliferative vitreoretinopathy (PVR) (OR, 2.88; 95% CI, 1.04–8.16; $p = 0.04$) were more at risk of developing CME 1 year after PPV. Endolaser retinopexy was associated with a greater risk of CME than cryotherapy retinopexy (OR, 3.06; 95% CI, 1.33–7.84; $p = 0.01$). Eyes undergoing cataract surgery within 6 months of the initial RRD repair were more likely to develop CME at 12 months (OR, 1.96; 95% CI, 1.06–3.63; $p = 0.03$). (4) Conclusions: CME is a common complication after PPV for primary RRD repair. Eyes with worse presenting VA, severe PVR at initial presentation, endolaser retinopexy, and cataract surgery within 6 months of initial RRD repair were risk factors for postoperative CME at 12 months.

**Keywords:** cystoid macular edema; rhegmatogenous retinal detachment; pars plana vitrectomy; vitreoretinal surgery; spectral-domain optical coherence tomography

## 1. Introduction

Rhegmatogenous retinal detachment (RRD) is a common and severe ocular condition affecting 6–18 patients per 100,000 each year [1,2]. Pars plana vitrectomy (PPV) has benefited from substantial technological advances in recent years, making this technique safe and effective for the treatment of RRD [3–6]. Functional recovery after RRD has now been widely studied, and cystoid macular edema (CME) is one of the main factors limiting functional recovery, along with epiretinal membrane formation (ERM) and photoreceptor alterations [7–12].

CME is a common retinal condition defined by an accumulation of fluid in the retina causing visual impairment [10–15]. CME is described in several ocular disorders, such as diabetic retinopathy or vascular occlusion, but it can also occur in postoperative situations, for example, cataract extraction or retinal detachment surgery [16,17]. Although large CMEs can be detected on fundus examination, retinal multimodal imaging provides a more refined diagnosis. The use of gold standard fluorescein angiography is continuously decreasing in favor of spectral-domain optical coherence tomography (SD-OCT). These

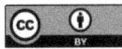

major advances in noninvasive retinal imaging have enabled a better detection and follow-up of CME [18,19].

The rate of CME after primary RRD repair ranges from 6% to 36%, regardless of the surgical technique used [8,9,20–22]. Age, lens status (pseudophakia and aphakia), macular status, and the severity of the retinal detachment, especially with proliferative vitreoretinopathy (PVR), are reported to be risk factors for CME after primary RRD repair [9,20,23,24]. Recently, Pole et al. showed a relationship in univariate analysis between the number of surgeries, macular status, PVR grading, and the occurrence of CME, but these parameters were no longer significant in multivariate analysis [23]. There are still limited data on the rate, risk factors, and outcomes of CME after RRD repair with PPV [24,25]. Therefore, we aimed to report the rate of CME after PPV for primary RRD repair, identify the risk factors, and describe the 12-month outcomes and characteristics of SD-OCT imaging.

## 2. Materials and Methods

### 2.1. Design and Setting

Participants in this study were adult patients who underwent 23-gauge (G) or 25 G PPV for RRD primary repair at the Dijon University Hospital Ophthalmology Department between 1 January 2015 and 31 December 2019. This was a retrospective consecutive case study. All patients underwent either 23 G or 25 G primary PPV for RRD repair using the Constellation Vision System (Alcon Laboratories, Inc., Fort Worth, TX, USA) or Stellaris Vision Enhancement System (Bausch and Lomb, Inc., Rochester, NY, USA); a wide-angle viewing system was used for surgery. Surgeries were performed under general or local anesthesia induced by peribulbar block. All patients received postoperative treatment including 1 month of a topical nonsteroidal anti-inflammatory drug (NSAID), either indomethacin (Indocollyre®, Laboratoire Chauvin, Bausch and Lomb, Montpellier, France) or bromfenac (Yellox®, Croma Pharma GmbH, Korneuburg, Austria; and Bausch and Lomb, Inc., Rochester, NY, USA), 1 month of topical dexamethasone (Dexafree®, Laboratoires Théa, Clermont-Ferrand, France), 7 days of topical dorzolamide/timolol (Cosidime®, Laboratoire Santen, Paris, France), and 5 days of oral acetazolamide (Diamox®, Coopération Pharmaceutique Française, Melun, France). Ethical approval from an institutional review board was not required for this study due to its retrospective design, in accordance with French regulations. This study adhered to the tenets of the Declaration of Helsinki and followed the STROBE statements for reporting observational studies [26].

### 2.2. Data Sources and Measurements

Data were obtained retrospectively from electronic medical records, preoperatively and at 1, 3, 6, and 12 months postoperatively (M0, M1, M3, M6, and M12, respectively). Only one eye from the same patient was considered for this study. Baseline characteristics and preoperative patient data were obtained, including gender, age, diabetes mellitus, the affected eye, lens status, axial length, and intraocular pressure-lowering therapy. Visual acuity and characteristics of retinal detachment were recorded (extent of RRD (1–4 quadrants), number of retinal tears, presence of vitreous hemorrhage, PVR grade, macular status, onset of symptoms). The following surgery characteristics were retrieved: tamponade agent (air, hexafluoride (SF6), hexafluoroethane (C2F6), octafluoropropane (C3F8), silicone oil (SO)); retinopexy type (laser, cryotherapy or combined); the presence of retinotomy; retinectomy; internal limiting membrane peeling; use of perfluorocarbon liquid; and surgeon experience (fellow or senior surgeon). The time between RRD repair surgery and phacoemulsification was recorded for patients benefiting from sequential cataract surgery during the follow-up period.

During follow-up, we collected data on best-corrected visual acuity (BCVA) measurements in decimals, recurrence of RRD, and the number of surgeries. BCVA was converted to the logarithm of the minimum angle of resolution (LogMAR) and Snellen BCVA for statistical analysis. Single-surgery anatomical success (SSAS) was defined as retinal reattachment 12 months after a single operation. Final anatomical success (FAS) was defined as retinal reattachment at 12 months, requiring one or additional surgeries for recurrent retinal detachment [6].

Postoperative SD-OCT imaging was performed using the Cirrus high-definition SD-OCT system (Carl Zeiss, Dublin, CA, USA). CME diagnosis was defined as hyporeflective spaces regardless of the retinal layer involved. CRT was not considered for analysis because of the varying degree of macular atrophy [23]. SD-OCT characteristics were collected, such as the presence of ERM, central retinal thickness (CRT), outer retinal layer alterations (inner and outer segment junction (IS/OS) and/or external limiting membrane disruption), and localization of cysts in the inner retinal layers (IRL) or outer retinal layers (ORL).

*2.3. Patient Selection and Groups*

Current procedural terminology codes 67108 and 67113 were used to screen adult patients who underwent PPV for primary repair of retinal detachment between 1 January 2015 and 31 December 2019. Only one eye per patient was included. Exclusion criteria were: a follow-up period of fewer than 6 months, any history of RRD or vitreoretinal surgery (macular hole surgery, epiretinal membrane peeling, PPV), non-rhegmatogenous retinal detachment, severe ocular trauma, uveitis, endophthalmitis, and macular edema (age-related macular degeneration, diabetic macular edema, uveitis, retinal vein occlusion, a history of macular edema).

Patients presenting with CME at the 12-month follow-up were classified into all CME patients (aCME) and patients with no CME (nCME patients). Patients presenting with CME within 1 year at any visit (M1, M3, M6, and/or M12) were grouped into transient CME (tCME) and chronic CME (cCME), as described in previous studies [23,25]. tCME was defined as CME that appeared within the first 6 months of surgery, lasted less than 6 months during the follow-up period, and resolved spontaneously or with topical medications only. cCME was defined as CME seen on OCT imaging at least 6 months apart and/or benefiting from more complex CME management with additional treatment such as systemic medication, intravitreal injection of dexamethasone implant, and/or surgery with ERM peeling. The management of CME was based on symptoms, visual acuity, and multimodal imaging at the discretion of the physician in consultation with the patient, thereby representing routine clinical practice.

*2.4. Outcomes*

The main outcome was the rate of CME at 12 months following primary RRD repair with PPV. We also examined risk factors for CME at 12 months and postoperative CME SD-OCT characteristics, SSAS rate, FAS rate, and visual outcomes at 12 months.

*2.5. Statistical Analysis*

Continuous variables are described as the median and interquartile range (IQR) or mean and standard deviation (SD) according to their distribution, while categorical variables are given by number and percentage. Risk factors for CME at 12 months were assessed through univariate and multivariate logistic regressions. Factors with a significance level lower than 20% in univariate regression and with less than 5% of missing values were retained for multivariate regressions. Results of regressions are expressed as odds ratios (ORs) with 95% confidence interval and $p$ values. Risk factors for chronic macular edema on SD-OCT imaging were assessed by univariate logistic regression. Missing values are reported in tables and were excluded from the analysis. The significance threshold was 5%. Boxplots were used to display the evolution of BCVA and CRT after surgery. All analyses were conducted using R Statistical Software version 4.0.1 (R Foundation for Statistical Computing, Vienna, Austria, 2021) with the gtsummary package (V 1.4.1).

## 3. Results

### 3.1. Study Participants

A total of 1042 patients underwent PPV surgery for primary retinal detachment repair between 1 January 2015 and 31 December 2019. Of these patients, 493 met the inclusion criteria (Figure 1). Baseline clinical and demographic characteristics are described in Table 1. Most patients were male (66%), the mean age was 63.0 (±10.9) years, and the mean BCVA at initial presentation was 1.23 (±0.93) LogMAR (20/400 Snellen VA chart).

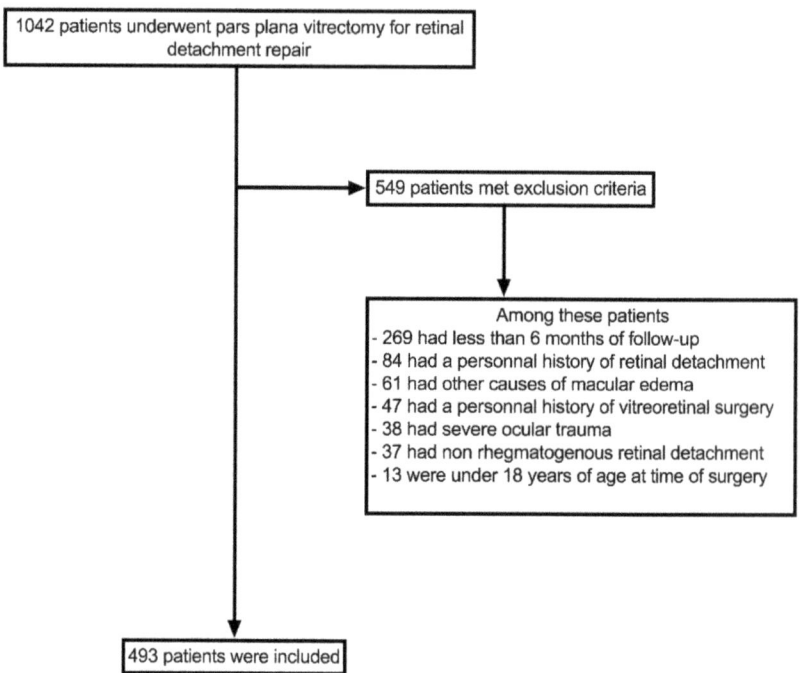

**Figure 1.** Flowchart of patient selection process.

**Table 1.** Population description.

|  | n = 493 |
|---|---|
| Age (year) | 63 (10.9) |
| Gender-Male | 324 (65.7%) |
| Lens status |  |
| Phakic | 304 (61.7%) |
| Pseudophakic | 187 (37.9%) |
| Aphakic | 2 (0.4%) |
| Axial length (mm) * | 24.78 (1.78) |
| Diabetes mellitus * | 43 (8.78%) |
| Initial BCVA (LogMAR) * | 1.23 (0.93) |
| Extent of RRD (1–4 quadrants) |  |
| 1 | 66 (13.4%) |
| 2 | 209 (42.4%) |
| 3 | 90 (18.2%) |
| 4 | 128 (26.0%) |

Table 1. Cont.

|  | n = 493 |
|---|---|
| Number of retinal tears * | |
| 0 | 23 (4.7%) |
| 1 | 253 (51.7%) |
| 2 | 101 (20.7%) |
| 3 | 57 (11.7%) |
| 4 and more | 55 (11.2%) |
| Proliferative vitreoretinopathy * | |
| Grade A | 101 (21.0%) |
| Grade B | 305 (63.6%) |
| Grade C | 74 (15.4%) |
| Macular status | |
| On | 138 (28.0%) |
| Off | 355 (72.0%) |
| Time to surgery after first symptoms (days) * | 17 (22) |
| Surgical procedure | |
| Pseudophakic-PPV only | 182 (36.9%) |
| Phakic-PPV only | 258 (52.3%) |
| Phakic-PPV with simultaneous PKE | 53 (10.8%) |
| Secondary cataract surgery | |
| Not applicable | 272 (55.2%) |
| Under 3 months | 51 (10.3%) |
| Between 3 and 6 months | 81 (16.4%) |
| Between 6 and 12 months | 89 (18.1%) |
| Single surgery anatomical success | 370 (75.0%) |
| Cystoid macular edema rate within the first 12 months *,† | 165 (33.9%) |
| Cystoid macular edema rate at 12 months * | 97 (28.1%) |

BCVA, best-corrected visual acuity; RRD, rhegmatogenous retinal detachment; PPV, pars plana vitrectomy; PKE, phacoemulsification; M6, 6 months after RRD repair; M12, 12 months after RRD repair. Categorical variables are described as $n$ (%); continuous variables are described as mean (SD). * Missing data ($n$): axial length (153); diabetes mellitus (3); initial BCVA (11); number of retinal tears (4); proliferative vitreoretinopathy (13); time to surgery after first symptoms (102); cystoid macular edema rate within the first 12 months (6); cystoid macular edema rate at M12 (148). † Patients that experienced at least one episode of CME at any visits within the first year.

### 3.2. Cystoid Macular Edema Rate and Risk Factors

Overall, 165 (34%, six missing data) patients experienced at least one episode of CME within the first year of follow-up. The rate of CME at 12 months was 28% (97 patients, 148 missing data). Baseline demographics and surgery characteristics are shown in Tables 2 and 3 for univariate and multivariate analysis, respectively. Due to missing data at 12 months, 345 patients were included in the univariate analysis and 327 in the multivariate analysis for risk factors of CME at 12 months. aCME and nCME patients were similar in age ($p = 0.86$), gender ($p = 0.52$), and axial length ($p = 0.73$) at baseline.

Table 2. Risk factors for cystoid macular edema at 12 months univariate analysis.

|  | nCME (n = 248) | aCME (n = 97) | OR * | 95% CI | p Value |
|---|---|---|---|---|---|
| Age (year) | 62 (56, 69) | 65 (57, 70) | 1.00 | 0.98–1.02 | 0.86 |
| Gender-Male | 165 (66.5%) | 61 (62.9%) | 0.85 | 0.52–1.40 | 0.52 |
| Lens status | | | | | |
| Phakic | 155 (62.5%) | 60 (61.9%) | — | — | |
| Pseudophakic | 92 (37.1%) | 37 (38.1%) | 1.04 | 0.64–1.68 | 0.88 |
| Aphakic | 1 (0.4%) | 0 (0.0%) | 0.00 | | >0.99 |
| Axial length (mm) † | 24.44 (23.68, 25.70) | 24.64 (23.95, 25.65) | 1.03 | 0.88–1.20 | 0.73 |
| Diabetes mellitus † | 22 (8.9%) | 10 (10.4%) | 1.19 | 0.52–2.55 | 0.67 |
| Initial BCVA (LogMAR) † | 0.85 (0.16, 2.30) | 2.30 (0.70, 2.30) | 1.72 | 1.32–2.27 | <0.001 |
| Macular status-Off | 175 (71.0%) | 79 (81.4%) | 1.80 | 1.02–3.28 | 0.048 |

Table 2. Cont.

| | nCME (n = 248) | aCME (n = 97) | OR * | 95% CI | p Value |
|---|---|---|---|---|---|
| Extent of RRD (1–4 quadrants) | | | 1.43 | 1.13–1.81 | 0.003 |
| 1 | 36 (14.5%) | 7 (7.2%) | | | |
| 2 | 107 (43.1%) | 36 (37.1%) | | | |
| 3 | 49 (19.8%) | 17 (17.6%) | | | |
| 4 | 56 (22.6%) | 37 (38.1%) | | | |
| Proliferative vitreoretinopathy [†] | | | | | |
| Grade A and B | 215 (89.2%) | 64 (67.4%) | — | — | |
| Grade C | 26 (10.8%) | 31 (32.6%) | 4.01 | 2.22–7.28 | <0.001 |
| Vitreous hemorrhage | 37 (14.9%) | 12 (12.4%) | 0.81 | 0.39–1.58 | 0.54 |
| Time to surgery after first symptoms (days) [†] | 10 (5, 20) | 8 (5, 14) | 1.01 | 1.00–1.02 | 0.19 |
| Surgical procedure | | | | | |
| Phakic-PPV only | 136 (54.8%) | 49 (50.5%) | — | — | |
| Pseudophakic-PPV only | 92 (37.1%) | 36 (37.1%) | 1.09 | 0.65–1.80 | 0.75 |
| Phakic-PPV with simultaneous PKE | 20 (8.1%) | 12 (12.4%) | 1.67 | 0.74–3.62 | 0.20 |
| Tamponade agent | | | | | |
| Hexafluoride (SF6) | 161 (64.9%) | 47 (48.5%) | — | — | |
| Air | 2 (0.8%) | 0 (0.0%) | 0.00 | | 0.98 |
| Hexafluoroethane (C2F6) | 45 (18.2%) | 20 (20.6%) | 1.52 | 0.81–2.81 | 0.18 |
| Octafluoropropane (C3F8) | 5 (2.0%) | 1 (1.0%) | 0.69 | 0.04–4.39 | 0.73 |
| Silicone oil | 35 (14.1%) | 29 (29.9%) | 2.84 | 1.57–5.13 | <0.001 |
| Retinopexy type [†] | | | | | |
| Cryotherapy | 65 (26.4%) | 9 (9.3%) | — | — | |
| Endolaser | 135 (54.9%) | 75 (77.3%) | 4.01 | 1.98–9.05 | <0.001 |
| Combined cryotherapy and endolaser | 46 (18.7%) | 13 (13.4%) | 2.04 | 0.81–5.33 | 0.13 |
| Retinotomy [†] | 66 (26.7%) | 28 (28.9%) | 1.11 | 0.65–1.86 | 0.69 |
| Retinectomy [†] | 2 (0.8%) | 5 (5.2%) | 6.66 | 1.41–47.1 | 0.02 |
| Internal limiting membrane peeling [†] | 27 (10.9%) | 26 (27.1%) | 3.03 | 1.65–5.54 | <0.001 |
| Use of PFCL [†] | 38 (15.5%) | 34 (35.4%) | 3.00 | 1.74–5.17 | <0.001 |
| Surgeon experience-fellow surgeon | 122 (49.2%) | 51 (52.6%) | 1.15 | 0.72–1.84 | 0.57 |
| Secondary cataract surgery within 6 months | 64 (25.8%) | 34 (35.1%) | 1.55 | 0.93–2.56 | 0.09 |
| Single surgery anatomical success | 194 (78.2%) | 60 (61.9%) | 2.22 | 1.33–3.68 | 0.002 |
| Number of RRD repair within 12 months [†] | | | 1.88 | 1.38–2.60 | <0.001 |
| 1 | 201 (81.1%) | 59 (61.5%) | | | |
| 2 | 33 (13.3%) | 21 (21.9%) | | | |
| 3 | 11 (4.4%) | 10 (10.4%) | | | |
| 4 | 3 (1.2%) | 6 (6.2%) | | | |
| Retinal re-detachment within 3 months [†] | 34 (13.7%) | 28 (29.2%) | 2.59 | 1.46–4.58 | 0.001 |

OR, odds ratio; CI, confidence interval; nCME, no cystoid macular edema group; aCME, cystoid macular edema group, BCVA, best-corrected visual acuity; RRD, rhegmatogenous retinal detachment; PPV, pars plana vitrectomy; PKE, phacoemulsification; PFCL, perfluorocarbon liquid. Categorical variables are described as $n$ (%), continuous variables are described as median (IQR). * Estimated from univariate logistic regression model. [†] Missing data (nCME; aCME): axial length (74; 28); diabetes mellitus (1; 1); initial BCVA (5; 2); proliferative vitreoretinopathy (7; 2); time to surgery after first symptoms (55; 17); retinopexy type (2; 0); retinotomy (1; 0); retinectomy (1; 0); internal limiting membrane peeling (1; 1); use of PCFL (2; 1); number of RRD repair within 12 months (0; 1); retinal re-detachment within 3 months (0; 1).

Table 3. Risk factors for cystoid macular edema at 12 months-multivariate analysis.

| | nCME (n = 236) | aCME (n = 91) | OR * | 95% CI | p Value |
|---|---|---|---|---|---|
| Initial BCVA (LogMAR) | 0.85 (0.16, 2.30) | 2.30 (0.81, 2.30) | 1.55 | 1.07–2.25 | 0.02 |
| Macular status-Off | 168 (71.2%) | 77 (84.6%) | 1.16 | 0.51–2.71 | 0.72 |
| Extent of RRD (1–4 quadrants) | | | 1.01 | 0.72–1.42 | 0.95 |
| 1 | 32 (13.6%) | 5 (5.5%) | | | |
| 2 | 103 (43.6%) | 34 (37.4%) | | | |
| 3 | 46 (19.5%) | 15 (16.5%) | | | |
| 4 | 55 (23.3%) | 37 (40.6%) | | | |

Table 3. Cont.

|  | nCME (n = 236) | aCME (n = 91) | OR * | 95% CI | p Value |
|---|---|---|---|---|---|
| **Proliferative vitreoretinopathy** |  |  |  |  |  |
| Grade A and B | 211 (89.4%) | 62 (68.1%) | — | — |  |
| Grade C | 25 (10.6%) | 29 (31.9%) | 2.88 | 1.04–8.16 | **0.04** |
| **Tamponade agent** |  |  |  |  |  |
| Hexafluoride (SF6) | 153 (64.8%) | 45 (49.4%) | — | — |  |
| Air | 2 (0.9%) | 0 (0.0%) | 0.00 |  | 0.99 |
| Hexafluoroethane (C2F6) | 43 (18.2%) | 17 (18.7%) | 0.80 | 0.36–1.70 | 0.57 |
| Octafluoropropane (C3F8) | 5 (2.1%) | 1 (1.1%) | 0.29 | 0.01–2.44 | 0.32 |
| Silicone oil | 33 (14.0%) | 28 (30.8%) | 0.65 | 0.22–1.78 | 0.41 |
| **Retinopexy type** |  |  |  |  |  |
| Cryotherapy | 63 (26,7%) | 8 (8.8%) | — | — |  |
| Endolaser | 128 (54.2%) | 70 (76.9%) | 3.06 | 1.33–7.84 | **0.01** |
| Combined cryotherapy and endolaser | 45 (19.1%) | 13 (14.3%) | 1.46 | 0.52–4.23 | 0.47 |
| Retinectomy | 2 (0.9%) | 4 (4.4%) | 1.86 | 0.31–15.0 | 0.51 |
| Internal limiting membrane peeling | 26 (11.0%) | 26 (28.6%) | 0.97 | 0.36–2.51 | 0.94 |
| Use of PFCL | 37 (15.7%) | 33 (36.3%) | 1.43 | 0.60–3.35 | 0.41 |
| Secondary cataract surgery within 6 months | 59 (25.0%) | 31 (34.1%) | 1.96 | 1.06–3.63 | **0.03** |
| Single surgery anatomical success | 189 (80.1%) | 57 (62.6%) | 0.67 | 0.18–2.15 | 0.51 |
| Number of RRD repair within 12 months |  |  | 2.09 | 1.00–4.67 | 0.06 |
| 1 | 196 (83.0%) | 57 (62.6%) |  |  |  |
| 2 | 29 (12.3%) | 21 (23.1%) |  |  |  |
| 3 | 9 (3.8%) | 8 (8.8%) |  |  |  |
| 4 | 2 (0.9%) | 5 (5.5%) |  |  |  |
| Retinal re-detachment within 3 months | 28 (11.9%) | 25 (27.5%) | 1.18 | 0.39–3.67 | 0.77 |

OR, odds ratio; CI, confidence interval; nCME, no cystoid macular edema group; aCME, cystoid macular edema group; BCVA, best-corrected visual acuity; RRD, rhegmatogenous retinal detachment; PFCL, perfluorocarbon liquid. Categorical variables are described as n (%), continuous variables are described as median (IQR). * Estimated from mutlivariate logistic regression model.

In univariate analysis, risk factors for CME at 12 months were lower initial BCVA (OR, 1.72; 95% CI, 1.32–2.27; $p < 0.001$), macula-off status (OR, 1.80; 95% CI, 1.02–3.28; $p = 0.048$), greater extent of RRD (OR, 1.43; 95% CI, 1.13–1.81; $p = 0.003$), severe grade C PVR (OR, 4.01; 95% CI, 2.22–7.28; $p < 0.001$), and SO tamponade (OR, 2.84; 95% CI, 1.57–5.13; $p < 0.001$). Eyes with early recurrence of RRD (within 3 months) and increased number of surgeries were at a greater risk of postoperative CME. Surgeon experience was not statistically associated with CME at 12 months ($p = 0.57$), nor were lens status ($p = 0.88$), vitreous hemorrhage at presentation ($p = 0.54$), and diabetes mellitus ($p = 0.67$).

In multivariate analysis, eyes with worse initial BCVA (OR, 1.55; 95% CI, 1.07–2.25; $p = 0.02$) and severe grade C PVR (OR, 2.88; 95% CI, 1.04–8.16; $p = 0.04$) had an increased risk of postoperative CME at 12 months (Table 3). Endolaser retinopexy was associated with an increased risk for postoperative CME at 12 months when compared to cryotherapy retinopexy (OR, 3.06; 95% CI, 1.33–7.84; $p = 0.01$). Post-vitrectomy cataract surgery within 6 months of the initial RRD repair was associated with CME at 12 months (OR, 1.96; 95% CI, 1.06–3.63; $p = 0.03$).

### 3.3. Visual and Anatomical Outcomes

SSAS was achieved in 370 (75%) patients, while the FAS rate was 98% ($n = 479$) at 12 months. A total of 116 patients experienced re-detachment during the study period, with 85 of these cases (73%) occurring within 3 months of initial surgery. An epiretinal membrane was found in 132 (38%) patients at 12 months. Median CRT was 282.5 (249.0–321.0) μm at 12 months. BCVA increased significantly after surgery until 1 month and remained stable until 12 months, with a median final BCVA of 0.22 (0.05–0.75) LogMAR (20/32 Snellen VA chart). Overall, 61 (16%) patients had a final BCVA of <20/200, 316 (84%) patients had a final BCVA of ≥20/200, and 209 (55%) patients achieved a final BCVA of ≥20/40.

During the study period, 156 (32%) patients received topical NSAIDs, 100 (20%) patients received oral acetazolamide. Dexamethasone injections (Ozurdex®, Allergan Pharmaceuticals Ireland, Dublin, Ireland) were used for 19 (4%) patients, and 17 (4%) patients underwent surgery for ERM peeling.

### 3.4. SD-OCT Characteristics of Postoperative CME

The CME characteristics were assessed using SD-OCT imaging for 161 patients and are shown in Table 4. Fifty-six patients were classified as having tCME, and 105 patients were classified as having cCME. Outer retinal layer alterations were present in 124 (77%) patients and more frequently in cCME patients ($p = 0.046$). Subretinal fluid was present in 15 (9%) patients and did not differ significantly between the tCME and cCME groups. CME localization in both the IRL and ORL (Figure 2) was a risk factor for cCME (OR, 6.44; 95% CI, 3.08–14.3; $p < 0.001$) in univariate analysis when compared to macular cysts located in the IRL only (Figure 3).

Table 4. Cystoid macular edema characteristics in SD-OCT imaging.

|  | tCME ($n = 56$) | cCME ($n = 105$) | OR * | 95% CI | $p$ Value |
|---|---|---|---|---|---|
| Outer retinal layer alteration | 38 (67.9%) | 86 (81.9%) | 2.14 | 1.01–4.56 | 0.046 |
| Macular cysts localization |  |  |  |  |  |
| IRL | 41 (73.2%) | 35 (33.3%) |  |  |  |
| ORL | 1 (1.8%) | 4 (3.8%) | 4.69 | 0.66–94.0 | 0.18 |
| IRL and ORL | 12 (21.4%) | 66 (62.9%) | 6.44 | 3.08–14.3 | <0.001 |
| Subretinal fluid | 3 (5.4%) | 12 (11.4%) | 2.28 | 0.69–10.3 | 0.22 |

SD-OCT, spectral-domain optical coherence tomography; tCME, transient cystoid macular edema group; cCME, chronic cystoid macular edema group; OR, odds ratio; CI, confidence interval; IRL, inner retinal layers; ORL, outer retinal layers. Categorical variables are described as $n$ (%). * Estimated from univariate logistic regression model.

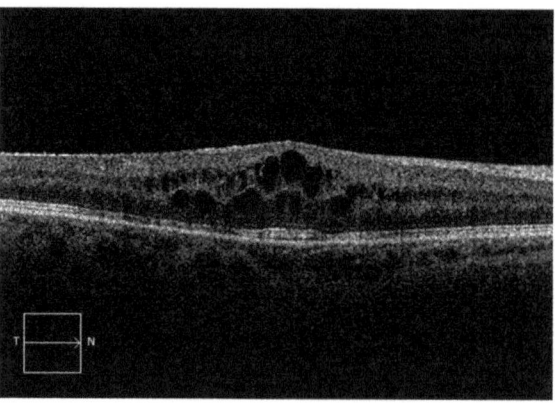

**Figure 2.** Spectral-domain optical coherence tomography showing cystoid macular edema in both inner and outer retinal layers after vitrectomy for rhegmatogenous retinal detachment.

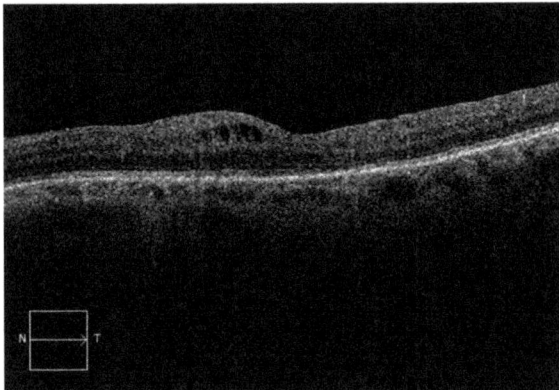

**Figure 3.** Spectral-domain optical coherence tomography showing cystoid macular edema in the inner retinal layers only after vitrectomy for rhegmatogenous retinal detachment.

## 4. Discussion

This study evaluated the rate of CME 1 year after PPV for primary RRD repair in routine clinical practice. Overall, 34% of patients ($n$ = 163) experienced at least one episode of CME within the first year of follow-up, while the rate of CME at 12 months was 28% (97 patients). When considering a CRT greater than 320 µm associated with macular cysts in SD-OCT for the diagnosis of CME, the rate of CME at 12 months decreased to 13% [27]. These findings are consistent with previous studies, although the range of CME rates varies greatly, primarily due to a difference in CME diagnostic criteria [27,28]. A recent single-center retrospective study with a smaller sample size but similar CME diagnostic criteria showed a CME rate of 25% among patients who underwent surgery with PPV or combined PPV and scleral buckling. Lower rates were previously reported, which may be explained by discrepancies in selection criteria with the exclusion of severe cases of RRD (PVR, SO tamponade, high myopia) or in follow-up time [8,22,24]. A study conducted by Yang et al. found a higher rate (36%) of postoperative CME, probably due to the severity of RRD in the eyes included in this study (SO tamponade only) [20]. Our rate might be overestimated owing to missing data ($n$ = 148, 30%) at 12 months, though no imputations were carried out, and patients with good anatomical and functional outcomes were more prone to resuming their follow-up outside of our academic institution.

Several risk factors for CME were described, such as age, pseudophakia and aphakia, macular status, severe PVR grade, retinectomy, number of surgeries, and RRD duration [9,23,24,28]. We found that eyes with worse BCVA and severe grade C PVR at baseline, and eyes that had endolaser retinopexy and cataract surgery within 6 months of primary RRD repair, were more likely to have CME 1 year after the primary repair. Severe PVR, lower initial BCVA, greater RRD extent, SO tamponade, recurrence within 3 months, retinectomy, and internal limiting membrane peeling are all RRD characteristics suggesting initial severity. They were associated with CME in univariate analysis, but only severe grade C PVR and initial BCVA remained significantly associated with CME at 12 months in the multivariate analysis. These findings confirm that inflammation is the leading process involved in CME development after RRD since PVR membranes form in response to a major increase in inflammatory cytokines following tissue damage caused by RRD and resultant inflammation. The use of endolaser retinopexy was associated with a significantly higher risk of postoperative CME than cryotherapy retinopexy, which was not previously described in earlier studies. In our institution, we believe that the initial severity of the RRD was a determinant of the retinopexy used, with cryotherapy mostly used for less severe or single-tear RRDs, which could explain the higher rate of CME in the endolaser retinopexy group. Moreover, 40% of patients had extensive endolaser retinopexy (360 degrees encircling) in the aCME group versus only 24% in the nCME group, which might increase the risk of ERM formation and CME occurrence in this group. Unfortunately, data on the average endolaser power and the total number of delivered spots were unavailable. Moreover, laser retinopexy was not performed in a standardized fashion in our study with several surgeons.

Lens status at baseline was not associated with CME at 12 months ($p = 0.88$). Lens status remains a controversial risk factor for CME in the literature. Meredith et al. and Chatziralli et al. found that pseudophakia was a risk factor for CME, although it was not confirmed in other studies [9,23,24,27,28]. Secondary cataract surgery within 6 months of initial surgery was not significantly associated with CME in univariate analysis, but the association was significant in multivariate analysis. Further analyses are needed to assess whether some patients could benefit from a postponed cataract surgery after RRD repair surgery.

Several studies investigated SD-OCT macular characteristics after RRD repair. Photoreceptor layer alterations are common and are associated with poor functional outcomes [8,11,27]. Similarly, CME was reported to alter BCVA in patients with a history of RRD [10]. Among patients presenting with CME, macular cysts were mainly localized in the IRL and, more precisely, in the INL. The distribution of macular cysts in both the IRL and ORL was associated with cCME. These findings are consistent with recent studies suggesting that cCME shares features with uveitic CME, whereas tCME might be a variant of pseudophakic CME [18,23,29].

Surgeon experience was not significantly associated with CME at 12 months in both univariate and multivariate analyses even though the SSAS rate was lower and more surgeries were needed to achieve FAS in the fellow surgeon group than the experienced surgeon group. The number of surgeries tended to influence CME formation but did not reach statistical significance in multivariate analysis ($p = 0.06$), as previously described [23]. The SSAS rate in our study (75%) at 12 months was in the lower range compared to previous studies (82–100%) [4,30–33]. As expected in a tertiary referral center, a majority of complex RRD cases were included. Indeed, 72% of patients had detached macula, 26% had RRD involving the four quadrants, and 15% had severe PVR (grade C). Almost half of the surgical procedures (49%) were performed by fellow vitreoretinal surgeons. Nevertheless, the FAS rate was high at the end of the follow-up period, showing the effectiveness of PPV for RRD repair.

Our study had several strengths. First, this real-world study had a large sample size with broad inclusion criteria incorporating complex RRD with severe PVR and SO tamponade, as well as a long follow-up period of 12 months. Anatomical and functional outcomes are within the range of previous studies in terms of CME, SSAS, and FAS rates. We acknowledged some weaknesses inherent in retrospective studies. The diagnosis of CME was based on the presence of hyporeflective space on SD-OCT imaging without dye angiography characteristics. Thus, the rate of CME might include both inflammatory CME with intraretinal leakage on dye angiography and macular cystoid degeneration without intraretinal leakage on dye angiography [34]. Nonetheless, CME after RRD repair may have distinct pathophysiology from other etiologies of CME [35]. Our department is a tertiary referral center, and more complex RRD cases may be referred to us. Some patients were referred to their ophthalmologists before the 6-month follow-up and were not included in this study. We also had missing data at 12 months, reducing our sample size for the analysis of risk factors. The study design did not allow us to use a Cox regression model to fix the onset of CME and adapt the monitoring of patients. Cataract formation or cataract surgery during the follow-up period might have influenced the visual outcomes. However, the final BCVA should not have been significantly impacted since, among our 304 phakic patients, only 30 were still phakic at the end of the follow-up period. Finally, the management of CME was made without reference to a guided protocol and is likely to differ among physicians (based on the anatomical and functional outcome of the surgery), which may have influenced the rate of CME at 12 months. Unfortunately, the study design did not allow us to assess and compare the outcome of a given treatment during the study period.

In conclusion, CME was a common complication 1 year after PPV for primary RRD repair in routine clinical practice. It might be helpful to address this matter with patients when explaining the surgical procedure, as CME might lead to repeated medical visits and chronic treatments. Localization of macular cysts in both the IRL and ORL on SD-OCT seemed to be a useful OCT biomarker of postoperative CME chronicity following RRD repair. Patients with low presenting VA and severe PVR should be monitored carefully for CME after RRD repair. Similarly, patients who had endolaser retinopexy and underwent cataract surgery within 6 months of RRD repair were more likely to have CME at 12 months. Further research is needed to determine whether patients may benefit from delayed cataract surgery.

**Author Contributions:** Conceptualization, M.M., F.B., C.M., C.C.-G., and P.-H.G.; methodology, M.M., F.V., F.B., L.A., I.B.G., A.M.B., and P.-H.G.; formal analysis, M.M., F.V., and P.E.; investigation, M.M. and F.V.; data curation, M.M.; writing—original draft preparation, M.M.; writing—review and editing, M.M., F.V., L.A., C.C.-G., and P.-H.G.; supervision, L.A., C.C.-G., and P.-H.G.; project administration, P.-H.G. All authors have read and agreed to the published version of the manuscript.

**Funding:** This research received no external funding.

**Institutional Review Board Statement:** The study was conducted in accordance with the Declaration of Helsinki, and ethical approval from an institutional review board was not needed for this study due to its retrospective design, in accordance with French regulations in force.

**Informed Consent Statement:** Patient consent was waived due to its retrospective design, in accordance with French regulations in force.

**Data Availability Statement:** Not applicable.

**Conflicts of Interest:** The authors declare no conflict of interest.

# References

1. Rowe, J.A.; Erie, J.C.; Baratz, K.H.; Hodge, D.O.; Gray, D.T.; Butterfield, L.; Robertson, D.M. Retinal detachment in Olmsted County, Minnesota, 1976 through 1995. *Ophthalmology* **1999**, *106*, 154–159. [CrossRef]
2. Steel, D.; Fraser, S. Retinal detachment. *BMJ Clin. Evid.* **2008**, *2008*, 710.
3. Ross, W.H. Visual recovery after macula-off retinal detachment. *Eye* **2002**, *16*, 440–446. [CrossRef]
4. Miller, D.M.; Riemann, C.D.; Foster, R.E.; Petersen, M.R. Primary repair of retinal detachment with 25-gauge pars plana vitrectomy. *Retina* **2008**, *28*, 931–936. [CrossRef] [PubMed]
5. Shinkai, Y.; Oshima, Y.; Yoneda, K.; Kogo, J.; Imai, H.; Watanabe, A.; Matsui, Y.; Suzuki, K.; Sotozono, C. Multicenter survey of sutureless 27-gauge vitrectomy for primary rhegmatogenous retinal detachment: A consecutive series of 410 cases. *Graefe's Arch. Clin. Exp. Ophthalmol.* **2019**, *257*, 2591–2600. [CrossRef] [PubMed]
6. Moinuddin, O.; Abuzaitoun, R.O.; Hwang, M.W.; Sathrasala, S.K.; Chen, X.D.; Stein, J.D.; Johnson, M.W.; Zacks, D.N.; Wubben, T.J.; Besirli, C.G. Surgical repair of primary non-complex rhegmatogenous retinal detachment in the modern era of small-gauge vitrectomy. *BMJ Open Ophthalmol.* **2021**, *6*, e000651. [CrossRef]
7. Okamoto, F.; Sugiura, Y.; Okamoto, Y.; Hiraoka, T.; Oshika, T. Metamorphopsia and optical coherence tomography findings after rhegmatogenous retinal detachment surgery. *Am. J. Ophthalmol.* **2014**, *157*, 214–220.e211. [CrossRef] [PubMed]
8. Delolme, M.P.; Dugas, B.; Nicot, F.; Muselier, A.; Bron, A.M.; Creuzot-Garcher, C. Anatomical and functional macular changes after rhegmatogenous retinal detachment with macula off. *Am. J. Ophthalmol.* **2012**, *153*, 128–136. [CrossRef]
9. Meredith, T.A.; Reeser, F.H.; Topping, T.M.; Aaberg, T.M. Cystoid macular edema after retinal detachment surgery. *Ophthalmology* **1980**, *87*, 1090–1095. [CrossRef]
10. Dormegny, L.; Jeanjean, L.C.; Liu, X.; Messerlin, A.; Bourcier, T.; Sauer, A.; Speeg-Schatz, C.; Gaucher, D. Visual Impairment and Macular Vascular Remodeling Secondary to Retrograde Maculopathy in Retinal Detachment Treated with Silicon Oil Tamponade. *Retina* **2021**, *41*, 309–316. [CrossRef]
11. Gharbiya, M.; Grandinetti, F.; Scavella, V.; Cecere, M.; Esposito, M.; Segnalini, A.; Gabrieli, C.B. Correlation between spectral-domain optical coherence tomography findings and visual outcome after primary rhegmatogenous retinal detachment repair. *Retina* **2012**, *32*, 43–53. [CrossRef] [PubMed]
12. Saber, E.E.; Bayoumy, A.S.M.; Elmohamady, M.N.; Faramawi, H.M. Macular microstructure and visual acuity after macula-off retinal detachment repair by 23-gauge vitrectomy plus silicone endotamponade. *Clin. Ophthalmol.* **2018**, *12*, 2005–2013. [CrossRef] [PubMed]
13. Augustin, A.; Loewenstein, A.; Kuppermann, B.D. Macular edema. General pathophysiology. *Dev. Ophthalmol.* **2010**, *47*, 10–26.

14. Bringmann, A.; Reichenbach, A.; Wiedemann, P. Pathomechanisms of cystoid macular edema. *Ophthalmic Res.* **2004**, *36*, 241–249. [CrossRef]
15. Tranos, P.G.; Wickremasinghe, S.S.; Stangos, N.T.; Topouzis, F.; Tsinopoulos, I.; Pavesio, C.E. Macular edema. *Surv. Ophthalmol.* **2004**, *49*, 470–490. [CrossRef]
16. Zur, D.; Loewenstein, A. Postsurgical Cystoid Macular Edema. *Dev. Ophthalmol.* **2017**, *58*, 178–190. [PubMed]
17. Daruich, A.; Matet, A.; Moulin, A.; Kowalczuk, L.; Nicolas, M.; Sellam, A.; Rothschild, P.R.; Omri, S.; Gélizé, E.; Jonet, L.; et al. Mechanisms of macular edema: Beyond the surface. *Prog. Retin. Eye Res.* **2018**, *63*, 20–68. [CrossRef] [PubMed]
18. Catier, A.; Tadayoni, R.; Paques, M.; Erginay, A.; Haouchine, B.; Gaudric, A.; Massin, P. Characterization of macular edema from various etiologies by optical coherence tomography. *Am. J. Ophthalmol.* **2005**, *140*, 200–206. [CrossRef]
19. Li, Y.; Xia, X.; Paulus, Y.M. Advances in Retinal Optical Imaging. *Photonics* **2018**, *5*, 9. [CrossRef]
20. Yang, J.Y.; Kim, H.K.; Kim, S.H.; Kim, S.S. Incidence and Risk Factors of Cystoid Macular Edema after Vitrectomy with Silicone Oil Tamponade for Retinal Detachment. *Korean J. Ophthalmol.* **2018**, *32*, 204–210. [CrossRef]
21. Sabates, N.R.; Sabates, F.N.; Sabates, R.; Lee, K.Y.; Ziemianski, M.C. Macular changes after retinal detachment surgery. *Am. J. Ophthalmol.* **1989**, *108*, 22–29. [CrossRef]
22. Ahmadieh, H.; Moradian, S.; Faghihi, H.; Parvaresh, M.M.; Ghanbari, H.; Mehryar, M.; Heidari, E.; Behboudi, H.; Banaee, T.; Golestan, B. Anatomic and visual outcomes of scleral buckling versus primary vitrectomy in pseudophakic and aphakic retinal detachment: Six-month follow-up results of a single operation—Report no. 1. *Ophthalmology* **2005**, *112*, 1421–1429. [CrossRef] [PubMed]
23. Pole, C.; Chehaibou, I.; Govetto, A.; Garrity, S.; Schwartz, S.D.; Hubschman, J.P. Macular edema after rhegmatogenous retinal detachment repair: Risk factors, OCT analysis, and treatment responses. *Int. J. Retin. Vitr.* **2021**, *7*, 9. [CrossRef] [PubMed]
24. Chatziralli, I.; Theodossiadis, G.; Dimitriou, E.; Kazantzis, D.; Theodossiadis, P. Macular Edema after Successful Pars Plana Vitrectomy for Rhegmatogenous Retinal Detachment: Factors Affecting Edema Development and Considerations for Treatment. *Ocul. Immunol. Inflamm.* **2021**, *29*, 187–192. [CrossRef]
25. Rossetti, L.; Chaudhuri, J.; Dickersin, K. Medical prophylaxis and treatment of cystoid macular edema after cataract surgery. The results of a meta-analysis. *Ophthalmology* **1998**, *105*, 397–405. [CrossRef]
26. Von Elm, E.; Altman, D.G.; Egger, M.; Pocock, S.J.; Gøtzsche, P.C.; Vandenbroucke, J.P. The Strengthening the Reporting of Observational Studies in Epidemiology (STROBE) statement: Guidelines for reporting observational studies. *J. Clin. Epidemiol.* **2008**, *61*, 344–349. [CrossRef]
27. Baudin, F.; Deschasse, C.; Gabrielle, P.H.; Berrod, J.P.; Le Mer, Y.; Arndt, C.; Tadayoni, R.; Delyfer, M.N.; Weber, M.; Gaucher, D.; et al. Functional and anatomical outcomes after successful repair of macula-off retinal detachment: A 12-month follow-up of the DOREFA study. *Acta Ophthalmol.* **2021**, *99*, e1190–e1197. [CrossRef]
28. Banker, T.P.; Reilly, G.S.; Jalaj, S.; Weichel, E.D. Epiretinal membrane and cystoid macular edema after retinal detachment repair with small-gauge pars plana vitrectomy. *Eur. J. Ophthalmol.* **2015**, *25*, 565–570. [CrossRef]
29. Han, J.V.; Patel, D.V.; Squirrell, D.; McGhee, C.N. Cystoid macular oedema following cataract surgery: A review. *Clin. Exp. Ophthalmol.* **2019**, *47*, 346–356. [CrossRef]
30. Kobashi, H.; Takano, M.; Yanagita, T.; Shiratani, T.; Wang, G.; Hoshi, K.; Shimizu, K. Scleral buckling and pars plana vitrectomy for rhegmatogenous retinal detachment: An analysis of 542 eyes. *Curr. Eye Res.* **2014**, *39*, 204–211. [CrossRef]
31. Bourla, D.H.; Bor, E.; Axer-Siegel, R.; Mimouni, K.; Weinberger, D. Outcomes and complications of rhegmatogenous retinal detachment repair with selective sutureless 25-gauge pars plana vitrectomy. *Am. J. Ophthalmol.* **2010**, *149*, 630–634.e631. [CrossRef] [PubMed]
32. Joseph, D.P.; Ryan, E.H.; Ryan, C.M.; Forbes, N.J.; Wagley, S.; Yonekawa, Y.; Mittra, R.A.; Parke, D.W.; Emerson, G.G.; Shah, G.K.; et al. Primary Retinal Detachment Outcomes Study: Pseudophakic Retinal Detachment Outcomes: Primary Retinal Detachment Outcomes Study Report Number 3. *Ophthalmology* **2020**, *127*, 1507–1514. [CrossRef] [PubMed]
33. Reeves, M.-G.R.; Afshar, A.R.; Pershing, S. Need for Retinal Detachment Reoperation Based on Primary Repair Method Among Commercially Insured Patients, 2003–2016. *Am. J. Ophthalmol.* **2021**, *229*, 71–81. [CrossRef]
34. Mohabati, D.; Hoyng, C.B.; Yzer, S.; Boon, C.J.F. Clinical characteristics and outcome of posterior cystoid macular degeneration in chronic central serous chorioretinopathy. *Retina* **2020**, *40*, 1742–1750. [CrossRef] [PubMed]
35. Romano, V.; Angi, M.; Scotti, F.; Del Grosso, R.; Romano, D.; Semeraro, F.; Vinciguerra, P.; Costagliola, C.; Romano, M.R. Inflammation and macular oedema after pars plana vitrectomy. *Mediat. Inflamm.* **2013**, *2013*, e971758. [CrossRef]

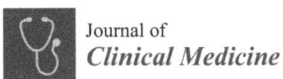

Article

# Encircling Scleral Buckling Surgery for Severe Hypotony with Ciliary Body Detachment on Anterior Segment Swept-Source Optical Coherence Tomography: A Case Series

Sławomir Cisiecki [1,2], Karolina Bonińska [1,2,*] and Maciej Bednarski [1,2]

1 Centrum Medyczne "Julianów", ul. Żeglarska 4, 91-321 Lodz, Poland
2 Miejskie Centrum Medyczne, ul. Milionowa 14, 93-113 Lodz, Poland
* Correspondence: karolina.boninska@gmail.com; Tel.: +48-607816193

**Abstract:** This study aimed to evaluate the usefulness of an encircling scleral buckling procedure to manage severe hypotony secondary to proliferative vitreoretinopathy (PVR)-induced retinal detachment. This retrospective study included six eyes of six patients (five women and one man) with hypotony (intraocular pressure [IOP] $\leq$ 6 mmHg) after multiple reattachment surgeries for PVR-induced retinal detachment. In patients with failure of hypotony resolution after conservative treatment (dexamethasone drops five times daily), 360° scleral buckling was performed under periocular anesthesia. The light perception was evaluated immediately postoperatively. The anatomic parameters were evaluated pre- and postoperatively observed on anterior segment swept-source optical coherence tomography. Ciliary body detachment (CBD) secondary to advanced cyclitic membranes associated with PVR grades C and D was detected in all eyes with hypotony. The mean IOP increased in all eyes (4.83 mmHg preoperatively vs. 10.17 mmHg postoperatively, $p = 0.006$), with subsequent improvement in best-corrected visual acuity (1.91 logMAR preoperatively vs. 1.50 logMAR postoperatively, $p = 0.034$). However, no eye showed any significant changes in CBD postoperatively. Scleral buckling surgery might be useful to increase IOP in eyes with persistent severe hypotonia secondary to PVR-induced CBD. Further studies are needed to improve outcomes in eyes with severe PVR-induced retinal detachment.

**Keywords:** ciliary body; hypotonia; intraocular pressure; optical coherence tomography; proliferative vitreoretinopathy; retinal detachment; scleral buckling

**Citation:** Cisiecki, S.; Bonińska, K.; Bednarski, M. Encircling Scleral Buckling Surgery for Severe Hypotony with Ciliary Body Detachment on Anterior Segment Swept-Source Optical Coherence Tomography: A Case Series. *J. Clin. Med.* **2022**, *11*, 4647. https://doi.org/10.3390/jcm11164647

Academic Editors: Georgios D. Panos and Shigeru Honda

Received: 25 June 2022
Accepted: 6 August 2022
Published: 9 August 2022

**Publisher's Note:** MDPI stays neutral with regard to jurisdictional claims in published maps and institutional affiliations.

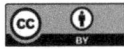

**Copyright:** © 2022 by the authors. Licensee MDPI, Basel, Switzerland. This article is an open access article distributed under the terms and conditions of the Creative Commons Attribution (CC BY) license (https://creativecommons.org/licenses/by/4.0/).

## 1. Introduction

Currently, ultrasound-guided biomicroscopy (UBM) and anterior segment optical coherence tomography (OCT) are the main tools available to visualize ciliary body structures. Ciliary body clefts can also be visualized using gonioscopy. Each of these methods has its limitations [1]. Recently, high-resolution anterior segment swept-source OCT (AS-SS-OCT), in which an increased laser wavelength allows the imaging of previously invisible structures, has become available for accurate diagnostic imaging. The opacity of optical media and short examination time are the advantages of this technique [2].

The condition of the ciliary body in patients with persistently low intraocular pressure (IOP) was assessed using AS-SS-OCT. This condition can lead to hypotonic maculopathy, choroidal detachment, and irreversible visual loss. The treatment options described in the literature include ciliary body suturing, external transconjunctival cryotherapy, direct cyclopexy, ciliochoroidal diathermy, scleral buckling, vitrectomy with gas, and injection of a high-molecular-weight viscoelastic substance into the anterior chamber. Such treatments have mostly been applied to traumatic cases with cyclodialysis cleft [3–7].

We describe outcomes of scleral buckling surgery, which may prevent and treat persistent hypotony secondary to PVR-induced ciliary body detachment by anatomical closure of the cleft and restoration of the apposition of the ciliary body to the sclera.

## 2. Materials and Methods

Ciliary body structures in patients were analyzed with severe hypotony following multiple surgeries to correct retinal detachment. Anatomical outcomes were assessed using AS-SS-OCT images (Figure 1).

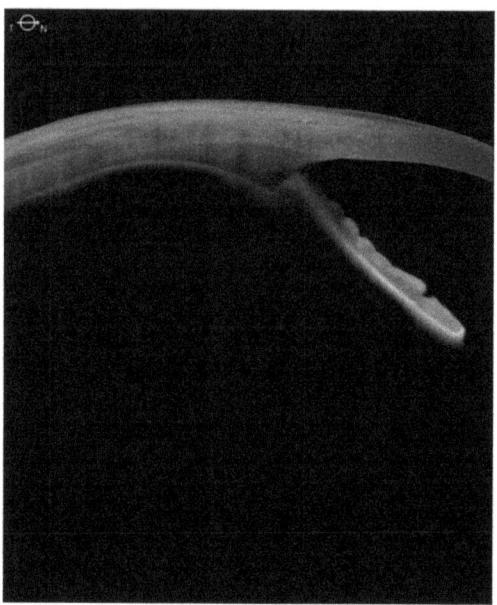

**Figure 1.** Anterior segment swept-source OCT with normal ciliary body structure.

This retrospective, single-center case series study was conducted at the Ophthalmology Department at Dr Jonscher Hospital in Lodz. The study was in accordance with the declarations of Helsinki and the institutional guidelines.

Data from six eyes of six patients (five women and one man) with hypotony (IOP ≤ 6 mmHg) after multiple reattachment surgeries for proliferative vitreoretinopathy (PVR)-induced retinal detachment were retrospectively analyzed. The mean age was 65.6 years (range 48–82 years). Complete ophthalmic examination was performed preoperatively at 1 week and at 1, 3, 6, 9, and 12 months after surgery. Detailed patient characteristics are shown in Table 1.

Numerical traits were depicted by their arithmetical mean, median, and standard deviation values. Normality of distribution was assessed by using the Shapiro–Wilk test. Considering the small size of the study group, the Quade test with bootstrapping was used to assess the significance of differences in preoperative versus postoperative logMAR and IOP. A level of $p < 0.05$ was deemed statistically significant. All the statistical procedures were performed using IBM® SPSS® Statistics, version 28 (Armonk, New York, NY, USA).

All patients underwent a complete ophthalmic examination. Visual acuity was assessed using the ETDRS charts, and IOP was measured using Goldmann applanation tonometry. The ciliary body was examined using SS-OCT ANTERION® (Heidelberg Engineering, Heidelberg, Germany).

Table 1. Patient data.

| Patient No. | Sex Age | BCVA before the Primary Surgery (Snellen, logMAR) | Final BCVA, 12 Months Post-Op. (Snellen, logMAR) | Primary Pathology and Previous Surgical Procedures | IOP Baseline | IOP Final, 12 Months Post-Op. | CB Baseline | CB Final, 12 Months Post-Op. |
|---|---|---|---|---|---|---|---|---|
| 1 | M 67 | HM (2.3 logMAR) | 0.01 (2.0 logMAR) | Globe injury with traumatic retinal detachment: 1. phacoppV+silicone oil 2. reppV+silicone oil exchange 3. 360° scleral buckling | 6 | 8 | CB detached in 3 quadrants | CB detached in 3 quadrants |
| 2 | F 65 | 0.05 (1.30 logMAR) | 0.05 (1.30 logMAR) | Retinal detachment with subretinal hemorrhage, VH: 1. plombage 2. phacoppV+gas 3. ppV+silicone oil 4. 360° scleral buckling | 4 | 8 | CB detached in 4 quadrants | CB detached in 4 quadrants |
| 3 | F 48 | HM (2.3 logMAR) | 0.03 (1.52 logMAR) | Retinal detachment: 1. phacoppV (BIL)+gas 2. 360° scleral buckling 3. ppV+silicone oil + IOL reposition 4. ppV+silicone oil removal | 6 | 14 | CB detached in 1 quadrant | CB detahced in 1 quadrant |
| 4 | F 66 | 0.1 (1.0 logMAR) | 0.25 (0.60 logMAR) | Retinal detachment: 1. phacoppV+silicone oil 2. ppV+silicone oil removal 3. ppV+silicone oil 4. 360° scleral buckling +silicone oil removal | 5 | 14 | CB detached in 3 quadrants | CB detached in 3 quadrants |
| 5 | F 82 | HM (2.3 logMAR) | HM (2.3 logMAR) | Retinal detachment: 1.ppV+gas 2.ppV+silicone oil 3.ppV+silicone oil removal 4.ppV+silicone oil 5.360° scleral buckling | 4 | 6 | CB detached in 4 quadrants | CB detached in 4 quadrants |
| 6 | F 66 | HM (2.3 logMAR) | 0.05 (1.30 logMAR) | Retinal detachment: 1.ppV+gas 2.360° scleral buckling | 4 | 11 | CB detached in 4 quadrants | CB detached in 4 quadrants |

No.—number, F—female, M—male, BCVA—best-corrected visual acuity, BIL—Bag in the Lens, phacoppV—phacovitrectomy, CB—ciliary body, HM—hand motion, plombage—the surgical protocol: drainage, filtered air injection to restore the tonus of the eye, followed by cryotherapy of single horseshoe tear and placing of primary radial sponge 3 mm-wide (FCI'S A.S, France) in inferior-temporal quadrant using Ethibond 5/0 mattress suture. VH—vitreous hemorrhage.

As the hypotony did not resolve after conservative treatment (dexamethasone drops five times daily), surgical intervention with periocular anesthesia was performed. All patients provided written informed consent prior to surgery.

*360° Scleral Buckling Surgery*

The eye was encircled with a #41 silicone band after placing mattress sutures using 6-0 polyester in all four quadrants. Broad sutures were placed over the portion of the buckle to provide optimal pressure. This was a nondrainage procedure. The silicone band was tied above the most detached ciliary body quadrant at the equator level. At the end of the procedure, the light perception was evaluated.

## 3. Results

Ciliary body detachment (CBD) secondary to the advanced cyclitic membrane associated with PVR grades C and D was detected in all eyes with hypotony (Table 1). We defined three patterns of CBD: (1) detachment between the longitudinal, circular, and oblique fibers (Figure 2a); (2) complete detachment with supraciliary fluid of varying thicknesses in all 4 quadrants (Figure 2b); (3) detachment in the *pars plicata* (Figure 2c).

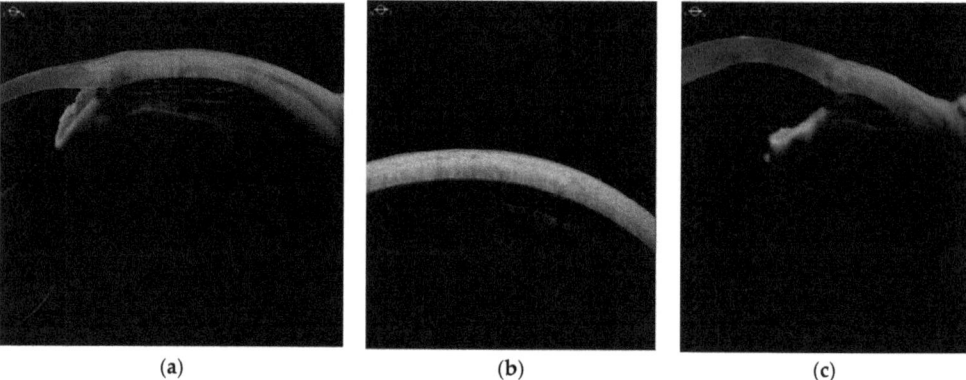

**Figure 2.** Anterior segment swept-source OCT. Ciliary body detachment between three types of fibers (**a**); supraciliary fluid in four quadrants in varying volume (**b**) and in the *pars plicata* (**c**).

We analyzed CBD before and after scleral buckling surgery (Figure 3a,b), and no eye showed any significant changes postoperatively (Figure 3c,d).

Next, we analyzed the effect of surgery on IOP and BCVA. The mean IOP increased in all eyes (4.83 mmHg preoperatively, Me = 4.50; SD = 0.98 vs. 10.17 mmHg postoperatively, M = 10.17, Me = 9.50; SD = 3.37; $p = 0.006$), with subsequent improvement in best-corrected visual acuity (1.91 logMAR preoperatively, Me = 2.28, SD = 0.59, vs. 1.50 postoperatively, Me = 1.41, SD = 0.59; $p = 0.034$) (Table 1).

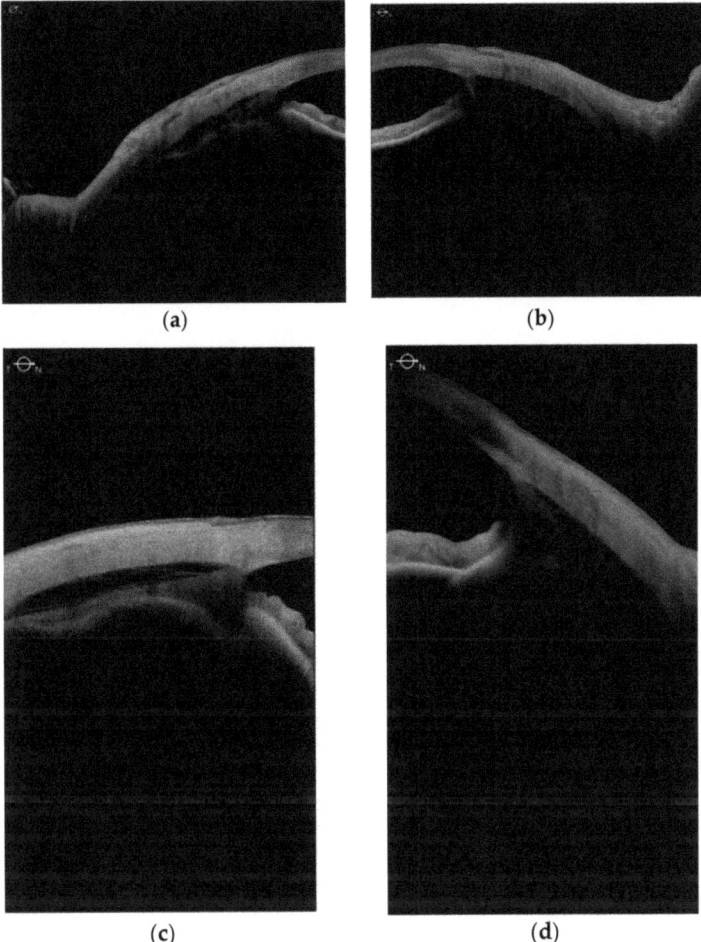

**Figure 3.** Anterior segment swept-source OCT demonstrates ciliary body detachment preoperatively (**a**,**b**) and postoperatively (**c**,**d**).

## 4. Discussion

Using AS-SS-OCT, we assessed the condition of the ciliary body and its correlation with decreased IOP. UBM, the alternative method, may not have allowed us to obtain the high-resolution images and quantitative data obtained in this study using AS-SS-OCT. UBM requires immersion of the eye and a qualified technician to obtain high-quality images. Although newer UBM devices do not require immersion, direct contact with the eye is still required and can cause artifacts [8].

Visualized CBD creates abnormal pathway for aequos homor drainage into the suprachoroidal space and leads to hypotony [9]. Surgical management in such cases is indicated when medical treatment of hypotony fails. There are a few different techniques described to treat this complication [3–7] but there is no effective method in the literature to treat hypotony after PVR-related CBD.

In our study, IOP increased after scleral buckling surgery despite persistent CBD. These results are similar to those obtained using UBM by Lávaque et al. [10], Xu W-W et al. [11], and Murta Fet al. [12]. Mandava et al. [13] utilized a sectorial and anterior buckle to abut the cyclodialysis cleft, 2 mm away from the limbus. After cleft closure, the scleral buckle was removed. Portney et al. used a sectorial and anterior buckle to abut the CBD with previous cryotherapy in the area where the buckle was going to be placed [14]. Inukai et al. also showed successful management of hypotonic maculopathy using 360° scleral buckling [15]. One reason for this might be that cerclage inhibits the posterior displacement of fluid from the suprachoroidal space, thereby decreasing flow through the uveoscleral pathway [10].

Differences between the traumatic clefts described by Lávaque et al. and PVR-induced CBD may affect the increase in IOP and may be more relevant in traumatic cleft cases. This is probably due to the relatively healthy condition of the detached ciliary body epithelium after trauma compared with that in PVR-induced CBD. The residual vitreous at the vitreous base provides a scaffold for membranes containing proliferating cells and a deposited extracellular matrix [16]. These membranes also incorporate the ciliary epithelium, which produces the aqueous humor, and prevent the reattachment of the ciliary body.

In the literature, there is no correlation between the extension of the cleft and the severity of hypotony to suggest that hypofunction of the ciliary body epithelium plays a significant role in persistent hypotony [9,17,18].

Our results suggest that scleral buckling surgery might increase IOP in eyes with persistent severe hypotonia and CBD caused by PVR or trauma; in some cases, the increase in IOP might be sufficient to eliminate or prevent postsurgical hypotony. Our work was based on a small case series. Further studies are needed to analyze ciliary body conditions after PVR-induced retinal detachment to improve outcomes in eyes with severe and currently untreatable end-stage PVR-induced retinal detachment.

**Author Contributions:** Conceptualization, S.C. and K.B.; methodology, M.B.; software, M.B.; validation, S.C., K.B. and M.B.; formal analysis, M.B.; investigation, S.C.; resources, M.B.; data curation, K.B.; writing—original draft preparation, K.B.; writing—review and editing, K.B.; visualization, KB; supervision, S.C.; project administration, M.B. All authors have read and agreed to the published version of the manuscript.

**Funding:** This research received no external funding.

**Institutional Review Board Statement:** The study was in accordance with the declarations of Helsinki and the institutional guidelines.

**Informed Consent Statement:** All patients provided written informed consent prior to surgery.

**Data Availability Statement:** The data presented in this study are available within this article.

**Conflicts of Interest:** The authors declare no conflict of interest.

## References

1. Ursea, R.; Silverman, R.H. Anterior-segment imaging for assessment of glaucoma. *Expert Rev. Ophthalmol.* **2010**, *5*, 59–74. [CrossRef] [PubMed]
2. Asam, J.S.; Polzer, M.; Tafreshi, A.; Hirnschall, N.; Findl, O. Anterior segment OCT. In *High Resolution Imaging in Microscopy and Ophthalmology: New Frontiers in Biomedical Optics*; Bille, J.F., Ed.; Springer: Cham, Switzerland, 2019; pp. 154–196.
3. Krohn, J. Cryotherapy in the treatment of cyclodialysis cleft induced hypotony. *Acta Ophthalmol. Scand.* **1997**, *75*, 96–98. [CrossRef] [PubMed]
4. Li, H.; Cai, J.; Li, X. Continuous ab interno repairing of traumatic cyclodialysis cleft using a 30-gauge needle in severe ocular trauma: A clinical observation. *BMC Ophthalmol.* **2019**, *19*, 266. [CrossRef] [PubMed]
5. Ioannidis, A.S.; Bunce, C.; Barton, K. The evaluation and surgical management of cyclodialysis clefts that have failed to respond to conservative management. *Br. J. Ophthalmol.* **2014**, *98*, 544–549. [CrossRef] [PubMed]
6. Selvan, H.; Gupta, V.; Gupta, S. Cyclodialysis: An updated approach to surgical strategies. *Acta Ophthalmol.* **2019**, *97*, 744–751. [CrossRef] [PubMed]
7. Sood, G.; Rajendran, V.; George, R.; Sharma, T.; Raman, R. Comparison of encirclage and cryotherapy with argon laser in the management of traumatic cyclodialysis cleft. *Int. J. Ophthalmol.* **2019**, *12*, 165–168. [PubMed]
8. Burés-Jelstrup, A.; Navarro, R.; Mateo, C.; Adan, A.; Corcóstegui, B. Detection of ciliary body detachment with anterior segment optical coherence tomography. *Acta Ophthalmol.* **2008**, *86*, 810–811. [CrossRef] [PubMed]
9. González-Martín-Moro, J.; Contreras-Martín, I.; Muñoz-Negrete, F.J.; Gómez-Sanz, F.; Zarallo-Gallardo, J. Cyclodialysis: An update. *Int. Ophthalmol.* **2017**, *37*, 441–457. [CrossRef] [PubMed]

10. Lávaque, E.B.; Iros, M.; Real, J.P.; Zambrano, A. Encircling scleral buckling for traumatic severe hypotony. *Ophthalmic Surg. Lasers Imaging Retin.* **2019**, *51*, 58–63. [CrossRef] [PubMed]
11. Xu, W.-W.; Huang, Y.-F.; Wang, L.-Q.; Zhang, M.-N. Cyclopexy versus vitrectomy combined with intraocular tamponade for treatment of cyclodialysis. *Int. J. Ophthalmol.* **2013**, *6*, 187–192. [PubMed]
12. Murta, F.; Mitne, S.; Allemann, N.; Paranhos Junior, A. Direct cyclopexy surgery for post-traumatic cyclodialysis with persistent hypotony: Ultrasound biomicroscopic evaluation. *Arq. Bras. Oftalmol.* **2014**, *77*, 50–53. [CrossRef] [PubMed]
13. Mandava, N.; Kahook, M.Y.; Mackenzie, D.L.; Olson, J.L. Anterior scleral buckling procedure for cyclodialysis cleft with chronic hypotony. *Ophthalmic Surg. Lasers Imaging* **2006**, *37*, 151–153. [CrossRef] [PubMed]
14. Portney, G.L.; Purcell, T.W. Surgical repair of cyclodialysis induced hypotony. *Ophthalmic Surg.* **1974**, *5*, 30–32. [PubMed]
15. Inukai, A.; Tanaka, S.; Hirose, A.; Tomimitsu, S.; Mochizuki, M. Three cases of hypotonic maculopathy due to blunt trauma, treated by 360-degree scleral buckling. *Nippon Ganka Gakkai Zasshi* **2003**, *107*, 337–342. [CrossRef] [PubMed]
16. Elner, S.G.; Elner, V.M.; Díaz-Rohena, R.; Freeman, H.M.; Tolentino, F.I.; Albert, D.M. Anterior proliferative vitreoretinopathy. Clinicopathologic, light microscopic, and ultrastructural findings. *Ophthalmology* **1988**, *95*, 1349–1357. [CrossRef]
17. Agrawal, P.; Shah, P. Long-term outcomes following the surgical repair of traumatic cyclodialysis clefts. *Eye* **2013**, *27*, 1347–1352. [CrossRef] [PubMed]
18. Malandrini, A.; Balestrazzi, A.; Martone, G.; Tosi, G.M.; Caporossi, A. Diagnosis and management of traumatic cyclodialysis cleft. *J. Cataract Refract. Surg.* **2008**, *34*, 1213–12161. [CrossRef] [PubMed]

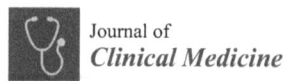 

Article

# Peripheral Circumferential Retinal Detachment after Pars Plana Vitrectomy: Complications and Management

Cherng-Ru Hsu [1,2] and Chung-May Yang [1,3,*]

1. Department of Ophthalmology, National Taiwan University Hospital, Taipei 100, Taiwan
2. Department of Ophthalmology, Tri-Service General Hospital, National Defense Medical Center, Taipei 114, Taiwan
3. Department of Ophthalmology, National Taiwan University College of Medicine, Taipei 100, Taiwan
* Correspondence: chungmay@ntu.edu.tw; Tel.: +886-2-23123456 (ext. 65181); Fax: +886-2-23934420

**Abstract:** Purpose: This study aimed to evaluate treatment outcomes and complications of peripheral circumferential retinal detachment (PCD) after successful vitrectomy. Methods: Eyes diagnosed with PCD after pars plana vitrectomy (PPV) were retrospectively reviewed. The patient demographic data, complications, management, and treatment outcomes were collected and analyzed. Results: The mean follow-up duration was 18.0 ± 11.9 months. BCVA ranged from light perception to 0.1 (median: counting fingers at 40 cm). Major complications included rubeosis iridis (seven eyes), vitreous hemorrhage (five eyes), hyphema (five eyes), corneal decompensation (three eyes), hypotony (two eyes), and neovascular glaucoma (two eyes). All eyes underwent peripheral retinectomy to remove the detached retina and release traction. Complete retinal reattachment was achieved in all eyes. The final BCVA ranged from hand motion to 0.1 (median: counting fingers at 30 cm). Conclusion: PCD may be associated with delayed-onset complications, causing severe loss of vision. Proper management, including peripheral retinectomy, may preserve visual function.

**Keywords:** anterior proliferative vitreoretinopathy; corneal opacity; hypotony; peripheral circumferential detachment; rubeosis iridis

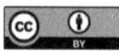

## 1. Introduction

Pars plana vitrectomy (PPV), with or without combined scleral buckle (SB), has been widely used to treat complicated rhegmatogenous retinal detachment (RRD). Many clinical variables, including choroidal detachment, significant hypotony, grade C proliferative vitreoretinopathy (PVR), four detached quadrants, and large or giant retinal breaks, have been identified as risk factors for surgical failure [1].

Recurrent retinal detachment (RD) usually occurs within 3 months after primary surgery [2]; recurrent RD that occurs 6 or more weeks postoperatively has been defined as late-onset recurrent RD [3]. Previous studies found that vitreous base traction was a major cause of recurrent RD [4]. With recent advancements in surgical techniques and tools, such as the use of small-gauge instruments and bimanual maneuvers to release tractional forces, the surgical outcome of post-vitrectomy retinal detachment has been enhanced; however, RD recurrence remains an important issue [5]. Among various patterns of recurrent RD, there is a specific form in which the RD is present circumferentially in the peripheral area. This peripheral circumferential detachment (PCD) is defined and characterized by its limitation to the periphery in a circumferential fashion. This unique configuration is generally attributed to the equatorial laser-induced chorioretinal scars obtained in previous surgeries, which prevent the RD from extending posteriorly [6]. PCD may initially be involved in the inferior periphery and may later extend circumferentially to form a tube-like configuration. In a manner distinct from classic re-detachment, which promptly or gradually advances toward the posterior retina or involves the macula, central vision remains unaffected due to the attachment of the posterior pole; however, specific late complications may occur, resulting in loss of late visual acuity (VA) [7].

In the present study, we evaluated the clinical characteristics and complications associated with PCD after successful vitrectomy and investigated the anatomical and functional treatment outcomes.

## 2. Materials and Methods

This retrospective case series study was conducted by reviewing the medical records of consecutive patients treated at National Taiwan University Hospital between January 2000 and December 2020. The study adhered to the tenets of the Declaration of Helsinki and was approved by the institutional review board of the National Taiwan University Hospital. The requirement for informed consent was waived.

We defined PCD as a form of recurrent RD limited to the periphery in a circumferential or tube-like fashion by old equatorial laser-induced chorioretinal scars. PCD was diagnosed mainly based on the findings of indirect ophthalmoscopy, B-scan ultrasonography, or optical coherence tomography (OCT). A standard three-port 23-gauge or 25-gauge PPV was performed for each patient by one senior surgeon (C.-M.Y.). The inclusion criteria were as follows: (1) recurrent RD after vitrectomy showing the distinct features of PCD and (2) development of late complications causing VA change. Patients were excluded if they had a follow-up duration of less than 6 months. Demographic data, including age, sex, number of previous surgeries, previous surgical procedures, onset time of symptoms, operation findings, complications, and follow-up duration, were recorded. Comprehensive ophthalmic examinations, including best-corrected visual acuity (BCVA) measurements, intraocular pressure (IOP) measurements, slit-lamp biomicroscopy, indirect ophthalmoscopy, and dilated color fundus photography (CR-DGi Image Viewer; Canon Inc., Tokyo, Japan), were performed. The outcome measurements were the anatomical outcome, indicated by whether the retina remained re-attached or not at the last visit, and the functional outcome, represented by the best-corrected visual acuity at the last visit. Successful re-attachment of PCD was defined as the attachment of the retina with or without endotamponade agents for at least 6 months of follow-up.

Statistical analyses were conducted using SPSS statistical software version 26 (SPSS Inc., IBM Company, Chicago, IL, USA). The mean and standard deviation were calculated for continuous variables. Categorical variables are expressed as frequencies and proportions. To quantify visual acuity in eyes with low vision, counting fingers' visual acuity was assigned the logMAR units of 1.7, 1.85, 1.90, and 2.00, based on the different distances of measurement and hand motion visual acuity of 2.30 [8].

## 3. Results

Nine eyes in nine patients (six men and three women) were included in the analysis. Patient ages ranged from 31 to 74 years (mean, $52.3 \pm 13.9$ years). The average follow-up duration was $19.6 \pm 12.5$ months (range: 6–48 months; median: 15 months). The mean number of previous operations was $2.3 \pm 0.47$ (range: 2–3). The average onset time of symptoms ranged from 3 to 96 weeks (mean, $130.4 \pm 155.7$ weeks). The preoperative BCVA was light perception in three eyes, hand motion in one eye, counting fingers in two eyes, and >0.01 in three eyes. The mean preoperative IOP was $17.1 \pm 15.3$ mmHg, including three eyes (22.2%) with an IOP $\leq 5$ mmHg and two eyes (22.2%) with an IOP > 30 mmHg (Table 1).

**Table 1.** Clinical characteristics of cases of peripheral circumferential retinal detachment.

| No. | Age | Sex | R/L | Pre Op VA (LogMAR) | Pre Op IOP | Hyphema | NVI | VH | Previous OP Procedures | Lens | Onset Time (Week) | OP Procedures | Findings | Ant. Adhesion | F/U (M) | Final VA (LogMAR) | Final IOP | Notes |
|---|---|---|---|---|---|---|---|---|---|---|---|---|---|---|---|---|---|---|
| 1 | 39 | M | R | LP(+) | 9 | + | + | + | PPV*2 | Dense cataract | 14 | PPL + 360° retinectomy + SO | 360° pRD | − | 9 | HM (2.3) | WNL | |
| 2 | 60 | M | R | CF/40 cm (1.85) | 1 | − | + | − | SB*1, PPV*1, Lens extraction | PC-IOL | 12 | 360° retinectomy + SO | 360° pRD | + | 12 | 0.1 (1.0) | 5 | |
| 3 | 46 | M | R | 0.05 (1.3) | 39 | − | + | − | PPV*2, SB + SO + PPL | Aphakia | 26 | 270° retinectomy + SO refill | 225° pRD | + | 6 | 0.1 (1.0) | WNL | |
| 4 | 40 | M | R | 0.025 (1.6) | WNL | − | + | − | PPV*1, SB + SO + PPL | Aphakia | 22 | 180° retinectomy + PI + SO refill | 180° pRD | − | 22 | 0.05 (1.3) | WNL | |
| 5 | 71 | F | R | CF/100 cm (1.7) | 6 | + | + | + | PPV*3, SO, Lens extraction | PC-IOL | 20 | 360° retinectomy + SO + IVIA | 360° pRD | + | 15 | HM (2.3) | 4 | IVIA*3, CO |
| 6 | 58 | F | S | HM (2.3) | 14 | + | + | + | PPV*2, SO, Lens extraction | PC-IOL | 416 | 270° retinectomy + SO removal + IVIA | 360° pRD | − | 30 | 0.1 (1.0) | WNL | IVIA*2, IVTA*2, mild CO, recurrent VH |
| 7 | 52 | F | R | LP(+) | 5 | + | + | + | SB, PPV for ERM | PC-IOL | 312 | 180° retinectomy + SO + IVIA | 180° pRD | − | 10 | HM (2.3) | 8 | |
| 8 | 74 | M | R | LP(+) | 45 | + | − | + | PPV*2 | AC-IOL | 312 | 150° retinectomy + IVIA + C3F8 | 150° pRD | − | 24 | CF/10 cm (2.0) | WNL | CO, DSAEK + IOL |
| 9 | 31 | M | R | 0.1 (1.0) | 18 | − | − | − | PPV*3, SB, SO | Aphakia | 40 | 210° retinectomy + ERM, ILM peeling + SO | 210° pRD, ERM, MH | − | 48 | CF/30 cm (1.9) | WNL | SO removal |

* Number of surgery; Ant., anterior; CF, counting fingers; CO, corneal opacity; DSAEK, Descemet's stripping endothelial keratoplasty; ERM, epiretinal membrane; F/U, follow-up; HM, hand motion; ILM, inner limiting membrane; IOP, intraocular pressure; IVIA, intravitreal injection of Avastin; IVTA, intravitreal injection of triamcinolone; LP, light perception; MH, macular hole; NVI, neovascularization of iris; OP, operation; PI, peripheral iridectomy; PPL, pars plana lensectomy; PPV, pars plana vitrectomy; pRD, peripheral rhegmatogenous retinal detachment; SB, scleral buckle; SO, silicone oil; VA, visual acuity; VH, vitreous hemorrhage; WNL, within normal limits.

The major complications included rubeosis iridis in seven eyes (77.8%), vitreous hemorrhage in five eyes (55.6%), hyphema in five eyes (55.6%), corneal decompensation in three eyes (33.3%), hypotony in two eyes (22.2%), and neovascular glaucoma in two eyes (22.2%). During surgical interventions for PCD, peripheral RD > 180° was noted in eight eyes (88.9%). Anterior PVR with retinal-ciliary adhesions was observed in three eyes (33.3%). Peripheral retinectomy to release the tractional tissue was performed in all nine eyes. Silicone oil (SO) was used for endotamponade in eight eyes (88.9%), and perfluoropropane (C3F8) was used as a gas tamponade in the remaining one eye (11.1%). Combined intravitreal anti-vascular endothelial growth factor (anti-VEGF) injection was performed in four eyes (44.4%), with either rubeosis iridis or hyphema with vitreous hemorrhage. After surgery, the retina was completely reattached with the regression of rubeosis iridis and resolution of neovascular glaucoma. One eye (case 6) had developed recurrent vitreous hemorrhage 30 months after the operation for PCD. Intravitreal injection of anti-VEGF and triamcinolone was prescribed initially, and one week later, and the vitreous hemorrhage had gradually resolved. The final BCVA at the last follow-up was hand motion in two eyes, counting fingers in three eyes, and ≥0.05 in four eyes. The mean final IOP was 5.7 ± 1.7 mmHg, including two eyes (22.2%) with IOP ≤ 5 mmHg and no eyes with IOP > 30 mmHg. Corneal decompensation was observed in three eyes during follow-up; among them, one eye (case 8) received corneal transplantation (Descemet stripping automated endothelial keratoplasty (DSAEK)) for severe corneal opacity (Tables 1 and 2). Corneal decompensation was related to recurrent hyphema and hypotony after multiple vitrectomies with SO tamponade in one patient (case 5), long-term SO-corneal touch before the development of PCD in one patient (case 6), and AC-IOL implantation and uveitis-glaucoma-hyphema syndrome in one patient (case 8). An example of PCD (case 6) is shown in Figure 1.

Table 2. Summary of patients' demographic data.

| Characteristics | n = 9 |
|---|---|
| Age, mean (range) | 52.3 (31–74) |
| Sex (M/F) | 6/3 |
| Pre-Op numbers, mean (range) | 2.3 (2–3) |
| Onset time, mean (range), (weeks) | 130.4 (12–416) |
| IOP (≤5 mmHg/>30 mmHg), (n) | 2/2 |
| BCVA (LS/HM/CF/>0.01), (n) | 3/1/2/3 |
| Lens status (Cataract/Pseudophakia/Aphakia), (n) | 1/5/3 |
| F/U, mean (range), (months) | 19.6 (6–48) |
| Iris rubeosis, (n) | 7 |
| Hyphema, (n) | 5 |
| Vitreous hemorrhage, (n) | 5 |
| Fundus change (pRD > 180°), (n) | 8 |
| OP procedures (Retinectomy/SO/IVIA), (n) | 9/7/3 |
| Complications | Corneal decompensation: 3; DSAEK: 1 |
| Final BCVA (LP/HM/CF/> 0.01), (n) | 0/3/2/4 |
| Final IOP (≤5 mmHg/>30 mmHg), (n) | 2/0 |

BCVA, beset-corrected visual acuity; CF, counting fingers; DSAEK, Descemet's stripping endothelial keratoplasty; F/U, follow-up; HM, hand motion; IOP, intraocular pressure; IVIA, intravitreal injection of Avastin; LP, light perception; OP, operation; pRD, peripheral rhegmatogenous retinal detachment; SO, silicone oil.

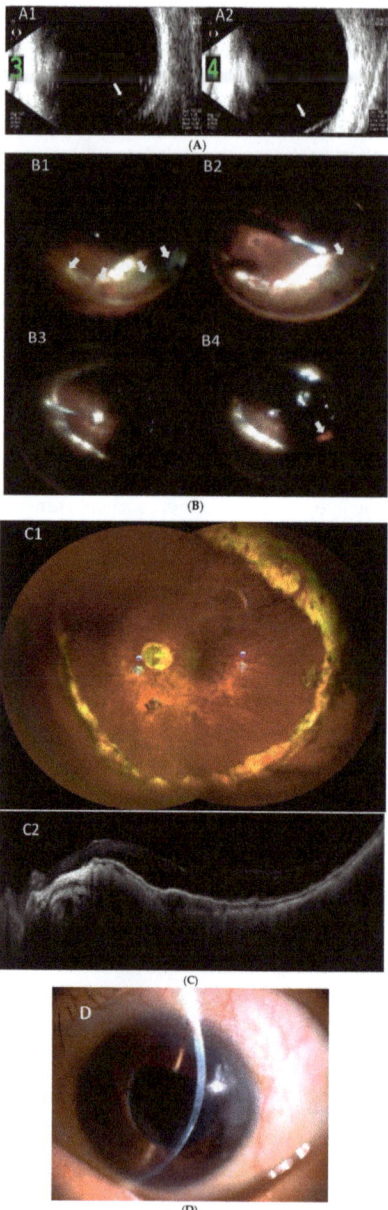

**Figure 1.** Representative imagings of peripheral circumferential retinal detachment (RD) in case 6. (**A**) Preoperative B-scan ultrasonography shows RD in inferior (**A1**) and (**A2**) nasal periphery (arrows); (**B**) intraoperative pictures show (**B1**) 270 degrees of peripheral RD (arrows), (**B2**) reti-nectomy of peripheral retina (arrow), (**B3**) fluid-air exchange, and (**B4**) supplementary laser pho-tocoagulation (arrow); (**C**) postoperative wide angle fundus photography shows attached retina under silicone oil (**C1**), and (**C2**) optical coherence tomography imaging shows the macula remained attached; (**D**) external eye photography shows superficial corneal scar from endothelial cell loss as a late-onset complication.

## 4. Discussion

In this study, the complications and treatment results of a unique pattern of recurrent RD after vitrectomy for RRD were reported. Recurrent postoperative RD was characterized by peripheral circumferential RD with a partial or complete tube-like configuration. Vision-affecting complications are usually late onset, including rubeosis iridis, vitreous hemorrhage, hyphema, corneal decompensation, hypotony, and neovascular glaucoma. The final vision was guarded in the majority of cases due to both anterior and posterior segment abnormalities despite careful removal of the peripheral detached retinal tissue, with or without SO tamponade.

A previous study observed that 10–13% of patients required additional interventions for recurrent RD despite initial anatomical success after a single operation [9,10]. For multiple recurrences of RD, Enders et al. found that patients with initial recurrent detachment were exposed to a 21–26% risk of recurrent RD after each additional surgical procedure aimed at RD repair [11]. Multiple surgical procedures increase intraocular inflammation and exacerbate the risk of PVR formation [12]. Preoperative anterior PVR and more severe PVR grades were associated with a higher incidence of RRD recurrence and worse visual outcomes [13,14]. In our series, all eyes underwent more than one vitreoretinal surgery for retinal attachment. Although PVR is usually associated with higher severity and macula involvement, RD is sometimes limited to the peripheral retina, as PVR is mainly anterior in its extent, and the peripheral circumferential heavy laser or SO in the vitreous cavity prevents the RD from advancing into the posterior retina. In our study, all nine eyes received supplemental laser retinopexy in the previous untreated peripheral retina during intraoperative management of PCD to achieve 360-degree laser retinopexy. As shown in a previous study [15], 360 degrees of laser retinopexy reduced the incidence of retinal detachment after silicone oil removal in vitrectomized eyes for rhegmatogenous retinal detachment. Although we did not remove all of the silicone oil in most SO-filled eyes during the last visit in our study, 360 degrees of laser retinopexy could prevent unseen breaks or avoid the formation of new breaks.

Unlike most major recurrent RDs, central vision remains initially unaffected in PCD due to the attachment of the macula. However, PCD may cause late onset complications. In this study, the main complications associated with late-onset PCD included rubeosis iridis, intraocular hemorrhage, chronic hypotony, and neovascular glaucoma. Rubeosis iridis in PCD may result from chronic ischemia and inflammation. Posterior segment ischemia and increased angiogenic factors resulting from RD are attributed to rubeosis iridis, which has been reported to occur as early as 3 weeks after PPV [7]. Ischemia may also induce NV in the peripheral retina. Chronic inflammation after multiple surgeries enhances the secretion and interaction of cytokines and angiogenic factors, which may contribute to and further worsen rubeosis iridis. A previous study reported the possibility of undetected peripheral retinal detachment or anterior PVR in the development of rubeosis iridis in eyes without retinal vascular disease [7]. Another possible factor leading to rubeosis may be the direct extension of fibrovascular tissue from the anterior PVR. The events that occur after rubeosis include obstruction of the trabecular meshwork and hyphema. In our cohort, 77.8% (7/9) of the patients had rubeosis iridis, and 55.6% (5/9) had hyphema. However, only two patients had glaucoma, while chronic hypotony occurred in two eyes in our series. Hypotony has been described in multiple operations, inflammation, and ciliary detachment, which are associated with inflow disturbance and outflow enhancement in RD [16]. The intraocular pressure depends on the balance between outflow obstruction and inflow production. Because NV and rubeosis take time to develop into PCD, the initial visual acuity may not decrease. Patients may seek help after sudden onset of vision loss due to intraocular hemorrhage or intraocular pressure change. The onset of complications varied among the study patients. The time of onset of PCD beyond one year was found in three patients (cases 6, 7, and 8) with poor baseline VA. In addition, vitreous hemorrhage with hyphema was noted in these three patients. It is possible that peripheral detachment occurred earlier than was noticed by major vision changes caused by hemorrhage in the eyes. The high complication rate may be due to the low patient numbers, as we only included patients with declined VA in our study. Eyes with a mild form of PCD that had a lesser extent of circumferential detachment of less than 150 degrees may not cause VA change and thus were not included. Therefore, the incidence of PCD may be underestimated. The more extensive the circumferential detachment, the higher the complication rate.

To prevent PCD, it is essential in the primary operation to release peripheral traction, trim, and support the vitreous base and properly seal the peripheral breaks. Once PCD complications occur, retinectomy of the detached and ischemic retina should be performed to eliminate neovascularization stimuli and release retino-ciliary traction. Intravitreal anti-VEGF injections may be administered at the end of surgery. Furthermore, SO injection to tamponade the retina may decrease hypotony-induced macular striae formation and prevent angiogenic factors from reaching the anterior segment. Scleral buckles may not be needed, as extended retinectomy alleviated the retinal-ciliary traction in our series. The combined PPV and encircling band reduced the traction within the vitreous base; however, this may cause anterior segment ischemia that aggravates the PCD-related complications, such as rubeosis iridis, vitreous hemorrhage, or hyphema.

After surgery, all nine eyes achieved retinal reattachment following extended retinectomy with SO-filled or C3F8 endotamponade at the end of the surgery. Intraocular silicone oil has previously been established as a long-term tamponade agent in treating severe vitreoretinal diseases as a last-resort option in selected patients. The recurrent vitreous hemorrhage observed in case 6 may reflect the unstable condition despite the successful re-attachment. Hence, SO tamponade may offer a more stable condition in these complicated cases. In our series, intraocular pressure was within the normal range in seven eyes, while two had hypotony at the last follow-up visit. Hypotony, which occurred in cases 2 and 5 despite an SO-filled vitreous cavity, may have been related to the 360° retinectomy that was performed and the annular anterior PVR before the operation. Decreased aqueous humor production secondary to ciliochoroidal effusion or ciliary body dysfunction secondary to anterior PVR with an increased posterior outflow of the subretinal fluid from retinectomy may account for this hypotony [17]. We reported four cases of PCD in our previous study [6]. Despite the lately improvement of modern surgical instruments, PCD developed with similar characteristics. In addition to a larger number of cases and a longer complication-onset time compared to our previous study, a significant feature of the present study was the development of corneal decompensation in one-third of the cases. Corneal abnormality is a complication of vitrectomy with gas or silicone oil tamponade [18]. Previous research has found that the development of corneal edema and keratopathy due to endothelial dysfunction is a consequence of insufficient nourishment from reduced aqueous humor circulation [19]. However, Banaee et al. did not find keratopathy to be more frequent in hypotonic eyes or in those with retained silicone oil. Instead, baseline corneal condition, multiple vitrectomies, and trauma history were significantly associated with the development of keratopathy [20]. Similarly, corneal opacity was noted in three patients in our series, and one of them (case 8) underwent DSAEK. AC IOL implantation, as in this patient, and older age may aggravate corneal decompensation. In addition, persistent hyphema after vitrectomy with corneal blood clot staining was observed in the three patients with corneal opacity.

Visual acuity improved in case 6 despite mild corneal opacity and in case 8 after corneal transplantation. Case 5 had corneal opacity and worse final visual acuity postoperatively despite reattachment of the retina. In contrast to cases 1–4, both cases 5 and 9 showed no improvement in VA after the operation. The predictability of functional outcomes remains poor because of the wide range in interindividual postoperative visual acuity. The relatively longer onset time found in cases 6–8 may have been due to several factors. The poor initial VA in these three patients might have delayed the awareness of vision change. In addition, it might take longer for the limited detachment area to generate sufficient angiogenic factors required for the development of neovascularization in the posterior and anterior segment structures. These possible reasons may explain the coexistence of hyphema and vitreous hemorrhage in cases 6–8. Although visual acuity of ultimate success in these extreme cases was limited, long-term follow-up demonstrated stable anatomical outcomes.

There were several limitations in this study. First, selection bias may exist due to the retrospective nature and monocentric setting of this study. Second, due to the rarity of PCD, despite the twenty-year interval, only a limited number of eyes were enrolled in our study. Furthermore, the follow-up time of individual patients was highly variable and was driven by subjective need rather than a regular follow-up time.

In conclusion, the results of this study suggest that prompt recognition and timely treatment of such late-onset complications in PCD are important to preserve a certain degree of visual function. However, functional outcomes in patients affected by PCD are very poor. Careful removal of the traction force in the vitreous base with retinectomy to release contractile tissue assists in restoring the retinal architecture and lowers the risk of persistent NV stimuli from the devitalized membrane.

**Author Contributions:** C.-R.H. and C.-M.Y., substantial contributions to the conception or design of the work; C.-R.H., the acquisition, analysis, or interpretation of data for the work; C.-R.H., drafting the work or revising it critically for important intellectual content; C.-M.Y., final approval of the version to be published; C.-R.H. and C.-M.Y., agreement to be accountable for all aspects of the work. All authors have read and agreed to the published version of the manuscript.

**Funding:** This research received no external funding.

**Institutional Review Board Statement:** The study adhered to the tenets of the Declaration of Helsinki and was approved by the institutional review board of the National Taiwan University Hospital (202202086RINC, date of approval: 25 March 2022).

**Informed Consent Statement:** The requirement for informed consent was waived.

**Data Availability Statement:** Data are available on reasonable request from the corresponding author on reasonable request. Email: chungmay@ntu.edu.tw.

**Conflicts of Interest:** The authors do not have any financial or proprietary interest in any material or methods mentioned in this article.

## References

1. Adelman, R.A.; Parnes, A.J.; Michalewska, Z.; Ducournau, D.; European Vitreo-Retinal Society (EVRS) Retinal Detachment Study Group. Clinical variables associated with failure of retinal detachment repair: The European vitreo-retinal society retinal detachment study report number 4. *Ophthalmology* **2014**, *121*, 1715–1719. [CrossRef] [PubMed]
2. Jia, L.Y.; Sun, Y.X.; Zhang, Y.P.; Ma, K. Risk Factors of Recurrent Retinal Detachment Following Surgical Treatment for Rhegmatogenous Retinal Detachment: A Retrospective Study. *Risk Manag. Healthc. Policy* **2020**, *13*, 3165. [CrossRef] [PubMed]
3. Benson, W.E. *Retinal Detachment: Diagnosis and Management*; Lippincott Williams & Wilkins: Philadelphia, PA, USA, 1988; Volume 270.
4. Foster, R.E.; Meyers, S.M. Recurrent Retinal Detachment More than 1 Year after Reattachment. *Ophthalmology* **2002**, *109*, 1821–1827. [CrossRef]
5. Mohamed, S.C.; Claes, C.; Tsang, C.W. Review of Small Gauge Vitrectomy: Progress and Innovations. *J. Ophthalmol.* **2017**, *2017*, 6285869. [CrossRef] [PubMed]
6. Lin, Y.C.; Chang, W.H.; Yang, C.M. Complications and management of post-vitrectomy circumferential retinal detachment. *J. Formos. Med. Assoc.* **2009**, *108*, 333–336. [CrossRef]
7. Barile, G.R.; Chang, S.; Horowitz, J.D.; Reppucci, V.S.; Schiff, W.M.; Wong, D.T. Neovascular complications associated with rubeosis iridis and peripheral retinal detachment after retinal detachment surgery. *Am. J. Ophthalmol.* **1998**, *126*, 379–389. [CrossRef]
8. Schulze-Bonsel, K.; Feltgen, N.; Burau, H.; Hansen, L.; Bach, M. Visual acuities "hand motion" and "counting fingers" can be quantified with the freiburg visual acuity test. *Investig. Ophthalmol. Vis. Sci.* **2006**, *47*, 1236–1240. [CrossRef] [PubMed]
9. Adelman, R.A.; Parnes, A.J.; Ducournau, D. European Vitreo-Retinal Society (EVRS) Retinal Detachment Study Group. Strategy for the management of uncomplicated retinal detachments: The European vitreo-retinal society retinal detachment study report 1. *Ophthalmology* **2013**, *120*, 1804–1808. [CrossRef] [PubMed]
10. Jackson, T.L.; Donachie, P.H.J.; Sallam, A.; Sparrow, J.M.; Johnston, R.L. United Kingdom National Ophthalmology Database study of vitreoretinal surgery: Report 3, retinal detachment. *Ophthalmology* **2014**, *121*, 643–648. [CrossRef] [PubMed]
11. Enders, P.; Schick, T.; Schaub, F.; Kemper, C.; Fauser, S. Risk of multiple recurring retinal detachment after primary rhegmatogenous retinal detachment repair. *Retina* **2017**, *37*, 930–935. [CrossRef] [PubMed]

12. Idrees, S.; Sridhar, J.; Kuriyan, A.E. Proliferative vitreoretinopathy: A review. *Int. Ophthalmol. Clin.* **2019**, *59*, 221. [CrossRef]
13. Wickham, L.; Ho-Yen, G.O.; Bunce, C.; Wong, D.; Charteris, D.G. Surgical failure following primary retinal detachment surgery by vitrectomy: Risk factors and functional outcomes. *Br. J. Ophthalmol.* **2011**, *95*, 1234–1238. [CrossRef] [PubMed]
14. Diddie, K.R.; Azen, S.P.; Freeman, H.M.; Boone, D.C.; Aaberg, T.M.; Lewis, H.; Radtke, N.D.; Ryan, S.J. Anterior proliferative vitreoretinopathy in the silicone study: Silicone Study Report Number 10. *Ophthalmology* **1996**, *103*, 1092–1099. [CrossRef]
15. Avitabile, T.; Longo, A.; Lentini, G.; Reibaldi, A. Retinal detachment after silicone oil removal is prevented by 360 laser treatment. *Br. J. Ophthalmol.* **2008**, *92*, 1479–1482. [CrossRef] [PubMed]
16. Van Meurs, J.C.; Bolt, B.J.; Mertens, D.A.; Peperkamp, E.; De Waardet, P. Rubeosis of the iris in proliferative vitreoretinopaty. *Retina* **1996**, *16*, 292–295. [CrossRef] [PubMed]
17. Wang, Q.; Thau, A.; Levin, A.V.; Lee, D. Ocular hypotony: A comprehensive review. *Surv. Ophthalmol.* **2019**, *64*, 619–638. [CrossRef] [PubMed]
18. Abrams, G.W.; Azen, S.P.; Barr, C.C.; Lai, M.Y.; Hutton, W.L.; Trese, M.T.; Irvine, A.; Ryan, S.J. The incidence of corneal abnormalities in the silicone study: Silicone Study Report 7. *Arch. Ophthalmol.* **1995**, *113*, 764–769. [CrossRef] [PubMed]
19. Hatton, M.P.; Perez, V.L.; Dohlman, C.H. Corneal oedema in ocular hypotony. *Exp. Eye Res.* **2004**, *78*, 549–552. [CrossRef] [PubMed]
20. Banaee, T.; Hosseini, S.M.; Eslampoor, A.; Abrishami, M.; Moosavi, M. Peripheral 360 retinectomy in complex retinal detachment. *Retina* **2009**, *29*, 811–818. [CrossRef] [PubMed]

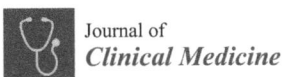

Article

# The Impact of the COVID-19 Pandemic and Lockdown on Macular Hole Surgery Provision and Surgical Outcomes: A Single-Centre Experience

Georgios D. Panos *, Olyvia Poyser, Humera Sarwar, Dharmalingam Kumudhan, Gavin Orr, Anwar Zaman and Craig Wilde

Department of Ophthalmology, Queen's Medical Centre Campus, Nottingham University Hospitals, Nottingham NG7 2UH, UK; olyviapoyser@hotmail.com (O.P.); humera.sarwar@nhs.net (H.S.); dharmalingam.kumudhan@nuh.nhs.uk (D.K.); gavin.orr@nuh.nhs.uk (G.O.); anwar.zaman@nuh.nhs.uk (A.Z.); craig.wilde@nuh.nhs.uk (C.W.)
* Correspondence: gdpanos@gmail.com; Tel.: +44-115-924-9924

**Abstract:** Purpose: We aimed to report the impact of the COVID-19 pandemic and related health policies and restrictions on the provision and efficacy of macular hole (MH) surgery. Methods: We carried out a retrospective cohort study. Two MH patient cohorts, those treated during the COVID-19 pandemic (12 months) and the pre-COVID-19 period (12 months before the lockdown) were reviewed and compared. Patient characteristics, time to consultation and surgery, MH size, baseline and postoperative visual acuity (VA) and failure rate were recorded and analysed. Results: A reduction of 43% in MH surgery occurred during the COVID-19 period (93 eyes vs. 53 eyes). Mean time to consultation and time to surgery increased significantly (52.7 days vs. 86.3 days, $p < 0.01$ and 51.3 days vs. 83.6 days, $p = 0.01$, respectively), while mean baseline and postoperative vision was significantly lower in the COVID-19 group (0.75 LogMAR vs. 0.63 LogMAR, $p < 0.01$ and 0.61 LogMAR vs. 0.44 LogMAR, $p < 0.01$, respectively). The median MH size was significantly larger in the COVID-19 group (296 μm vs. 365 μm, $p = 0.016$), and the failure rate increased from 7.6% to 15.4% (odds ratio 2.2 (95% CI: 0.72–6.8)). Conclusions: Our findings suggest the COVID-19 pandemic caused a significant reduction in MH surgery, increased waiting times and led to poorer surgical outcomes. For future pandemics, better strategies are required that allow semi-elective and elective surgery to continue in a timely fashion. Health providers should preserve the delivery of ophthalmological care, with enhanced encouragement to seek medical help for acute symptoms.

**Keywords:** macular hole surgery; COVID-19; pandemic; lockdown; policies; retinal surgery

## 1. Introduction

Since coronavirus disease 2019 (COVID-19) was declared a pandemic by the World Health Organization (WHO), many countries, including the United Kingdom (UK), have imposed national lockdowns. The related restrictions significantly affected healthcare services and the provision of patient care due to cancellations of routine outpatient appointments and surgery. In order to minimise the risk of COVID-19 transmission, patients were discouraged to attend hospital visits, unless critically necessary.

A study from Moorfield's Eye Hospital, London, UK, reported a significant reduction in clinical and surgical activities, including in the A&E department (>50% reduction), the medical retinal service (did not attend (DNA) rate increased to 24.9%) and vitreoretinal (VR) service (average drop of 62% in retinal detachment (RD) surgery) [1]. Audits from our department demonstrate during the first UK lockdown (late March–June 2020), outpatient and surgical activities were reduced by 63% and 67%, respectively, compared to the same period the previous year. This resulted in increased breaches of the 18-week referral to treatment (RTT) target in outpatient appointments (by 75%) and surgeries (by 471%) [2].

Moreover, during this period, patients with RD presented with a longer duration of symptoms, with the proportion of macula-off detachments and proliferative vitreoretinopathy (PVR) increasing, resulting in an escalated risk of worse outcomes in surgery [3].

This study reports the effect of the COVID-19-related policies and restrictions on the efficacy of the macular hole (MH) surgery at Queen's Medical Centre (QMC), which is one of the largest hospitals in the UK.

## 2. Materials and Methods

This study was performed in accordance with institutional guidelines and the ethical standards of the Declaration of Helsinki. The institutional review board approved the protocol (reference no. 21-219C).

This is a single-centre, retrospective cohort study. Consecutive patients who underwent MH surgery during the first year of the COVID-19 pandemic (April 2020–March 2021) were included in the study (study/COVID-19 group), while patients who underwent MH surgery one year before the pandemic (April 2019–March 2020) were included to serve as the control group (pre-COVID-19 group). Only the first eye of each patient was included in the case both eyes underwent surgery, either in the COVID-19 or pre-COVID-19 period, in order not to violate the statistical assumption of independence of observations. Eyes which developed postoperative complications not related to the delay of the surgery (i.e., RD, choroidal neovascularisation) were excluded from analysis.

The study protocol included collection of demographic data including age, gender, recorded **symptom duration** at clinical presentation, **time to consultation** in calendar days from day of referral (either from eye casualty, or optician or general practitioner (GP) or other hospital/clinic) to the VR clinic appointment, **time to surgery** in calendar days from the day of listing in the VR clinic, **lens status** (phakic, aphakic or combined in the case patient had combined surgery), **best corrected visual acuity (BCVA)** in LogMAR units at baseline and 3 months postsurgery, MH **size** and **need for further MH surgery** in the case of failure/nonclosure.

### 2.1. Visual Acuity

BCVA was recorded on LogMAR charts with a score of 0.02 equal to 1 letter. Postoperative BCVA was recorded at 3 months since this period is sufficient for anatomical and functional recovery following MH surgery and gas dispersion, while the effect of cataract formation in phakic eyes is minimal.

### 2.2. Macular Hole Size

Macular hole size was measured manually on the optical coherence tomography (OCT) with the Heidelberg Spectralis software caliper as a line drawn roughly parallel to the retinal pigment epithelium, at the narrowest distance between the hole edges.

### 2.3. Time to Consultation and Time to Surgery

Any delays not related to the pandemic or to normal waiting, such as cancellations/rescheduling by the patient, incorrect booking or other unforeseen circumstances, were taken into account to reflect the real waiting time.

### 2.4. Surgical Technique

The same experienced consultant vitreoretinal surgeons (GO, AZ, DK, CW) operated on the patients of both groups. All patients underwent pars plana vitrectomy (core and peripheral) with three 23-gauge ports. Posterior vitreous detachment was induced, unless it was present. The internal limiting membrane (ILM) was stained with MembraneBlue Dual (DORC, Zuidland, The Netherlands) and peeled with end-gripping forceps. Following internal 360-degree search with indentation, air–fluid exchange (AFX) was performed with Charles flute followed by air–gas exchange. For all MH patients, perfluoropropane ($C_3F_8$) 12% (Alchimia, Ponte San Nicolò, Italy) was used as tamponade. Patients were advised to lie facing down for 10 days and attended regular follow-up appointments (week 1, week 3, week 6 and month 3) for the first 3 months after surgery.

### 2.5. Statistical Analysis

Statistical analysis was performed with MedCalc Statistical Software, version 18.2 (MedCalc Software bvba, Ostend, Belgium; http://www.medcalc.org; accessed on 19 March 2022). Data distribution was checked with the Shapiro–Wilk test and Q–Q plots. Parametric and non-parametric tests were applied accordingly. Data are presented as mean ± standard deviation or median (range). Values of $p$ less than 0.05 were considered statistically significant.

## 3. Results

A total of fifty-three (53) eyes of 52 patients underwent MH surgery during the COVID-19 period, whereas 93 eyes of 91 patients underwent MH surgery during the pre-COVID-19 period, suggesting a reduction of 43% due to the lockdown secondary to the pandemic. A total of 52 (52) eyes of 52 patients in the COVID-19 period and 79 eyes of 79 patients in the pre-COVID-19 period met the inclusion criteria and were included in the analysis as the study and control group, respectively. The two groups were similar in terms of age, sex ratio and lens status; however, the mean symptom duration in the study group was longer by 1.5 months compared to the control group (5 months ± 3.4 vs. 3.5 months ± 2.0, $p = 0.01$). Demographic characteristics of both groups are depicted in Table 1.

**Table 1.** Demographic characteristics of the groups.

|  | Control Group (Pre-COVID-19) | Study Group (COVID-19) | $p$ Value |
|---|---|---|---|
| Total number of eyes/patients operated on | 93/91 | 53/52 |  |
| Number of eyes/patients included | 79/79 | 52/52 |  |
| Age (years, mean ± SD) | 67.6 ± 7.3 | 68.6 ± 6.6 | 0.48 |
| M:F | 28:51 (35.4% M, 64.6% F) | 16:36 (30.8% M, 69.2% F) | 0.57 |
| Lens status | 64.9% phakic | 60.4% phakic | 0.60 |
|  | 18.2% pseudophakic | 18.8% pseudophakic | 0.93 |
|  | 16.9% combined surgery | 20.8% combined | 0.57 |
| Symptom duration (at VR clinic appointment) | Median: 3 months (1–8) Mean: 3.5 months ± 2.0 | Median: 4 months (1–12) Mean: 5 months ± 3.4 | 0.01 |

### 3.1. Time to Consultation

Mean time to consultation in the study group was significantly longer compared to the control group (86.3 days ± 71.7 vs. 52.7 days ± 25.7; Welch test, $p < 0.01$, Figure 1A), suggesting a significantly increased waiting time from the day of the referral to the VR clinic appointment.

### 3.2. Time to Surgery

Similarly, the mean waiting time to surgery from the day of listing at the VR clinic appointment increased by approximately a month during the pandemic, (83.6 days ± 90.1 vs. 51.3 days ± 22.5; Welch test, $p = 0.01$, Figure 1B).

### 3.3. Visual Acuity

Mean baseline BCVA in the study group was 0.75 LogMAR ± 0.27, whereas the baseline BCVA in the control group was 0.63 LogMAR ± 0.20; this difference was statistically significant (Welch test, $p < 0.01$, Figure 1C). Similarly, mean postoperative BCVA in the study group was significantly worse compared to the postoperative BCVA of the control group (0.61 LogMAR ± 0.31 vs. 0.44 LogMAR ± 0.23; Welch test, $p < 0.01$, Figure 1D). However, the difference in the BCVA improvement between the groups was not statistically significant (0.138 LogMAR ± 0.29 vs. 0.185 LogMAR ± 0.24; t-test, $p = 0.33$, Figure 1E).

An improvement of at least 2 lines on the LogMAR chart was observed in 47.05% of the patients in the study group, and an improvement of at least 3 lines was observed in 31.37% of the study group patients following MH surgery. For the patients in the control group, the same proportions were 52.6% and 38.15%, respectively (Figure 2A,B).

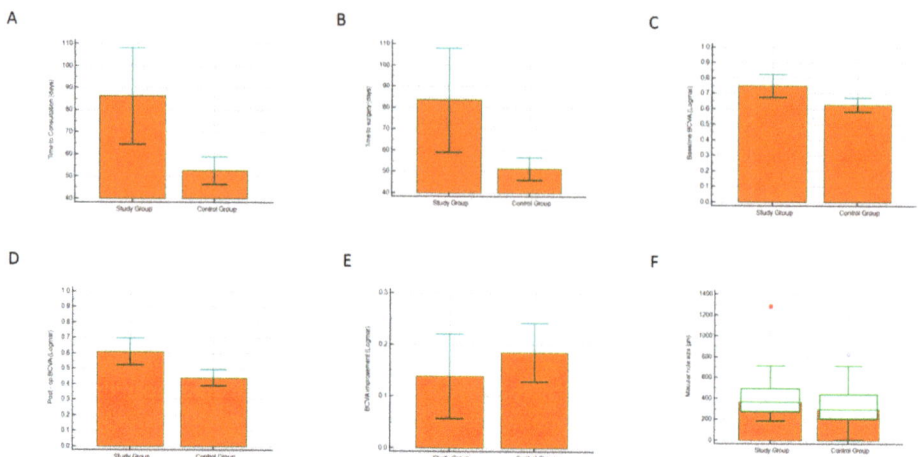

**Figure 1.** (**A**) Time to consultation (days), (**B**) time to surgery (days), (**C**) baseline best corrected visual acuity (LogMAR units), (**D**) post-op best corrected visual acuity (LogMAR units), (**E**) best corrected visual acuity improvement (LogMAR units), (**F**) macular hole size (μm).

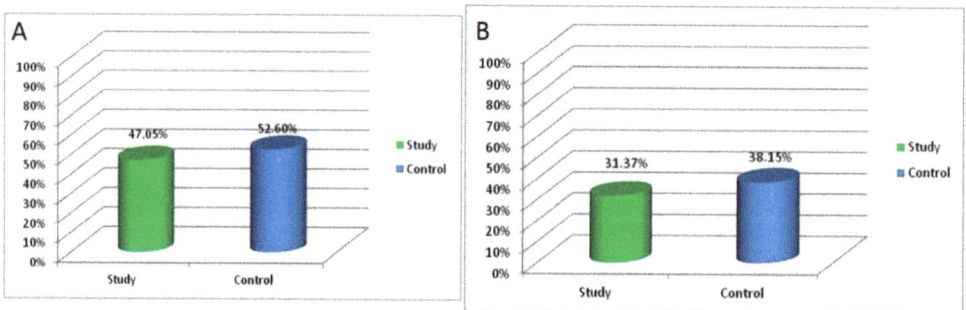

**Figure 2.** (**A**) Proportion of patients with an improvement of at least 2 lines on the LogMAR chart (**B**). Proportion of patients with an improvement of at least 3 lines on the LogMAR chart.

*3.4. Macular Hole Size*

Median MH size in the study group was 365 μm (range: 182–1283) while in the control group the median MH size was 296 μm (range: 50–829); this difference was found to be statistically significant (Mann–Whitney U test, $p = 0.016$, Figure 1F).

*3.5. Failure Rate*

Eight eyes (15.4%) in the study group required further surgery due to non-closure of the MH during the first attempt, whereas the MH surgery failed at the first attempt in the control group in only six eyes (7.6%) (odds ratio 2.2 (95% CI: 0.72–6.8)).

## 4. Discussion

The COVID-19 pandemic has greatly impacted patients and healthcare workers, both directly and indirectly. It created challenges for the NHS, resulting in a sharp decline in referrals to secondary care and a drop in hospital activity. We investigated whether these changes altered surgical outcomes of MH patients during the COVID-19 pandemic. We found a significant reduction in MH surgery during the COVID-19 pandemic with an associated suggestion of delayed presentation and increased waiting times from the day of referral to the day of the clinical and surgical appointments. These delays appear cumulative to such an extent that an increased mean MH size was noted among patients presenting during the pandemic. These changes are known to pose a significant risk for worse functional outcomes, and we demonstrated worse vision at presentation during the pandemic, with worse surgical outcomes postoperatively. Failure of anatomical closure was twice as high among patients operated on during the pandemic, compared to those who were treated the preceding year.

For the purposes of this study, we considered the first year of the pandemic as the COVID-19 period, commencing in April 2020 at the start of the national lockdown in the UK. During this year, wider social restrictions and hospital policies varied, depending on the epidemiological status of the country. Periods of strict full lockdown and significantly reduced clinical and surgical activity were followed by periods of partial lockdown or near normality with only slight reductions in clinical and surgical activity. We defined the pre-COVID-19 period as the same period of the previous year (April 2019–March 2020).

Although MH surgery is not considered an emergency, it is well-documented that successful outcomes and the level of visual recovery are affected by the duration of the MH [4,5]. A recent study by the BEAVRS macular hole outcome group demonstrated that an MH duration longer than 4 months reduces the chance of visual success by 50% [6]. During the first year of the pandemic, patients presented in our VR clinic with longer symptom durations. The reasons for this are complex and varied, but are likely secondary to patients being reluctant to attend (or failure to gain adequate or prompt access to) eye casualty or GP/optometry appointments, owing to the perceived risk of coronavirus infection. Hospitals treating COVID-19 patients were perhaps considered high-risk environments and avoided by some, particularly the predominantly elderly ophthalmic populations. During the national lockdown, where the message was to 'stay at home, protect the NHS, save lives', many patients may have deferred seeking help for other health conditions, particularly ones that were considered minor. Intense media coverage of the pandemic, frequently reporting worrying stories, such as shortages of personal protective equipment (PPE) and hospital capacity issues, may have confounded the issue. Healthcare workers and hospitals were possibly substandard in reassuring patients to attend for non-COVID-19-related disease. Significant delays in clinical appointments were caused by reduced non-urgent clinical activity that followed the NHS England and Royal College of Ophthalmologists Directives, in order to tackle the spread of the virus. Outpatient clinic capacity was reduced to allow enhanced cleaning and to comply with social distancing rules within clinical waiting areas. Time to treatment was further delayed secondary to reduced theatre capacity. Operating lists were cancelled, and lists had to be shared across ophthalmic subspecialties, secondary to redeployment of doctors (particularly anaesthetists and trainees) and nursing staff to medical wards, intensive care units or dedicated COVID-19 wards. Staff sickness from COVID-19 was high, and staff absences secondary to shielding among those with COVID-19-positive contacts or those deemed high risk if they were to suffer from COVID-19 infection also contributed. Clinicians often had no influence on top-down policies instituted by the government and enacted through senior hospital management without debate or discussion. Pathways were changed and staff redeployed in ways that ultimately prioritised COVID-19, but significantly compromised other patient cohorts. The cumulative effect was the development of larger MHs, worse baseline and postoperative visual acuity and increased failure rate (over two times) in patients who were referred, seen in clinic, listed for surgery and operated on for MH during the first year of the pandemic.

There have been numerous studies investigating the effect of the first 3 months of the lockdown period on ophthalmic surgeries and consultations [3,7–10], most of which focus on retinal detachment surgery [3,9,10]. To the best of our knowledge, this is the first study to report the longer-term impact of COVID-19-related policies and lockdown restrictions on MH surgery.

In a recent study, Awan et al. reported a 45.5% reduction in retinal surgeries during the first lockdown in Pakistan (March–June 2020) [7]. During this period, no MH surgery was performed. A retrospective analysis from six ophthalmology departments in Italy reported a reduction of 77% in MH surgery during the first month of the national lockdown (10 March–9 April 2020) compared to the month before (43 cases vs. 10 cases) [8]. Awad et al. reported a statistically significant increase in retinal detachment cases presenting with PVR during the first 2 months of the lockdown period in Nottingham, UK (March–May 2020) [3], while in Scotland, the weekly mean number of rhegmatogenous retinal detachments reduced from 18.2 before lockdown to 8.6 during the first 5 weeks of lockdown, decreasing the annual incidence from 17.37/100,000/year to 8.21. Simultaneously, macula-off retinal detachments increased at presentation by 10% [9]. Similarly, a study from Beijing, China, reported a 55.9% reduction in retinal detachment surgery during the COVID-19 pandemic but showed no significant difference in the severity of PVR and in surgery outcomes [10].

## 5. Conclusions

In summary, we report a cohort of MH patients treated during the first year of the COVID-19 pandemic. Significant disruption to healthcare service provision caused a reduction in MH surgery and longer waiting times, leading to poorer anatomical and functional outcomes. For future pandemics, better strategies are required that allow semi-elective and elective surgery to continue in a timely fashion. Health providers should preserve the delivery of ophthalmological care, with enhanced encouragement to seek medical help for acute symptoms. Massive investment within the NHS with additional resources will be required.

**Author Contributions:** Data curation, G.D.P., O.P. and H.S.; Formal analysis, G.D.P.; Methodology, G.D.P.; Supervision, C.W.; Writing – original draft, G.D.P.; Writing – review & editing, D.K., G.O., A.Z. and C.W. All authors have read and agreed to the published version of the manuscript.

**Funding:** This research received no specific grant from any funding agency in the public, commercial or not-for-profit sectors.

**Institutional Review Board Statement:** This study was performed in accordance with institutional guidelines and the ethical standards of the Declaration of Helsinki. The institutional review board approved the protocol (reference no. 21-219C).

**Informed Consent Statement:** Informed consent was obtained from all subjects involved in the study.

**Data Availability Statement:** Data are available from the authors upon reasonable request.

**Conflicts of Interest:** The authors have no conflicts of interest to declare.

## References

1. Wickham, L.; Hay, G.; Hamilton, R.; Wooding, J.; Tossounis, H.; da Cruz, L.; Siriwardena, D.; Strouthidis, N. The impact of COVID policies on acute ophthalmology services-experiences from moorfields eye hospital nhs foundation trust. *Eye* **2020**, *34*, 1189–1192. [CrossRef] [PubMed]
2. Ting, D.S.J.; Deshmukh, R.; Said, D.G.; Dua, H.S. The impact of COVID-19 pandemic on ophthalmology services: Are we ready for the aftermath? *Ther. Adv. Ophthalmol.* **2020**, *12*, 2515841420964099. [CrossRef] [PubMed]
3. Awad, M.; Poostchi, A.; Orr, G.; Kumudhan, D.; Zaman, A.; Wilde, C. Delayed presentation and increased prevalence of proliferative vitreoretinopathy for primary rhegmatogenous retinal detachments presenting during the COVID-19 pandemic lockdown. *Eye* **2021**, *35*, 1282–1283. [CrossRef] [PubMed]
4. Willis, A.W.; Garcia-Cosio, J.F. Macular hole surgery. Comparison of longstanding versus recent macular holes. *Ophthalmology* **1996**, *103*, 1811–1814. [CrossRef]
5. Jaycock, P.D.; Bunce, C.; Xing, W.; Thomas, D.; Poon, W.; Gazzard, G.; Williamson, T.H.; Laidlaw, D.A. Outcomes of macular hole surgery: Implications for surgical management and clinical governance. *Eye* **2005**, *19*, 879–884. [CrossRef] [PubMed]
6. Steel, D.H.; Donachie, P.H.J.; Aylward, G.W.; Laidlaw, D.A.; Williamson, T.H.; Yorston, D. Factors affecting anatomical and visual outcome after macular hole surgery: Findings from a large prospective uk cohort. *Eye* **2021**, *35*, 316–325. [CrossRef] [PubMed]

7. Awan, M.A.; Shaheen, F.; Mohsin, F. Impact of COVID-19 lockdown on retinal surgeries. *Pak. J. Med. Sci.* **2021**, *37*, 1808–1812. [CrossRef] [PubMed]
8. Dell'Omo, R.; Filippelli, M.; Semeraro, F.; Avitabile, T.; Giansanti, F.; Parmeggiani, F.; Romano, M.R.; Strianese, D.; Romano, V.; Virgili, G.; et al. Effects of the first month of lockdown for COVID-19 in italy: A preliminary analysis on the eyecare system from six centers. *Eur. J. Ophthalmol.* **2021**, *31*, 2252–2258. [CrossRef] [PubMed]
9. Shams, F.; El-Abiary, M.; Goudie, C.; Yorston, D. Effects of lockdown on retinal detachment incidence in scotland. *Eye* **2021**, *35*, 1279–1280. [CrossRef] [PubMed]
10. Li, J.; Zhao, M.; She, H.; Chandra, A. The impact of the COVID-19 pandemic lockdown on rhegmatogenous retinal detachment services-experiences from the tongren eye center in beijing. *PLoS ONE* **2021**, *16*, e0254751. [CrossRef] [PubMed]

MDPI
St. Alban-Anlage 66
4052 Basel
Switzerland
www.mdpi.com

*Journal of Clinical Medicine* Editorial Office
E-mail: jcm@mdpi.com
www.mdpi.com/journal/jcm

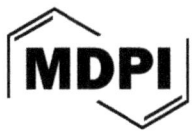

Disclaimer/Publisher's Note: The statements, opinions and data contained in all publications are solely those of the individual author(s) and contributor(s) and not of MDPI and/or the editor(s). MDPI and/or the editor(s) disclaim responsibility for any injury to people or property resulting from any ideas, methods, instructions or products referred to in the content.

www.ingramcontent.com/pod-product-compliance
Lightning Source LLC
LaVergne TN
LVHW070634100526
838202LV00012B/805